ENVIRONMENTAL TOBACCO SMOKE

Measuring Exposures and Assessing Health Effects

Committee on Passive Smoking
Board on Environmental Studies and Toxicology
National Research Council

NATIONAL ACADEMY PRESS
Washington, D.C. 1986

National Academy Press • 2101 Constitution Avenue, NW • Washington, DC 20418

NOTICE: The project that is the subject of this report was approved by the Governing Board of the National Research Council, whose members are drawn from the councils of the National Academy of Sciences, the National Academy of Engineering, and the Institute of Medicine. The members of the committee responsible for the report were chosen for their special competences and with regard for appropriate balance.

This report has been reviewed by a group other than the authors according to procedures approved by a Report Review Committee consisting of members of the National Academy of Sciences, the National Academy of Engineering, and the Institute of Medicine.

The National Research Council was established by the National Academy of Sciences in 1916 to associate the broad community of science and technology with the Academy's purposes of furthering knowledge and of advising the federal government. The Council operates in accordance with general policies determined by the Academy under the authority of its congressional charter of 1863, which establishes the Academy as a private, nonprofit, self-governing membership corporation. The Council has become the principal operating agency of both the National Academy of Sciences and the National Academy of Engineering in the conduct of their services to the government, the public, and the scientific and engineering communities. It is administered jointly by both Academies and the Institute of Medicine. The National Academy of Engineering and the Institute of Medicine were established in 1964 and 1970, respectively, under the charter of the National Academy of Sciences.

This study was prepared under EPA Contract #68-02-4073 and Department of Health and Human Services, Public Health Services Grant #ASU000001-06-S1. The content of this publication does not necessarily reflect the views or policies of the U.S. Environmental Protection Agency or the Department of Health and Human Services, and an official endorsement should not be inferred.

INTERNATIONAL STANDARD BOOK NUMBER 0-309-03730-1

LIBRARY OF CONGRESS CATALOG CARD NUMBER 86-28622

Printed in the United States of America

First Printing, November 1986
Second Printing, January 1987
Third Printing, March 1987
Fourth Printing, May 1987

BOARD ON ENVIRONMENTAL STUDIES AND TOXICOLOGY

COMMITTEE ON PASSIVE SMOKING

BARBARA S. HULKA, University of North Carolina, Chapel Hill, North Carolina, *Chairman*
OLAV AXELSON, University Hospital, Linkoping, Sweden
JOSEPH BRAIN, Harvard School of Public Health, Boston, Massachusetts
PATRICIA BUFFLER, University of Texas at Houston, Houston, Texas
A. SONIA BUIST, Oregon Health Sciences University, Portland, Oregon
DIETRICH HOFFMANN, American Health Foundation, Valhalla, New York
BRIAN LEADERER, Yale University, New Haven, Connecticut
GENEVIEVE MATANOSKI, Johns Hopkins University, Baltimore, Maryland
JAMES ROBINS, Harvard School of Public Health, Boston, Massachusetts
JOHN SPENGLER, Harvard School of Public Health, Boston, Massachusetts
NICHOLAS WALD, Medical College of St. Bartholomew's Hospital, London, England

National Research Council Staff

DEVRA LEE DAVIS, Acting Director, BEST
DIANE K. WAGENER, Project Director
MARVIN SCHNEIDERMAN, Senior Staff Officer
RICHARD E. MORRIS, Editor
EDNA W. PAULSON, Information Specialist
MARY ELLEN SCHECKENBACH, Staff Assistant
JULIETTE L. WALKER, Senior Secretary

Preface

The Office of Air and Radiation of the Environmental Protection Agency and the Office on Smoking and Health of the Department of Health and Human Services asked the National Research Council to evaluate methods for assessing exposure to environmental tobacco smoke and to review the literature on the health consequences from such exposures. The National Research Council responded to this request by appointing 11 scientists to serve on the Committee on Passive Smoking, in the Board on Environmental Studies and Toxicology, under the Commission on Life Sciences. The committee membership represented the disciplines of toxicology, biochemistry, atmospheric science, epidemiology, biostatistics, and pulmonary physiology.

The committee's charge was to review the existing scientific literature and to identify the current state of knowledge with respect to known facts and areas of uncertainty. Many more of the latter were found than the former. To the extent that they could be justified scientifically, conclusions have been stated and recommendations proposed. Many of the recommendations are for future research, rather than for public policy. The latter were for the most part avoided on two grounds: the data were frequently not sufficiently secure and the charge to the committee was primarily for scientific review.

The committee conducted a public hearing on scientific studies relevant to its charge on January 29, 1986. Furthermore, it reviewed the published scientific literature and received testimony from professional societies; medical, industry, consumer, and public interest groups; academic scientists; and others involved in the generation and interpretation of scientific evidence on the health consequences of exposure to cigarette smoking. Pursuance of these activities was followed by the preparation of individual chapters by committee members and consultants. Thereafter, chapters were discussed, revised, and integrated with each other for the full report.

In producing this report, the committee confronted a complex charge under severe time constraints. That it completed its task well and on time is a credit both to its members and the scientific staff of the National Research Council. I would like to express my personal appreciation to every one of the committee members, all of whom donated their time, intellect, and knowledge to the substance of this report. Dr. Diane Wagener of the National Research Council assumed the difficult task of coordinating, translating, and negotiating ideas and insights among committee members, consultants, and reviewers. Drs. Devra Davis and Marvin Schneiderman worked with Dr. Wagener in ensuring the thoughtful and timely completion of this report.

While the committee restricted itself to analysis of the scientific data, it was not unmindful of the fact of modern life that smokers and nonsmokers have taken strong positions regarding the right to smoke on the one hand and a rejection of being exposed to other people's smoke on the other. Persons on each side of the issue may wish to infer information from this report that the committee did not intend. Our strategy has been to synthesize information, present judgments and conclusions wherever possible, and to recognize inadequacies in existing data in order to provide a focus for future research. We have not taken the stance of a public policy board that necessarily has to make decisions on less-than-adequate information. Rather, we have chosen to prepare a scientifically responsible report that will be intelligible to a lay audience and useful to a scientific one.

BARBARA S. HULKA, *Chairman*
Committee on Passive Smoking

Acknowledgments

The preparation of this report by the Committee on Passive Smoking would not have been possible without assistance from a large number of people.

The committee consulted with a number of experts about various topics. We would like to thank the Office on Smoking and Health, particularly Clarisse Brown, who provided us with the many statistics and data that were requested by various members of the committee. We would also like to thank William Cain and Edward LaVoie for their contributions. Other individuals who gave special assistance in the preparation of the report include Leslie Waters Barger, Kiran Nanchahal, Simon Thompson, Christopher Frost, and Don Blevins.

The committee thanks all the peer reviewers of the report. Their constructive remarks contributed to the improvement of presentations of technical information and its readability.

We would like to express our thanks to the NRC staff for their work in supporting the committee. We would especially like to thank Edna W. Paulson and the staff of the Toxicology Information Center, who were of great assistance.

Contents

EXECUTIVE SUMMARY 1
Introduction, 1
Environmental Tobacco Smoke, 2
Measures of Exposure, 3
In Vivo and In Vitro Studies, 7
Health Effects, 7

1 INTRODUCTION 13
Definitions, 14
Trends in Cigarette Usage, 15
Organization, 20
References, 21

Part I
PHYSICOCHEMICAL AND TOXICOLOGICAL STUDIES OF ENVIRONMENTAL TOBACCO SMOKE

2 THE PHYSICOCHEMICAL NATURE OF SIDESTREAM SMOKE AND ENVIRONMENTAL TOBACCO SMOKE 25
Introduction, 25
Sidestream Smoke, 28
Principal Chemical Constituents of Environmental Tobacco Smoke, 36
Radioactivity of Environmental Tobacco Smoke, 37
Toxic and Carcinogenic Agents in Tobacco Smoke, 44
Summary and Recommendations, 45
References, 48

3 IN VIVO AND IN VITRO ASSAYS TO ASSESS THE HEALTH EFFECTS OF ENVIRONMENTAL TOBACCO SMOKE.................54
Introduction, 54
In Vivo Assays on Environmental Tobacco Smoke, 55
In Vitro Assays on Environmental Tobacco Smoke, 58
Summary and Recommendations, 59
References, 61

Part II
ASSESSING EXPOSURES TO ENVIRONMENTAL TOBACCO SMOKE

4 INTRODUCTION..65

5 ASSESSING EXPOSURES TO ENVIRONMENTAL TOBACCO SMOKE IN THE EXTERNAL ENVIRONMENT 69
Tracers for Environmental Tobacco Smoke, 70
Personal Monitoring, 76
Concentrations of Environmental Tobacco Smoke in Indoor Environments, 79
Modeling, 81
Summary and Recommendations, 94
References, 97

6 ASSESSING EXPOSURES TO ENVIRONMENTAL TOBACCO SMOKE USING QUESTIONNAIRES.......101
Exposure Histories Derived from Questionnaires, 102
Environmental Tobacco Smoke Exposure Data for Studies of Acute and Chronic Health Effects, 107
Data Quality, 108
Other Variables, 115
Summary and Recommendations, 116
References, 118

7 EXPOSURE-DOSE RELATIONSHIPS FOR ENVIRONMENTAL TOBACCO SMOKE................120
Estimating Dose, 120
Particle Size, 121
Breathing Pattern, 122
Deposition of Cigarette Smoke Particles, 123
Particle Retention in the Lungs, 126
Gases in Environmental Tobacco Smoke, 127
Summary and Recommendations, 129
References, 131

8 ASSESSING EXPOSURES TO ENVIRONMENTAL TOBACCO SMOKE USING BIOLOGICAL MARKERS................................133
Biological Markers in Physiological Fluids, 134
Genotoxicity of the Urine, 148
Future Needs, 152
Summary and Recommendations, 152
References, 154

Part III
HEALTH EFFECTS POSSIBLY ASSOCIATED WITH EXPOSURE TO ENVIRONMENTAL TOBACCO SMOKE BY NONSMOKERS

9 INTRODUCTION..163

10 SENSORY REACTIONS TO AND IRRITATION EFFECTS OF ENVIRONMENTAL TOBACCO SMOKE..166
Odor, 166
Irritation, 172
Hypersensitive Individuals, 176
Summary and Recommendations, 177
References, 179

11 EFFECTS OF EXPOSURE TO ENVIRONMENTAL TOBACCO SMOKE ON LUNG FUNCTION AND RESPIRATORY SYMPTOMS 182
Lung Function and Symptoms in Active Smokers, 182
Plausibility for an Effect Due to Passive Smoking, 184
Methodologic Considerations for Epidemiologic Studies, 185
Cross-sectional Studies, 188
Longitudinal Studies of Lung Function in Children and Adults, 200
The Effect of Passive Smoking on Respiratory Infections, 202
When Do Pulmonary Effects of Passive Smoking Occur?, 209
Studies of Acute Pulmonary Effects, 212
Summary and Recommendations, 216
References, 218

12 EXPOSURE TO ENVIRONMENTAL TOBACCO SMOKE AND LUNG CANCER 223
Using Biological Markers to Estimate Risk, 224
Assessing the Risk From Epidemiologic Studies of Lung Cancer and Exposure to ETS, 227
Corrections to Estimates for Systematic Errors, 231
Other Considerations, 242
Summary and Recommendations, 245
References, 246

13 CANCERS OTHER THAN LUNG CANCER 250
Smoking-Related Cancers, 250
Cancers Not Related to Smoking, 252
Interpretation, 254
Summary and Recommendations, 255
References, 255

14 CARDIOVASCULAR SYSTEM 257
Acute Cardiovascular Effects of Environmental Tobacco Smoke Exposure, 257
Cardiovascular Disease Morbidity and Mortality, 262
Summary and Recommendations, 265
References, 266

15 OTHER HEALTH CONSIDERATIONS IN CHILDREN 269
Environmental Tobacco Smoke Exposure by Nonsmoking Pregnant Women, 269
Growth in Children, 271
Chronic Ear Infections, 272
Summary and Recommendations, 273
References, 274

APPENDIXES
A. Guidelines for Public and Occupational Chemical Exposures to Materials That Are Also Found in Environmental Tobacco Smoke 279

B. Method of Combining Data From Studies of Environmental Tobacco Smoke Exposure and Lung Cancer 284
Case-Control Studies, 284
Prospective (or Cohort) Studies, 286
Summing Over Studies, 287
References, 288

C. Adjustments to Epidemiologic Estimates of Excess Lung Cancer in Persons Exposed to Environmental Tobacco Smoke 289
Using Cotinine Measurements to Correct Misreporting, 290
References, 293

D. Risk Assessment—Exposure to Environmental Tobacco Smoke and Lung Cancer 294
James Robins
Introduction, 294
D-1 Estimation of the True Relative Risk, 297
D-2 The Carcinogen-Equivalent Number of Actively Smoked Cigarettes Inhaled Daily by Passive Smokers: Comparisons of Epidemiologic with Dosimetric Estimates, 301
D-3 Estimating the Number of Lung Cancer Deaths in Nonsmokers in 1985 Attributable to ETS, 304
D-4 Lifetime Risk of Death From Lung Cancer Attributable to ETS, 306
Discussion, 311
Technical Discussions, 313
References, 336

Executive Summary

INTRODUCTION

A Committee of the National Research Council's (NRC's) Board on Environmental Studies and Toxicology prepared this report in response to requests from two federal government agencies, the Office of Air and Radiation of the Environmental Protection Agency (EPA) and the Office of Smoking and Health of the Department of Health and Human Services. The report evaluates methodologies in epidemiologic and related studies for obtaining measurements of exposure to environmental tobacco smoke (ETS) by nonsmokers and also outlines the possible health effects of such exposures as reported in the published literature. This committee was asked to review original research data and identify research needs but was not charged with preparing policy statements or recommendations for public health actions. In particular, the NRC was asked to:

- review the chemical and physical characterizations of the constituents of ETS;
- include a toxicological profile of sidestream and environmental tobacco smoke;
- review the epidemiologic and related literature on the health effects of exposure to ETS; and
- recommend future exposure monitoring, modeling, and epidemiologic research.

To address these and related issues, the NRC formed the Committee on Passive Smoking in the Board on Environmental Studies and Toxicology of the Commission on Life Sciences. The committee consists of professionals in a variety of fields, including epidemiology, toxicology, biochemistry, atmospheric science, biostatistics, and pulmonary physiology.

The subject of the committee's report is the use of epidemiology and related disciplines for the study of possible health effects of exposure to ETS by nonsmokers. Smokers are also exposed to ETS, but the health effects of this exposure, which are likely to be less intense than those of active smoking, are not the subject of this report. The primary goal of the studies reviewed in this report is to determine whether there is a relationship between health outcomes in human populations and ETS-exposure of nonsmokers. It is a formidable task to assess exposure to the complex mixture of ETS with enough precision to permit use in analytic studies, including quantitative risk estimation. For some health outcomes the relevant duration of exposure may be minutes, for others it may be decades. Numerous factors, in addition to exposure to smoke, can influence the risk of illness. These other factors must be taken into account if the magnitude of the effects of exposure to ETS is to be evaluated.

ENVIRONMENTAL TOBACCO SMOKE

More than 3,800 compounds have been identified in cigarette smoke. The major source, by far, for ETS is sidestream smoke (SS) which is emitted from the burning end of a cigarette in between puffs. The remainder of ETS consists of exhaled mainstream smoke (MS), smoke which escapes from the burning end during puff-drawing, and gases which diffuse during smoking through the cigarette paper. Each of the mixtures, MS, SS, and ETS, is an aerosol consisting of a particulate phase and a vapor phase. However, the smokes of MS, SS, and ETS differ, as the result of changes in the concentrations of individual constituents, the phase (particulate or vapor) in which the constituents are present, and various secondary reactions that chemically and physically alter ("age") the composition of the smoke. Undiluted SS contains higher concentrations of some toxic compounds than undiluted MS, including ammonia, volatile amines, volatile nitrosamines, nicotine decomposition products, and aromatic amines. However, concentrations of these SS emissions are considerably diluted in the indoor space where ETS exposures take place. The hydrophobic vapor phase constituents of ETS are likely to enter the lung of the exposed individual, while the hydrophilic vapor phase constituents are likely to be absorbed in the upper respiratory tract. Particles <2.5 μm (in this report referred to as respirable suspended particulates [RSP]) dominate the particulate phase of ETS and can be inhaled deeply into the lung.

Standard laboratory procedures have been established to assess the physicochemical properties of SS and MS. *Research is needed to standardize both the collection and evaluation of ETS so that the effects of ETS can be studied in laboratories and in human populations.*

The changes in distribution of particular constituents of ETS as the smoke ages in the indoor environment are largely unknown. For example, it is known that almost all of the nicotine shifts from the particulate phase in MS and fresh SS to the vapor phase in ETS. Consequently, indoor air-cleaning systems designed to remove particles will not greatly alter the nicotine exposure, but may alter the concentrations of other noxious or toxic components. *Research is needed to determine the distribution of constituents in the particulate and vapor phases of aged ETS. Also, the efficiency of air-cleaning systems in removing the constituents needs to be studied.*

Indoor radon comes from sources in the environment and decays to short-lived radon daughters, which may become bound to the RSP in ETS. However, some long-lived radon daughters come from tobacco itself. *Research should be conducted on possible interactions between ETS and radon daughters, especially as radon daughters can adhere to RSP and increase the potential hazard of ETS.*

MEASURES OF EXPOSURE

There are currently no direct measures of the *dose* absorbed of ETS in a population under study. *Exposures* to ETS, however, can be assessed by questionnaires, air monitoring, modeling of concentrations, or biological markers. *Future epidemiologic studies should incorporate into their design several of these exposure assessment methods in order to assess exposures to ETS more accurately and to estimate dose.*

Questionnaires

The simplest measure of ETS exposure is contained in the reply to the questions: "Are you a cigarette smoker?" and "If you are a nonsmoker, do you live with, or work with, or have regular contact with persons who are smokers?" There are great difficulties in developing uniform questions that elicit unambiguous replies and, more particularly, in using these replies to make firm quantitative estimates of exposure. They can be used, however, as a basis for classifying individuals into broad categories of exposure, recognizing the problems such as incorrectly estimating exposure through errors in reporting of current smoking habits, neglecting exposure to ETS in other environments like workplaces or public places, and reporting an exsmoker as a nonsmoker. Reports of whether or not the subject has smoked can be obtained with reasonable reliability from surrogate respondents. However, quantification of integrated exposure over many years is not likely to be fully reliable or precise. At best, such quantification provides an approximation of exposure, whether the information is obtained from the individual himself or from a surrogate. *To estimate integrated exposure to ETS, future studies need to estimate a long-term ETS exposure history, including what fraction of the day is spent in the presence of ETS and at what ages these exposures occurred. The data from such a history should be entered into a specific time-place model, from which cumulative exposure can be estimated.*

Monitoring

The use of air monitoring (personal or indoor space) is handicapped by the lack of a clear definition of the physicochemical nature of ETS and the identification of the individual, or target, constituents of ETS associated with the health or comfort effects under study. Proxy, or surrogate, constituents have been measured in a number of studies as indicators of ETS exposure in both personal and indoor space monitoring. RSP, carbon monoxide, nicotine, nitrogen oxides, acrolein, nitroso-compounds, and benzo[*a*]pyrene are some of the compounds or classes of air contaminants that have been measured under field conditions as indicators of ETS exposure. While some of the ETS constituents, particularly nicotine and RSP, have proved to be useful surrogates for ETS, no single measure has completely met all the criteria for an ideal ETS surrogate. To facilitate the study of the health effects of ETS exposure, an ideal marker or tracer of exposure to ETS should be unique (or nearly unique) to tobacco smoke, should be a constituent of tobacco smoke that is present in sufficient quantity so it can be measured even at low ETS levels, and should stand in a fairly constant ratio across brands of cigarettes to other tobacco smoke constituents (or contaminants) of interest. *Reliable information needs to be obtained on the quantity, transport, and fate of such chemicals in ordinary indoor environments.*

A majority of field studies have used RSP as an indicator of exposure to ETS because of the substantial emission of RSP in indoor spaces from tobacco combustion. ETS is the dominant contributor to the indoor levels of RSP. The total RSP, as measured by personal monitors, has been found to be substantially elevated for individuals who reported being exposed to ETS as compared with those who reported no such exposure. Both air monitoring and modeling clearly indicate that RSP concentrations will be elevated over background levels in indoor spaces when even low smoking rates occur. *The importance of variation in the input parameters–such as room size, temperature, humidity, air exchange rate, and numbers of cigarettes smoked—should be noted when interpreting the data on the constituents of ETS obtained from personal monitors and indoor space monitors.*

Biological Markers

In theory, dose of ETS to the tissues or organs could be measured directly through the use of biological markers that accurately indicate uptake in the tissues or organs. Optimal assessment of exposure to ETS should derive from measures made on physiological fluids of exposed persons. Several chemicals found in such fluids may be able to serve as biological markers of recent exposures. The criteria for acceptable biological markers are similar to those for measuring ETS in the external environment.

The biological markers that have been most useful for assessing recent exposures to ETS are nicotine and its metabolite, cotinine. Nicotine and cotinine derive virtually exclusively from tobacco products, of which tobacco smoke is the most important direct source. They can be identified and quantified in saliva, blood, or urine. Generally, the mean concentrations of nicotine and cotinine in the plasma or urine of nonsmokers exposed to ETS are about 1 percent of the mean values observed in active smokers. Several studies have indicated that urinary cotinine concentrations in infants and children increase as the numbers of reported smokers increase in the home. At present, there may be difficulty in interpreting the relative cotinine levels in nonsmokers compared with smokers because of the reported slower clearance of cotinine in nonsmokers. *Absorption, metabolism, and excretion of ETS constituents, including nicotine, need to be carefully studied in order to evaluate whether there are differences between smokers and nonsmokers in these factors. Further epidemiologic studies using biological markers are needed to quantify exposure-dose relationships in nonsmokers.*

Thiocyanate, as measured in saliva, serum, or urine, does not appear to be sufficiently sensitive as an indicator of ETS exposure. Similarly, exhaled carbon monoxide and carboxyhemoglobin are not sufficiently sensitive to moderate or low levels of ETS exposure and thus are not particularly useful biological markers for exposure to ETS, except in experimental, acute exposure situations. There are several other sources of carbon monoxide in the environment that equal or exceed the concentrations of carbon monoxide attributable to ETS.

Other suggested biological markers of exposure are *N*-nitrosoproline, nitrosothioproline, and some of the aromatic amines that are present in high concentrations in SS. However, data on sensitivity and reliability of laboratory procedures for these markers are not sufficient to recommend their use at this time in epidemiologic studies of ETS.

Laboratory assays have shown mutagenic activity in the urine of smokers and ETS-exposed nonsmokers. The mutagenicity of urine is a function of many factors—such as dietary constituents, occupational exposures, and other environmental factors—which render any findings of mutagenicity nonspecific. *Research is needed to clarify the appropriate methods for estimating mutagenicity and to isolate and identify the active agents in body fluids of ETS-exposed nonsmokers.*

DNA adducts derived from tobacco-related chemicals can be measured in the blood. However, these chemicals, such as benzo[*a*]pyrene, are not unique to ETS. *Studies are needed that can measure adducts of tobacco-specific chemicals.*

IN VIVO AND IN VITRO STUDIES

Laboratory studies can contribute to a better understanding of the factors and mechanisms involved in the induction of disease by environmental agents. There have been numerous bioassays conducted on MS. In examining the effects of MS, many research workers have used condensates of the smoke painted on the shaved skin of mice. This contrasts with the human exposure that is mainly in the respiratory tract. Nonetheless, these skin-painting studies have been useful in examining the carcinogenicity of different tobacco constituents and thus advancing knowledge of the actions of MS on a gross exposure level. *Similar work with skin painting has not been done with ETS and would be of value for assessing the differential toxicity of ETS and MS.*

In constrast to MS exposure, ETS exposure involves proportionately more exposure to gas phase than to particulate phase constituents. There have not, however, been studies of the effects of exposure to aged ETS. *The relative in vivo toxicity of MS, SS, and ETS needs to be assessed.*

Some studies have attempted to evaluate the gas phase of MS, SS, and ETS in short-term, in vitro assays. A solution of the gas phase of MS has been shown to induce dose-dependent increases in sister-chromatid exchanges in cultured human lymphocytes. Mutagenic activity has been found in the particulate matter of SS and in condensates of ETS. However, the work done to date is too sparse to permit any estimates of the mutagenicity of ETS per se, even though most of ETS consists of SS. *Further in vitro assays of ETS are needed.*

HEALTH EFFECTS

This report reviews both chronic and acute health effects associated with ETS exposure in nonsmokers. Most epidemiologic studies of chronic health effects have been conducted on persons who have had long-term exposures to ETS from household members. The studies do not directly address chronic health effects in individuals who are exposed at work or have occasional exposures in the home or elsewhere.

Because the physicochemical nature of ETS, MS, and SS differ, the extrapolation of health effects from studies of MS or of active smokers to nonsmokers exposed to ETS may not be appropriate. However, chemicals known to be toxic and carcinogenic in MS are also present in ETS. *Laboratory studies in conjunction with epidemiologic investigations are needed to help clarify possible health effects of exposure to ETS in nonsmokers.*

Acute, Noxious Effects

The most common acute effects associated with exposure to ETS are eye, nose, and throat irritation, and objectionable smell of tobacco smoke. Tobacco smoke has a distinct and persistent odor, making control through ventilation particularly difficult. In closed rooms where smoking is allowed, a ventilation rate of greater than 50 cubic feet per minute per occupant is necessary to achieve air quality that is acceptable to more than 80% of adults entering the room as contrasted with rates of less than 10 cubic feet per minute per occupant when there is no smoking or other pollution. Annoyance with noxious tobacco odor largely governs the reactions of visitors, while occupants of smoky rooms are more likely to complain about irritating effects to the eye, nose, or throat. Particle filtration appears to lead to little or no decline in odor and irritation, suggesting that the effects are produced by gas-phase constituents. During exposure to ETS, eye blink rate is correlated with sensory irritation, such as burning eyes and nasal irritation. For some persons, eye tearing can be so intense as to be incapacitating. There is some evidence that nonsmokers are more sensitive to the noxious qualities of cigarette smoke than are smokers. *Objective physiological or biochemical indices should be sought to validate reports of noxious reactions and chronic irritation associated with ETS.*

Smoke contains immunogens, that is, substances that can activate the immune system. Approximately half of atopic (allergy prone) individuals react to various extracts of tobacco leaf or smoke presented in skin tests. However, the components of the extract that are responsible for this reaction have not been isolated. There is little correlation between positive reactions to skin tests and self-reported complaints of tobacco smoke sensitivity. *Research is needed to evaluate the medical importance in atopic persons of these positive reactions to skin tests using ETS extracts and to relate immune response on skin tests to subjective complaints about the noxious, irritating properties of tobacco smoke.*

Respiratory Symptoms and Lung Function

Respiratory symptoms, such as wheezing, coughing, and sputum production, are increased in children of smoking parents. These symptoms are more common in children of smokers than children of nonsmokers. The largest studies place the increased risk of 20 to 80%, depending on the symptom being assessed and number of smokers in the household. Also, respiratory infections manifested as pneumonia and bronchitis are significantly increased in infants of smoking parents. Some studies have reported that infants of smoking parents are hospitalized for respiratory infections more frequently than children of nonsmokers. Among children aged under 1 year, studies are remarkably consistent in showing an increased risk of respiratory infections among children living in homes where parents smoke. There is a dose-response relationship that relates more to maternal smoking than paternal smoking. The association persists after allowing for possible confounding factors such as occupational data, respiratory illness in the parents, and birthweight. The mechanisms of the increased risk may either be a direct effect of ETS or due to a higher risk of cross-infection in such homes. Regardless of the mechanism, the exposure of small children to smoking in the home appears to put them at risk of respiratory illness.

Since children exposed to ETS from parental smoking have an increased frequency of pulmonary symptoms and respiratory infections, *it is prudent to eliminate ETS exposure from the environments of small children.*

There is some evidence that parental smoking may affect the rate of lung growth in children. In children with one or more parents who smoke, lung function increase, which is a normal growth phenomenon, shows a small decrease in the rate of growth. An important issue currently unresolved is whether a child who is affected by exposure to ETS from parental smoking may be at an increased risk for the development of chronic airflow obstruction in adult life. In all studies of children, it is difficult to distinguish between the role of ETS exposure in utero and postnatally. *Research is needed to address the issues of ETS exposure during childhood and fetal life and its possible relationship with airway hyperresponsiveness and pulmonary diseases in adult life.*

Three studies have shown a small reduction in pulmonary function in normal adults exposed to ETS. Interpretation of these findings is difficult because pulmonary effects in normal adults are likely to reflect the cumulative burden of many environmental and occupational exposures and other insults to the lung. Thus, the effects of ETS on the lungs of adults are likely to be confounded by many other factors, making it difficult to attribute any portion of the effect solely to ETS.

In some studies of asthmatics, in whom pulmonary reactions to ETS should be more readily produced, no effects on lung function were reported. In other studies, asthmatics reported complaints upon exposure to ETS and showed significant pulmonary function changes after experimental smoke exposure. ***Future studies of asthmatics exposed to ETS should be designed so as to limit the distortion produced by heterogeneous patient groups, varying medication schedules, and psychogenic effects of ETS.***

Lung Cancer

Considering the evidence as a whole, exposure to ETS increases the incidence of lung cancer in nonsmokers. Estimates of the magnitude of the increased risk vary. Among studies of various populations in Europe, Asia, and North America, the risk of lung cancer is roughly 30% higher for nonsmoking spouses of smokers than it is for nonsmoking spouses of nonsmokers. There is consistency among the studies in that all of the studies individually include the 30% increased risk within the 95% confidence intervals. Patterns and extent of exposure may vary in different communities and countries. Based on presently available epidemiologic data, the estimate of the increased risk from the American studies is lower than the average for all the studies, though not significantly so. These estimates are almost exclusively derived from the comparison of persons identified as exposed, or unexposed, on the basis of their spouse's smoking habits.

Certain errors in the reporting of smoking habits have probably contributed to the risks observed in the epidemiologic studies. Misclassification of current or exsmokers as nonsmokers would tend to produce an observed relative risk that is larger than the true risk. This effect was studied in detail using estimates of the extent of the errors involved and judged to contribute only a portion of the excess risk. Underestimation of the increased risk might also be introduced because the supposedly unexposed population had some exposure to ETS, although they were classified as unexposed in the studies. Taking both types of errors into account produces an estimate of the excess lung cancer risk for nonsmokers married to smokers compared with completely unexposed individuals that is similar to the relative risk observed in the epidemiologic studies considered.

Since carcinogenic agents contained in ETS are inhaled by nonsmokers, in the absence of a threshold for carcinogenic effects, an increased risk of lung cancer due to ETS exposure is biologically plausible. ***Laboratory studies would be important in determining the concentrations of carcinogenic constituents of ETS present in typical daily environments. The use of biological markers in epidemiologic studies is recommended to more precisely quantify dose-response relationships between ETS exposure and lung cancer occurrence.***

Other Cancers

There have been few studies of risk for cancers other than lung in nonsmokers exposed to ETS. Some of the sites considered have been brain, hematopoetic, and all sites combined. The results of these studies have been inconsistent. ***Whether or not there is an association between ETS exposure and cancers of any site other than lung is an important topic for future epidemiologic inquiries.***

Cardiovascular Disease

Since active smoking has an adverse effect on cardiovascular disease morbidity and mortality, ETS exposure has also become suspect. Reports have noted an excess risk of cardiovascular disease in ETS-exposed nonsmokers; however, methodologic problems in the designs and analyses of these studies preclude any firm conclusions about the results. Studies reporting that ETS can precipitate the onset of angina pectoris among people who already have this condition are subject to the same precautionary note. Exposure to ETS produced no statistically significant effects on heart rate or blood pressure in school-aged children or healthy adult subjects, either during exercise or at rest. Data are not available as to possible adverse cardiovascular effects in susceptible populations, such as infants, elderly, or diseased individuals.

Further experimental and observational studies should be conducted to assess the effect of long-term and acute ETS exposure on cardiac function, blood pressure, and angina in nonsmokers.

Other Health Considerations in Children

Several other health outcomes have been studied that relate to the growth and health of children. For all postnatal outcomes, it is often not possible to differentiate the effect of in utero exposure to ETS from subsequent childhood exposures to ETS.

Nonsmoking pregnant women exposed to smoking spouses have been reported to produce babies of lower birthweight than nonsmoking women with nonsmoking spouses. Some studies have noted a dose-response relationship between the number of cigarettes smoked by fathers and birthweight of the offspring. *Additional studies of intrauterine fetal growth retardation associated with ETS exposure of nonsmoking mothers need to be conducted with better assessments of the magnitude of ETS exposure.*

Several studies have examined possible relationships between chronic exposure to ETS by children and parameters of growth and development. Growth is an especially difficult phenomenon to study since many factors—such as genetics, nutrition, social class, and ethnicity—play important roles. It is difficult to assign proportional causality to each factor. Moreover, height and weight ratios and other growth measures are not reliably obtained in standard pediatric surveys. A few studies have shown that children of smokers have reduced growth and development, and one study reported a dose-response relationship between reduced height and increasing numbers of cigarettes smoked in the home by either the mother or the father. *Further work is needed to determine the nature of this association.*

Otitis media is a common occurrence in young children. In several studies, parental smoking, along with several other risk factors, has been linked to increased risk of chronic ear infections in children. *Further work is needed to determine whether the association is causal.*

1
Introduction

Environmental tobacco smoke (ETS) occurs in homes, at workplaces, and in public places. The acute irritating and noxious effects of involuntary exposure to ETS, or "passive smoking," are well established. Based in part on these irritating properties of ETS, a recent report of the NRC recommended a ban on smoking in the small enclosed spaces of airliner cabins (National Research Council, 1986). More than 20 states and numerous local governments have enacted legislation and policies restricting smoking (1985 information obtained from the Office on Smoking and Health, personal communications). Such public information campaigns and other actions have convinced a large portion of the population that active cigarette smoking is dangerous to health. To many, this also implies that exposure to ETS can affect health. This report, in part, evaluates whether the latter beliefs are warranted. It also makes recommendations for future exposure monitoring and epidemiologic research.

The issues are complex. In some cases the conclusions are uncertain, because much of the scientific data necessary to shed light on these concerns does not exist. This report addresses the following major issues pertaining to ETS:

- *The nature of the smoke.* What constitutes ETS? What are the chemicals in ETS and what are the dilutions therein? There are two physical phases of smoke: particulate phase and vapor phase. What chemicals are in each phase? Are any of these chemicals carcinogenic or toxic, as determined in bioassays?

• *Factors affecting exposure and the assessment of exposure.* To what extent is the nonsmoker exposed to harmful chemicals that can be measured in ETS? How can we measure exposure to ETS? Can ambient monitoring be used in epidemiological studies? How reliable is questionnaire information? What constitutes the dose a person may receive? Are there objective measures of dose received, such as tobacco-smoke-specific biological markers? What choices and reasons for choice are there among the markers?

• *Effects of exposure.* What are the health effects, if any, consequent to exposure to ETS? Are these health effects related to discomfort or irritant effects only, or more serious disease? Are the potential health effects reversible when exposure ceases? What are the data from human studies? Do interactions with other environmental agents at workplaces or in homes need to be considered? Are there biologically plausible explanations for the various effects ascribed to ETS exposure?

The report considers sensitive populations such as children, pregnant women, older persons, and those with persisting respiratory illnesses. It does not consider the established effects on the fetus carried by a pregnant, smoking woman because this is not an instance in which a nonsmoking individual *breathes* ETS generated by other people. However, a pregnant, nonsmoking woman might be affected by exposure to ETS, as may her fetus.

The health effects considered include respiratory symptoms and lung function, and other respiratory ailments (especially in children), such as asthma and allergic responses, cancer at various sites, and cardiovascular disease, among others. Some attention is paid to irritation, annoyance, and associated responses.

DEFINITIONS

Environmental tobacco smoke (ETS) originates from the smoldering end of the tobacco product in between puffs, known as sidestream smoke (SS), and from the smoker's exhaled smoke. [The smoke that the smoker inhales is known as mainstream smoke (MS).] Other contributors to ETS include minor amounts of smoke that escape during the puff-drawing from the burning cone and some vapor-phase components that diffuse through the cigarette paper into the environment. These various components are released into the environment and are diluted by ambient air. They may also aggregate with pollutants already in the environment and thereby change character. The composition of this complex mixture, known as ETS, has different physicochemical characteristics than the MS.

There are various terms in the literature that refer to the inhalation of ETS by nonsmokers, e.g., "passive smoking," "involuntary smoking," and "breathing other people's smoke." We will refer to the inhalation of ETS by using the terms "passive smoking" and "exposure to ETS by nonsmokers" interchangeably.

TRENDS IN CIGARETTE USAGE

Exposure of nonsmokers to ETS is a function of several variables, one of which is the number of active smokers with whom the nonsmoker comes into contact throughout some period of time. The percent of the population who smoke steadily increased over the first two-thirds of this century but has declined more recently. In 1980, 32% of the adult population considered themselves to be cigarette smokers (U.S. Department of Commerce, 1984). This percentage, now roughly equal for men and for women, reflects a reduction of almost one-third in men since the publication of the first *Surgeon General's Report on Smoking and Health* in 1964 (U.S. Public Health Service, 1964). Figure 1-1 shows the trends in cigarette usage between 1955 and 1985 for males and females. Table 1-1 gives cigarette consumption since 1900. Table 1-2 illustrates an overall increase in cigar and pipe smoking, followed by a decline during the past decade. The actual probability of exposure to ETS is complex, affected by ventilation rates, size of houses, restrictions on where tobacco products may be smoked, and changes in the cigarette itself. The consequence of Figure 1-1 is that the general probability of being exposed to some ETS for the nonsmoker has increased until quite recently.

The magnitude of exposure to ETS will depend upon the number of cigarettes and/or cigars and pipes smoked in a given environment, as well as other factors such as ventilation. Light smokers are more likely to stop smoking than heavy smokers, which might explain why over the past 30 years the number of cigarettes per smoker and the total consumption (Figure 1-2) have not declined as rapidly as the percentage of people who smoke (see also cigar and loose tobacco consumption in Table 1-2). From a peak consumption in the early 1960s, there has been a decline of

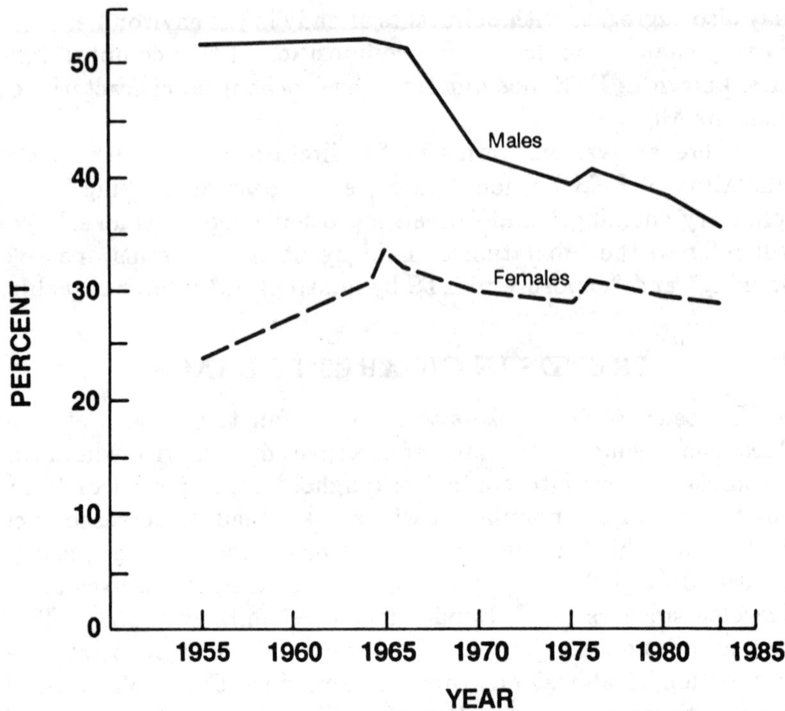

FIGURE 1-1 Percentage of current smokers in the United States. Adult population, by sex, 1955-1983. From Shopland and Brown (1985).

20% in the per capita (U.S.) consumption of cigarettes (Shopland and Brown, 1985). These data, however, are averaged over the total U.S. population, including smokers and nonsmokers. Among persons who consider themselves smokers, the cigarette consumption per adult smoker actually has increased from 27.3 to 30.0 cigarettes per day. Table 1-3 demonstrates that, for both sexes, the percent of smokers who are heavy smokers has steadily increased over the past 30 years. Therefore, the consumption per active smoker indicates that the nonsmoker who has close contact with a smoker may be exposed to greater amounts of smoke in 1985 than in 1955, although the total number of hours a nonsmoker is exposed to ETS would have declined.

Counteracting this trend of increased exposure has been the trend of reduction in amount of tobacco used to fill each cigarette. Physical changes of the leaf due to modern methods of processing, the use of filter tips (United States, >90% of all cigarettes since

TABLE 1-1 U.S. Cigarette Consumption, 1900 to 1985[a]

Year	Total Billions	Number Per Capita, 18 Years and Older	Year	Total Billions	Number Per Capita, 18 Years and Older	Year	Total Billions	Number Per Capita, 18 Years and Older
1900	2.5	54	1930	119.3	1,485	1960	484.4	4,171
1901	2.5	53	1931	114.0	1,399	1961	502.5	4,266
1902	2.8	60	1932	102.8	1,245	1962	508.4	4,265
1903	3.1	64	1933	111.6	1,334	1963	523.9	4,345
1904	3.3	66	1934	125.7	1,483	1964	511.3	4,195
1905	3.6	70	1935	134.4	1,564	1965	528.8	4,259
1906	4.5	86	1936	152.7	1,754	1966	541.3	4,287
1907	5.3	99	1937	162.8	1,847	1967	549.3	4,280
1908	5.7	105	1938	163.4	1,830	1968	545.6	4,186
1909	7.0	125	1939	172.1	1,900	1969	528.9	3,993
1910	8.6	151	1940	181.9	1,976	1970	536.5	3,985
1911	10.1	173	1941	208.9	2,236	1971	555.1	4,037
1912	13.2	223	1942	245.0	2,585	1972	566.8	4,043
1913	15.8	260	1943	284.3	2,956	1973	589.7	4,148
1914	16.5	267	1944	296.3	3,039	1974	599.0	4,141
1915	17.9	285	1945	340.6	3,449	1975	607.2	4,123
1916	25.2	395	1946	344.3	3,446	1976	613.5	4,092
1917	35.7	551	1947	345.4	3,416	1977	617.0	4,051
1918	45.6	697	1948	358.9	3,505	1978	616.0	3,967
1919	48.0	727	1949	360.9	3,480	1979	621.5	3,861
1920	44.6	665	1950	369.8	3,522	1980	631.5	3,851
1921	50.7	742	1951	397.1	3,744	1981	640.0	3,840
1922	53.4	770	1952	416.0	3,886	1982	634.0	3,753
1923	64.4	911	1953	408.2	3,778	1983	600.0	3,502
1924	71.0	982	1954	387.0	3,546	1984	600.4[b]	3,461[b]
1925	79.8	1,085	1955	396.4	3,597	1985	595.0[c]	3,384[c]
1926	89.1	1,191	1956	406.5	3,650			
1927	97.5	1,279	1957	422.5	3,755			
1928	106.0	1,366	1958	448.9	3,953			
1929	118.6	1,504	1959	467.5	4,073			

[a]Includes overseas forces, 1917–1919 and 1940 to date. Commodity Economics Division, Economic Research Service, USDA.

[b]Subject to revision.

[c]Estimated.

SOURCE: U.S. Department of Agriculture, 1985.

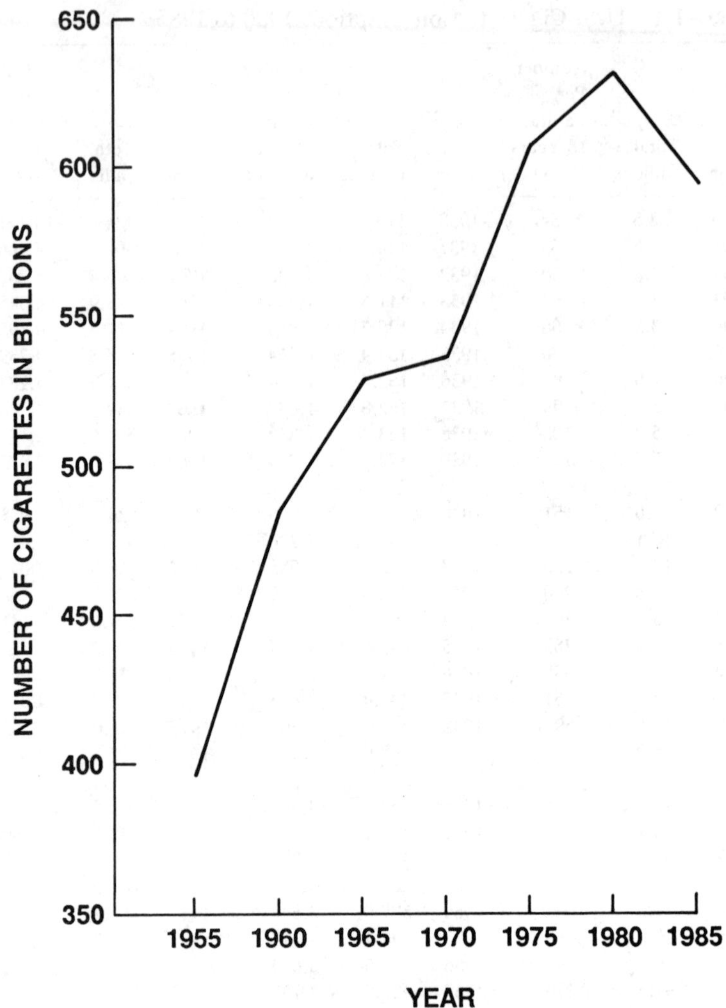

FIGURE 1-2 Total cigarette consumption (domestic sales), 1955- 1985.

1978; Griese, 1984), and variations in the composition of tobacco blends for cigarettes (Norman, 1982) have made this reduction possible.

In 1956, the U.S. average tar and nicotine yields were 38.4 mg and 2.69 mg, respectively. Since then, tar and nicotine yields have steadily decreased to 13.2 mg tar and 0.95 mg nicotine in 1980 (The Tobacco Institute, 1981). However, tar and nicotine yields in the SS of cigarettes have not significantly changed except

TABLE 1-2 U.S. Consumption of Cigars and Tobacco for Pipes and Hand-rolled Cigarettes

Year	Cigars, millions	Tobacco, Mn. lb[a]	Year	Cigars, millions	Tobacco, Mn. lb[a]	Year	Cigars, millions
1920	8,609	—	1950	5,608	104.3	1980	5,386
1921	7,435	—	1951	5,778	97.4	1981	5,231
1922	7,527	—	1952	6,037	92.9	1982	4,901
1923	7,505	—	1953	6,107	84.3	1983	4,884
1924	7,189	—	1954	6,024	81.2		
1925	6,949	—	1955	6,078	77.8		
1926	7,008	—	1956	6,039	70.0		
1927	7,008	—	1957	6,194	68.9		
1928	6,874	—	1958	6,586	74.4		
1929	6,972	—	1959	7,377	71.9		
1930	6,272	—	1960	7,434	72.2		
1931	5,656	—	1961	7,083	72.7		
1932	4,724	—	1962	7,103	69.8		
1933	4,553	—	1963	7,434	69.7		
1934	4,818	—	1964	9,899	81.7		
1935	4,943	—	1965	8,949	69.8		
1936	5,362	—	1966	8,610	68.6		
1937	5,516	—	1967	8,403	66.4		
1938	5,294	—	1968	8,331	69.6		
1939	5,469	—	1969	8,579	68.3		
1940	5,491	—	1970	8,881	74.0		
1941	5,933	—	1971	8,830	69.5		
1942	6,339	—	1972	11,125	66.8		
1943	5,350	—	1973	11,126	59.5		
1944	4,878	—	1974	9,339			
1945	5,027	—	1975	8,663			
1946	5,929	—	1976	7,492			
1947	5,706	—	1977	6,792			
1948	5,860	—	1978	6,231			
1949	5,625	—	1979	5,706			

[a]Tobacco for pipes and hand-rolled cigarettes, not available prior to 1950.

SOURCES: Lee, 1975; *Tobacco Reporter*, 1984.

TABLE 1-3 Number of Cigarettes Smoked per Day, as a Percentage of Current Smokers, by Sex

	Less Than 15	15–24	25 or More
Males			
1965	30.1	45.7	24.1
1976	24.9	44.4	30.7
1980	24.2	41.7	34.2
1983	23.5	42.9	33.6
Females			
1965	46.2	40.8	13.0
1976	37.6	43.4	19.0
1980	34.7	42.0	23.0
1983	33.8	45.6	20.6

SOURCE: Shopland and Brown, 1985.

in the case of cigarettes designed for ultralow yields of tar and nicotine. Certain other components, in particular volatile, toxic components, are released into SS in significantly greater amounts than into MS. Furthermore, ETS contains significantly smaller particles than MS, and nicotine, and perhaps other smoke constituents, is volatilized to a greater extent in SS than in MS. This means that the gas-phase composition of SS differs substantially from that of MS.

The health implications to nonsmokers of exposure to ETS may not be a simple extrapolation from the studies of active smokers. The complexities of such extrapolations will be discussed.

Children represent a large population of nonsmokers who may be exposed to environmental smoke. Several cohort studies of children are reviewed in Chapter 11. Although there is some variation among these studies, they indicate, mainly through questionnaires, that between 50 and 65 percent of the children have been exposed to tobacco smoke in the home during the past 20 years. Health implications of this exposure for the developing child will be discussed.

ORGANIZATION

This report begins with a discussion of the components of ETS (Chapter 2) and what in vivo and in vitro studies have determined about ETS (Chapter 3). Various methods of exposure assessment are considered in Chapters 4 through 8, including physical effects, questionnaires, and biological markers. Chapters 9 through 15 review epidemiologic studies of possible health effects of these exposures. The health consequences examined range from irritation and allergic reactions to cancer and cardiovascular disease. Only studies that assess exposures under experimental conditions or in the home are included. ETS potentially interacts with constituents of the ambient air. This makes the evaluation of possible health effects due to workplace exposure complex and specific to each situation because of the varying nature of contaminants. Each chapter concludes with a summary of what is currently known, the strength of that knowledge, and what additional information would further clarify the relationship of ETS and possible health effects. Some recommendations for additional research are also given.

REFERENCES

Griese, V.N. Market growth of reduced tar cigarettes. Recent Adv. Tob. Sci. 10:4-14, 1984.

Lee, P.N., Ed. Tobacco Consumption in Various Countries, pp. 82-84. London, England: Tobacco Research Council, 1975.

National Research Council, Committee on Airliner Cabin Air Quality. Airliner Cabin Environment: Air Quality and Safety. Washington, D.C.: National Academy Press, 1986. 303 pp.

Norman, V. Changes in smoke chemistry of modern day cigarettes. Recent Adv. Tob. Sci. 8:141-177, 1982.

Shopland, D.R., and C. Brown. Changes in cigarette smoking prevalence in the U.S.: 1955-1983. Ann. Behav. Med. 7:5-8, 1985.

The Tobacco Institute. U.S. tar/nicotine levels dropping. The Tob. Observ. 6:1, 1981.

Tobacco Reporter. Cigars in the U.S.: Is the upturn real? Tob. Rep. 111:43-46, 1984.

U.S. Department of Agriculture. Tobacco: Outlook and Situation Report. DOA Publ. No. TS-129. Washington, D.C.: U.S. Government Printing Office, 1985.

U.S. Department of Commerce. Statistical Abstract of the United States: 1985. Washington, D.C.: U.S. Department of Commerce, Bureau of the Census, 1984. 119 pp.

I

PHYSICOCHEMICAL AND TOXICOLOGICAL STUDIES OF ENVIRONMENTAL TOBACCO SMOKE

2
The Physicochemical Nature of Sidestream Smoke and Environmental Tobacco Smoke

INTRODUCTION

Mainstream smoke (MS) is the aerosol drawn into the mouth of a smoker from a cigarette, cigar, or pipe. Sidestream smoke (SS) is the aerosol emitted in the surrounding air from a smoldering tobacco product between puff-drawing. SS is a major source of environmental tobacco smoke (ETS), i.e., air pollution caused by the burning of tobacco products. Other contributors to ETS are the exhaled portion of MS and the smoke that escapes from the burning part of a tobacco product during puff-drawing. In addition, some volatile components (e.g., carbon monoxide) diffuse through cigarette paper and contribute to ETS.

Tobacco smoke aerosols are diluted with air by the time they are inhaled as ETS air pollutants. Furthermore, the physical characteristics and chemical composition of ETS change as the pollutants "age": nicotine is volatilized; particle sizes decrease; nitrogen oxide gradually oxidizes to nitrogen dioxide; various components of the ambient air (e.g., radon daughters) can be adsorbed on the particles; and other physicochemical changes can occur.

In the scientific literature, the terms "passive smoke," "passive smoking," and "involuntary smoking" are used often. These terms do not adequately describe ETS and its inhalation, but they are used interchangeably with "ETS" in this report.

Most of the reported data on MS, SS, and ETS pertain to cigarette smoking. Few comparative data on smoke pollutants from other tobacco products are available.

In the laboratory, cigarettes, cigars, and pipes are smoked by machines under standardized conditions (Wynder and Hoffmann, 1967) to obtain reproducible data for the determination of various individual constituents of undiluted MS and SS. Such data provide a scientific basis for comparing tobacco products and brands. The standardized machine-smoking conditions were developed 3 decades ago to simulate human smoking behavior (Wartman et al., 1959). However, these can differ substantially from those of today's cigarette smokers, especially in the case of filter-tipped products that are designed to deliver low yields of tar and nicotine (Herning et al., 1981).

For cigarettes and cigarette-like cigars weighing up to 1.5 g, the most widely used machine-smoking conditions in the test laboratory are as follows: one 35-ml puff lasting 2 seconds taken once a minute. The butt length for nonfilter cigarettes is 23 mm. For filter-tipped cigarettes, the total length is increased 3 mm for filter tip plus overwrap (Pillsbury et al., 1969; Brunnemann et al., 1976). For cigars, the conditions are as follows: a 30-ml puff taken once every 40 seconds and a butt length of 33 mm (International Committee for Cigar Smoke Study, 1974). For pipe smoking the test calls for a bowl filled with 1 g of tobacco and for a 50-ml puff lasting 2 seconds to be taken every 12 seconds (Miller, 1964).

Several devices have been used for generating SS from cigarettes and cigars (Dube and Greene, 1982). Among them, the Neurath and Ehmke chamber or modification thereof have been used for chemical analytic work on SS (Neurath and Ehmke, 1964; Brunnemann and Hoffmann, 1974). When SS is generated, a stream of air is sent through a chamber at 25 ml/second. At this rate, the tar and nicotine yields in the MS of cigarettes and cigars smoked in the chamber are similar to those obtained by smoking cigarettes or cigars in the open air. However, the velocity of the airstream through the chamber has considerable influence on the yields of individual compounds in SS (Rühl et al., 1980; Klus and Kuhn, 1982). In order to collect the particulate matter of MS and SS, the aerosols are directed through a glass-fiber filter that traps more than 99% of all the particles with diameters of 0.1 μm or more (Wartman et al., 1959). The portion of the smoke that passes through the filter is designated as the vapor phase. This arbitrary separation into particulate phase and vapor phase does not necessarily reflect the physicochemical conditions prevailing in MS and

SS. However, it does reflect specific trapping systems and analytic methods that have been developed for the standardized determination of individual components or groups of components in MS or SS (Brunnemann and Hoffmann, 1982; Dube and Greene, 1982).

Standardized machine-smoking conditions do not exactly duplicate the smoking patterns of an individual, which depend on many factors. For example, low nicotine delivery in cigarette smoke generally induces a smoker to puff more frequently (up to 5 puffs/minute), to draw larger volumes (up to 55 ml/puff), and to inhale more deeply. Puffing more frequently increases the amount of tobacco consumed during generation of MS and thus diminishes the amount of tobacco burned between puffs. This, in turn, affects the release of combustion products in SS, so an increase in puff frequency diminishes the production of SS and ETS. Also, smoking behavior appears to depend strongly on the blood concentration of nicotine that the smoker desires to reach (Krasnegor, 1979; Grabowski and Bell, 1983).

The smoker, because of proximity to the source, usually inhales more of the SS and ETS originating from the burning of the tobacco product than a nonsmoker; however, we do not know the exact amount and we do not know the degree to which inhaled SS and ETS aerosols are retained in the smoker's respiratory tract. Model studies with MS have shown that more than 90% of some hydrophilic volatile components (e.g., acetaldehyde) is retained after inhalation by the smoker (Dalham et al., 1968a). Therefore, one may assume that a large proportion of the hydrophilic agents in the vapor phase of SS and ETS is also retained when smoke-polluted ambient air is inhaled. In the case of hydrophobic components of the vapor phase of MS (e.g., carbon monoxide), the retained fraction depends on the depth of inhalation, but it hardly ever exceeds 50% (Dalham et al., 1968b). An active smoker generally retains 90% or more of MS particles (Dalham et al., 1968b; Hiller, 1984), whereas a nonsmoker exposed to ETS appears to retain a smaller percentage of ETS particles. It has been calculated that, depending on the degree of SS pollution, a nonsmoker exposed to ETS can retain 0.014 to 1.6 mg of particles per day from ETS (Hiller, 1984).

SIDESTREAM SMOKE

The SS generated between puffs originates from a strongly reducing atmosphere. Therefore, undiluted SS contains more combustion products that result from oxygen deficiency and thermal cracking of molecules than does MS. In addition, SS formation involves generation of higher amounts of compounds from nitrosation reactions. Consequently, SS differs substantially from MS.

Table 2-1 compares MS and SS from nonfilter cigarettes. During the consumption of one whole cigarette under standard smoking conditions, the formation of cigarette MS generated during 10 puffs (each 2 seconds) of a blended nonfilter cigarette requires 20 s and consumes 347 mg of tobacco. The formation of SS from the same cigarette smoldering requires 550 seconds and consumes 411 mg of tobacco. However, as shown with experimental cigarettes, the amounts of tobacco consumed during and between puffs depend greatly on the type of tobacco (Johnson et al., 1973a). In addition, MS and SS are generated at different temperatures. For example, under laminar atmospheric conditions, the SS of a smoldering cigarette enters the surrounding atmosphere about 3 mm in front of the paper burn line, at about 350°C (Baker, 1984).

The pH of the MS of a blended American cigarette ranges from 6.0 to 6.5, whereas the pH of SS is 6.7 to 7.5. Above a pH of 6.0, the proportion of unprotonated nicotine in undiluted smoke increases; therefore, SS contains more free nicotine in the gas phase than MS. The pH of SS of cigars is 7.5 to 8.7; pH values for pipe smoke have not been reported (Brunnemann and Hoffmann, 1974). Under conditions prevailing in MS, SS, and ETS, unprotonated nicotine is primarily present in the vapor phase; its absorption through the mucous membranes is faster; thus, its pharmacologic effect is different from that of unprotonated nicotine in the particulate matter (Armitage and Turner, 1970).

About 300-400 of the more than 3,800 compounds identified in tobacco smoke have been measured in MS and SS. Table 2-2 lists the amounts of selected substances reported to occur in the MS and in SS from the burning of a whole nonfilter cigarette and the range of the ratio of their amounts in SS/MS. A ratio greater than unity means that more of a substance is released in SS than in MS. The separation of the compounds in Table 2-2 into vapor phase and particulate phase constituents reflects the conditions

TABLE 2-1 Some Physiocochemical Characteristics of Fresh, Undiluted Mainstream and Sidestream Smoke from a Nonfilter Cigarette[a]

Characteristics	MS	SS	Reference
Duration of smoke production, s	20	550	Neurath and Horstmann, 1973
Tobacco burned, mg	347	411	Neurath and Horstmann, 1973
Peak temperature during formation, °C	900	600	Wynder and Hoffmann, 1967
pH	6.0-6.2	6.4-6.6	Brunnemann and Hoffmann, 1974
Number of particles per cigarette	10.5×10^{12}	3.5×10^{12}	Scassellatti-Sforzoline and Savino, 1968
Particle size, μm	0.1-1.0	0.01-0.8	Carter and Hasegawa, 1975; Hiller et al., 1982
Particle mean diameter, μm	0.4	0.32	Carter and Hasegawa, 1975; Hiller et al., 1982
Gas concentration, vol.%			
Carbon monoxide	3-5	2-3	Keith and Derrick, 1960
Carbon dioxide	8-11	4-6	Wynder and Hoffmann, 1967
Oxygen	12-16	1.5-2	Baker, 1984
Hydrogen	3-15	0.8-1.0	Hoffmann et al., 1984a,b

[a]Data were obtained under standard laboratory smoking conditions of one puff per minute, lasting 2 s, and having volume of 35 ml. Mainstream smoke collected directly from end of cigarette. Sidestream smoke was measured 4 mm from burning cone (gas temperature, 350°C).

prevailing in MS and does not apply to the distribution of these compounds in the vapor phase and particulate phase of SS.

The ratio of the amount of tobacco burned during SS generation to that burned during MS generation is 1.2:1 to 1.5:1 (see Table 2-1 for data on nonfilter cigarettes). Therefore, if one assumed that the combustion process is the same during the generation of the two kinds of smoke, the ratios of their various constituents would also be between 1.2:1 and 1.5:1. That is not the case, as indicated by the higher SS/MS values in Table 2-2. For instance, in the first part of Table 2-2, which lists volatile compounds, the ratios for carbon monoxide range from 2.5 to 4.7, for carbon dioxide from 8 to 11, for acrolein from 8 to 15, and for benzene about 10.

TABLE 2-2 Distribution of Constituents in Fresh, Undiluted Mainstream Smoke and Diluted Sidestream Smoke from Nonfilter Cigarettes[a]

Constituent	Amount in MS	Range in SS/MS
Vapor phase[b]		
Carbon monoxide	10-23 mg	2.5-4.7
Carbon dioxide	20-40 mg	8-11
Carbonyl sulfide	18-42 μg	0.03-0.13
Benzene[c]	12-48 μg	5-10
Toluene	100-200 μg	5.6-8.3
Formaldehyde	70-100 μg	0.1-≈50
Acrolein	60-100 μg	8-15
Acetone	100-250 μg	2-5
Pyridine	16-40 μg	6.5-20
3-Methylpyridine	12-36 μg	3-13
3-Vinylpyridine	11-30 μg	20-40
Hydrogen cyanide	400-500 μg	0.1-0.25
Hydrazine[d]	32 ng	3
Ammonia	50-130 μg	40-170
Methylamine	11.5-28.7 μg	4.2-6.4
Dimethylamine	7.8-10 μg	3.7-5.1
Nitrogen oxides	100-600 μg	4-10
N-Nitrosodimethylamine[e]	10-40 ng	20-100
N-Nitrosodiethylamine[e]	ND-25 ng	<40
N-Nitrosopyrrolidine[e]	6-30 ng	6-30
Formic acid	210-490 μg	1.4-1.6
Acetic acid	330-810 μg	1.9-3.6
Methyl chloride	150-600 μg	1.7-3.3
Particulate phase[b]		
Particulate matter[c]	15-40 mg	1.3-1.9
Nicotine	1-2.5 mg	2.6-3.3
Anatabine	2-20 μg	<0.1-0.5
Phenol	60-140 μg	1.6-3.0
Catechol	100-360 μg	0.6-0.9
Hydroquinone	110-300 μg	0.7-0.9
Aniline	360 ng	30
2-Toluidine	160 ng	19
2-Naphthylamine[c]	1.7 ng	30
4-Aminobiphenyl[c]	4.6 ng	31
Benz[*a*]anthracene[e]	20-70 ng	2-4
Benzo[*a*]pyrene[d]	20-40 ng	2.5-3.5
Cholesterol	22 μg	0.9
γ-Butyrolactone[e]	10-22 μg	3.6-5.0
Quinoline	0.5-2 μg	8-11
Harman[f]	1.7-3.1 μg	0.7-1.7
N′-Nitrosonornicotine[e]	200-3,000 ng	0.5-3
NNK[g]	100-1,000 ng	1-4
N-Nitrosodiethanolamine[e]	20-70 ng	1.2

TABLE 2-2 *Continued*

Constituent	Amount in MS	Range of SS/MS
Cadmium	100 ng	7.2
Nickel[d]	20-80 ng	13-30
Zinc	60 ng	6.7
Polonium-210[e]	0.04-0.1 pCi	1.0-4.0
Benzoic acid	14-28 μg	0.67-0.95
Lactic acid	63-174 μg	0.5-0.7
Glycolic acid	37-126 μg	0.6-0.95
Succinic acid	110-140 μg	0.43-0.62

[a]Data from Elliot and Rowe (1975); Schmeltz et al. (1979); Hoffmann et al. (1983); Klus and Kuhn (1982); Sakuma et al. (1983, 1984a,b); Hiller et al. (1982). Diluted SS is collected with airflow of 25 ml/s, which is passed over the burning cone.

[b]Separation into vapor and particulate phases reflects conditions prevailing in MS and does not necessarily imply same separation in SS.

[c]Human carcinogen (U.S. Department of Health and Human Services, 1983).

[d]Suspected human carcinogen (U.S. Department of Health and Human Services, 1983).

[e]Animal carcinogen (Vainio et al., 1985).

[f]1-methyl-9*H*-pyrido[3,4-*b*]-indole.

[g]NNK = 4-(*N*-methyl-*N*-nitrosamino)-1-(3-pyridyl)-1-butanone.

The high SS/MS values of carbon monoxide and carbon dioxide show that more of each of these constituents is generated in the oxygen-deficient cone during smoldering than during puff-drawing. After passing briefly through the hot cone, most of the carbon monoxide is oxidized to carbon dioxide, probably because of the high temperature gradient and sudden exposure to air.

The high SS/MS values of volatile pyridines are thought to be due to the fact that these compounds are formed from the alkaloids during smoldering (Schmeltz et al., 1979). Hydrogen cyanide is formed primarily from protein at temperatures above 700°C (Johnson and Karg, 1971). Thus, smoldering of tobacco at 600°C does not favor the pyrosynthesis of hydrogen cyanide to the extent that it occurs during MS generation.

With regard to the carcinogenic potential of SS, it is important to consider the SS/MS ratio of NO_x—4 to 10. More than 95% of the NO_x inhaled by the smoker is in the form of nitric oxide, and only a small portion is oxidized to the powerful nitrosating agent, nitrogen dioxide. Only a small fraction of nitric oxide is expected to be retained in the respiratory system by being bound to hemoglobin. NO_x released into the environment in SS is partially oxidized to nitrogen dioxide (Vilicins and Lephardt, 1975). Thus, environments polluted with SS are expected to contain increased concentrations of the hydrophilic nitrosating agent, nitrogen dioxide.

Perhaps the most remarkable data in this portion of Table 2-2 are the very high SS/MS values of ammonia, nitrogen oxide, and the volatile *N*-nitrosamines. Studies with [^{15}N]nitrate have shown that, during burning of tobacco, nitrate is reduced to ammonia, which is released to a greater extent in SS than in MS during puff-drawing (Just et al., 1972). An extreme example is the case of a cigarette made exclusively from burley tobacco, a variety generally rich in nitrate (2.0-5.0% in U.S. survey); ammonia is released in SS at 8,500 μg/cigarette (SS/MS 170, according to Johnson et al., 1973b). (In the case of a blended cigarette, the greater generation of ammonia in SS causes an increased pH, which can be above 7, whereas the pH of MS is about 6.)

The ranges of high SS/MS ratios of the highly carcinogenic volatile *N*-nitrosamines (such as *N*-nitrosodimethylamine—20 to 100) have been well established (Brunnemann et al., 1977, 1980; Rühl et al., 1980).

The second part of Table 2-2 lists some constituents of particulate matter, their amounts reported to occur in MS during the burning of one cigarette, and ranges of the relative amounts in SS/MS. The increases in SS of tobacco-specific *N*-nitrosamines, such as 4-(*N*-methyl-*N*-nitrosamino)-1-(3-pyridyl)-1-butanone (NNK), *N*-nitrosodiethanolamine, and *N'*-nitrosonornicotine, are up to fourfold. Presently we do not know whether the tobacco-specific *N*-nitrosamines are present in the particulate phase or in the vapor phase of ETS (Hoffmann and Hecht, 1985).

Constituents of the vapor phase would be less likely to settle with the smoke particles, but would remain in the ambient air for longer spans of time. Research is needed to evaluate this distribution, which is important with respect to the carcinogenic potential of SS. The meaning of the abundant release of amines in SS (SS/MS, to 30-fold)—as indicated by the data in aniline, 2-toluidine, and the alkaloids—should also be examined. Some amines are readily nitrosated to *N*-nitrosamines, but analytic data on secondary reactions of amines in polluted environments are lacking.

TABLE 2-3 Relative Concentrations (SS/MS) of Selected Components in Fresh, Undiluted Smoke of Four 85-mm Commercial American Cigarettes[a]

	Constituent Concentrations in Smoke[b]							
	Cigarette A, NF		Cigarette B, F		Cigarette C, F		Cigarette D, PF	
Constituent[c]	SS	SS/MS	SS	SS/MS	SS	SS/MS	SS	SS/MS
Tar, mg/g	22.6	1.1	24.4	1.6	20.0	2.9	14.1	15.6
Nicotine, mg/g	4.6	2.2	4.0	2.7	3.4	4.2	3.0	20.0
CO, mg/g	28.3	2.1	36.6	2.7	33.2	3.5	26.8	14.9
NH_3, mg/g	524	7.0	893	46	213.1	6.3	236	5.8
Catechol, μg/g	58.2	1.4	89.8	1.3	69.5	2.6	117	12.9
BaP, ng/g	67	2.6	45.7	2.6	51.7	4.2	448	20.4
NDMA, ng/g	735	23.6	597	139	611	50.4	685	167
NPYR, ng/g	177	2.7	139	13.6	233	7.1	234	17.7
NNN, ng/g	857	0.85	307	0.63	185	0.68	338	5.1

[a]Data from Adams et al. (1985). Tar values for MS: cigarette A, 20.1 mg; cigarette B, 15.6 mg; cigarette C, 6.8 mg; cigarette D, 0.9 mg.

[b]NF = nonfilter cigarette; F = filter cigarette; PF = cigarette with perforated filter tip; B*a*P = benzo[*a*]pyrene.

[c]NDMA = *N*-nitrosodimethylamine; NPYR = *N*-nitrosopyrrolidine; NNN = *N'*-nitrosonornicotine.

To comprehend the data in Table 2-2 fully, some aspects should be emphasized. First, the data are based on analyses of nonfilter cigarettes that were smoked under standard laboratory conditions. Second, those conditions, established according to smoking patterns observed 3 decades ago, have been shown not to reflect today's smoking behavior. The difference is especially evident in the case of filter cigarettes designed for low smoke yields. Most consumers inhale the smoke of such cigarettes more intensely than the smoke of nonfilter cigarettes (Hill and Marquardt, 1980; Herning et al., 1981). This difference affects the yield of SS. Conventional cigarette filter tips primarily influence the yield of MS, but have little impact on SS yield. However, highly active filter tips, especially those with perforations, also affect the yield of SS (Adams et al., 1985). It is apparent in Table 2-3 that for all cigarettes studied the SS/MS values are greater than 1 for many toxic and carcinogenic constituents.

TABLE 2-4 Measured Concentrations of Carbon Monoxide in ETS[a]

Location	Tobacco Burned	Ventilation	Carbon Monoxide Concentrations, ppm				References
					Nonsmoke Controls		
			Mean	Range	Mean	Range	
Rooms	—	—	—	4.3–9	2.2 ± 0.98	0.4–4.5	Coburn et al., 1965
Train	1–18 smokers	Natural	—	0–40	—	—	Harmsen and Effenberger, 1957
Submarines (66 m^3)	157 cigarettes/day	Yes	<40	—	—	—	Cano et al., 1970
	94–103 cigarettes/day	Yes	<40	—	—	—	
18 military aircraft	—	Yes	<2–5	—	—	—	U.S. Department of Transportation, 1971
8 commercial aircraft	—	Yes	<2	—	—	—	U.S. Department of Transportation, 1971
Rooms	—	—	—	5–25	—	—	Porthein, 1971
14 public places	—	—	<10	—	—	—	Perry, 1973
Ferry boat	—	—	18.4 ± 8.7	—	3.0 ± 2.4	—	Godin et al., 1972
Theater foyer	—	—	3.4 ± 0.8	—	1.4 ± 0.8	—	Godin et al., 1972
Intercity bus	23 cigarettes	15 changes/h	32	—	—	—	Seiff, 1973
	3 cigarettes	15 changes/h	18	—	—	—	
2 conference rooms	—	8 changes/h	—	8 (peak)	1–2	—	Slavin and Hertz, 1975
Office	—	236 m^3/h	—	<2.5–4.6	—	—	Harke, 1974
	—	Natural	—	<2.9–9.0	—	—	—
Automobile	2 smokers (4 cigarettes)	Natural	—	42 (peak)	—	13.5 (peak)	Harke and Peters, 1974
		Mechanical	—	32 (peak)	—	15.0 (peak)	
9 night clubs	—	Varied	13.4	6.5–41.9	—	—	Sebben et al., 1977
14 restaurants	—	—	9.9 ± 5.5	—	9.2 (outdoor)	3.0–35	Sebben et al., 1977
45 restaurants	—	—	8.2 ± 2.2	7.1 ± 1.7	—	—	Sebben et al., 1977

33 stores	—	—	10.0 ± 4.2	11.5 ± 6.5	11.5 ± 6.5	—	Sebben et al., 1977
3 hospital lobbies	—	—	—	4.8	—	—	Sebben et al., 1977
6 coffee houses	Varied	—	2–23	—	—	—	Badre et al., 1978
Room	18 smokers	—	50	—	—	—	Badre et al., 1978
Hospital lobby	12–30 smokers	—	5	—	—	—	Badre et al., 1978
2 train compartments	2-3 smokers	—	—	4-5	—	—	Badre et al., 1978
Automobile	3 smokers	Natural, open	14	—	—	—	Badre et al., 1978
	2 smokers	Natural, closed	20	—	—	—	
10 offices	—	—	2.5 ± 10	1.5-1.0	2.5 ± 1.0	1.5 ± 4.5	Chappell and Parker, 1977
15 restaurants	—	—	4.0 ± 2.5	1.0-9.5	2.5 ± 1.5	1.0-5.0	Chappell and Parker, 1977
14 night clubs and taverns	—	—	13.0 ± 7.0	3.0-29.0	3.0 ± 2.0	1.0-5.0	Chappell and Parker, 1977
Tavern	—	Artificial	8.5	—	—	—	Chappell and Parker, 1977
	—	None	—	35 (peak)	—	—	
Office	—	Natural, open	1.0	10.0 (peak)	—	—	Chappell and Parker, 1977
Restaurant	—	Mechanical	5.1	2.1-9.9	4.8 (outdoors)	—	Fischer et al., 1978
Restaurant	—	Natural	2.6	1.4-3.4	1.5 (outdoors)	—	Fischer et al., 1978
Bar	—	Natural, open	4.8	2.4-9.6	1.7 (outdoors)	—	Weber et al., 1976
Cafeteria	—	11 changes/h	1.2	0.7-1.7	0.4 (outdoors)	—	Weber et al., 1976
44 offices	—	—	1.1	6.5 (max)	—	—	Weber, 1984
25 offices	—	—	2.78 ± 1.42	—	2.59 ± 2.33	—	Szadkowski et al., 1976
Tavern	—	6 changes/h	11.5	10–12	2 (outdoors)	—	Cuddeback et al., 1976
Tavern	—	1-2 changes/h	12.0	3-22	—	—	Cuddeback et al., 1976

[a]Time-weighted average (TWA) of carbon monoxide, 50 ppm (55 mg/m^3). TWA = average concentration to which worker may be exposed continuously for 8 h without damage to health (National Institute for Occupational Safety and Health, 1971).

PRINCIPAL CHEMICAL CONSTITUENTS OF ENVIRONMENTAL TOBACCO SMOKE

Air dilution physicochemically changes SS and other contributors to ETS. Depending on the degree of air dilution of SS, the concentration of particles in ETS can range from a few micrograms to 300-500 mg/m^3. A high degree of air dilution can reduce this yield to a few micrograms per cubic meter. At the same time, the median diameter of the particles will decrease from 0.32 μm to 0.14 or 0.098 μm (Keith and Derrick, 1960; Wynder and Hoffmann, 1967; Ingebrethsen and Sears, 1985). Another change caused by air dilution of SS is the volatilization of nicotine. In ETS, nicotine is present almost exclusively in the vapor phase (Eudy et al., 1985). In addition, redistributions of other constituents in SS due to air dilution might account for the presence of other semivolatile chemicals in the vapor phase of ETS, but we lack data on such effects.

The scientific literature contains an abundance of data on indoor air pollution by ETS (U.S. Public Health Service, 1979; National Research Council, 1981). We limit our review here to measurements made under field conditions and have excluded data from experimental studies. Most of the published data, summarized in Tables 2-4 through 2-9, do not exclude the possibility that, even though the respiratory environments analyzed were polluted largely by ETS, some other sources of pollution contributed to the reported concentrations of individual agents. (Many studies have dealt with the measurement of particulate matter in environments polluted by tobacco smoke. Chapter 5 discusses the measurement of particulate matter, and the results of the studies are summarized in Table 5-1.)

Table 2-4 shows concentrations of carbon monoxide measured in a variety of indoor spaces with and without occupancy by smokers. Carbon monoxide concentrations were generally higher in spaces where smoke was present. They were highly variable, however, and collected data on each space were insufficient (e.g., number of cigarettes smoked and volume of space) to show a consistent relationship.

Tobacco is the only known source of nicotine, so the *Nicotiana* alkaloid is a specific indicator for tobacco smoke pollution. Nicotine concentrations in smoke-polluted rooms were generally found to be 5-50 μg/m^3 and much higher (up to 500 μg/m^3) in heavily polluted environments (Table 2-5). In small interior compartments, such as automobiles, occupants who smoke tobacco have generated nicotine concentrations of 1,010 $\mu g/m^3$ (Badre et al., 1978).

Freshly generated tobacco smoke contains nitric oxide, but not nitrogen dioxide. On release into the environment, nitric oxide is gradually oxidized to nitrogen dioxide. The estimated half-life of nitric oxide is 10-20 minutes, depending on the degree of air dilution. Table 2-6 shows concentrations of nitric oxide and nitrogen dioxide in smoke-polluted environments and indicates means ranging from 9 to 195 ppb for nitric oxide and 21 to 76 ppb for nitrogen dioxide. Generally, the nitrogen oxide values reported in Table 2-6 are significantly in excess of those observed for outdoor atmospheres. However, some severe air pollution episodes in industrial areas have reportedly caused levels of 100 ppb, which persisted over several hours or even for several days (Goldsmith and Friberg, 1977). As a constituent of the respiratory environment, nitrogen dioxide conceivably contributes to endogenous nitrosation, which leads to the presence of nitrosamines in exposed subjects. Whereas it has been clearly demonstrated that inhaled cigarette smoke increases the endogenous formation of *N*-nitrosamines (Hoffmann and Brunnemann, 1983; Ladd et al., 1984; Lu et al., 1986; Tsuda et al., 1986), the endogenous formation of *N*-nitrosamines in nonsmokers exposed to ETS has so far not been demonstrated (Brunnemann et al., 1984).

Tables 2-7 and 2-8 show concentrations of acrolein and acetone in ETS. These volatile carbonyl compounds are known to affect mucociliary function and thus inhibit the clearance of smoke particles from the lung (Wynder and Hoffmann, 1967).

Table 2-9 shows concentrations of some additional toxic agents in ETS. Benzene, *N*-nitrosodimethylamine, *N*-nitrosodiethylamine, and the polynuclear aromatic hydrocarbons, represented by benzo[*a*]pyrene, are of concern, because they are known carcinogens (Vainio et al., 1985).

RADIOACTIVITY OF ENVIRONMENTAL TOBACCO SMOKE

The radioactive isotopes of lead (Pb-210), bismuth (Bi-210), and polonium (Po-210), known as long-lived radon daughters in the decay chain of uranium via radium and radon (Radford and

TABLE 2-5 Measured Concentrations of Nicotine in ETS[a]

Location	Tobacco Burned	Ventilation	Nicotine Concentrations, $\mu g/m^3$		References
			Mean	Range	
Train	—	Natural, closed	—	0.7–3.1	Harmsen and Effenberger, 1957
6 coffee houses	Smokers varied	—	—	25–52	Badre et al., 1978
Room	18 smokers	—	500	—	Badre et al., 1978
Hospital lobby	12–30 smokers	—	37	—	Badre et al., 1978
2 train compartments	2–3 smokers	—	—	36–50	Badre et al., 1978
Automobile	3 smokers	Natural, open	65	—	Badre et al., 1978
		Natural, closed	1,010	—	
Submarines	157 cigarettes/day	Yes	32	—	Cano et al., 1970
(66 m^3)	94–103 cigarettes/day	Yes	15–35	—	
Train	—	—	4.9	—	Hinds and First, 1975
Bus	—	—	6.7	—	Hinds and First, 1975
Bus waiting room	—	—	1.0	—	Hinds and First, 1975
Airline waiting room	—	—	3.1	—	Hinds and First, 1975
Restaurant	—	—	5.2	—	Hinds and First, 1975
Cocktail lounge	—	—	10.3	—	Hinds and First, 1975
Student lounge	—	—	2.8	—	Hinds and First, 1975
44 offices	—	—	0.9 ± 1.9	13.8 (peak)	Weber and Fischer, 1980

[a]Time-weighted average (TWA) of nicotine, 500 $\mu g/m^3$. TWA = average concentration to which worker may be exposed continuously for 8 h without damage to health (National Institute for Occupational Safety and Health, 1971).

TABLE 2-6 Measured Concentrations of Nitrogen Oxides in ETS[a]

Location	Tobacco Burned	Ventilation	Nitrogen Oxides Concentrations, ppb			References
			Mean	Range	Nonsmoke Control, Mean	
Restaurant	—	Mechanical	NO_2 76	59–105	63 (outdoors)	Fischer et al., 1978
			NO 120	36–218	115 (outdoors)	
Restaurant	—	Natural	NO_2 63	24–99	50 (outdoors)	Weber, 1984
			NO 80	14–121	11 (outdoors)	
Bar	—	Natural, open	NO_2 21	1–61	48 (outdoors)	Weber et al., 1979
			NO 195	66–414	44 (outdoors)	
Cafeteria	—	11 changes/h	NO_2 58	35–103	27	Weber et al., 1979
			NO 9	2–38	5	
44 offices	Varied	Varied	NO_2 24 ± 22	115 (peak)	—	Weber and Fischer, 1980
			NO 32 ± 60	200 (peak)	—	

[a]Time-weighted averages (TWAs): nitric oxide, 25 ppm; nitrogen dioxide, 1 ppm. TWA = average concentration to which worker may be exposed continuously for 8 h without damage to health (National Institute for Occupational Safety and Health, 1971).

TABLE 2-7 Measured Concentrations of Acrolein in ETS[a]

Location	Tobacco Burned	Ventilation	Acrolein Concentrations		References
			Mean	Range	
Coffee houses	Varied	—	—	0.03–0.10 mg/m^3	Badre et al., 1978
Room	18 smokers	—	0.185 mg/m^3	—	Badre et al., 1978
Hospital lobby	12–30 smokers	—	0.02 mg/m^3	—	Badre et al., 1978
2 train compartments	2–3 smokers	—	—	0.02–0.12 mg/m^3	Badre et al., 1978
Automobile	3 smokers	Natural, open	0.03 mg/m^3	—	Badre et al., 1978
	2 smokers	Natural, closed	0.3 mg/m^3	—	
Restaurant	—	Mechanical	7 ppb	—	Fischer et al., 1978
	—	Natural	8 ppb	—	
Bar	—	Natural, open	10 ppb	—	Weber et al., 1976
Cafeteria	—	11 changes/h	6 ppb	—	Weber et al., 1976

[a]Time-weighted average (TWA) of acrolein, 0.1 ppm. TWA = average concentration to which worker may be exposed continuously for 8 h without damage to health (National Institute for Occupational Safety and Health, 1971).

TABLE 2-8 Measured Concentrations of Acetone in ETS[a]

Location	Tobacco Burned	Ventilation	Acetone Concentrations, mg/m^3		References
			Mean	Range	
6 coffee houses	Varied	—	—	0.91–5.88	Badre et al., 1978
Room	18 smokers	—	0.51	—	Badre et al., 1978
Hospital lobby	12–30 smokers	—	1.16	—	Badre et al., 1978
2 train compartments	2–3 smokers	—	—	0.36–0.75	Badre et al., 1978
Automobile	3 smokers	Natural, open	0.32	—	Badre et al., 1978
	2 smokers	Natural, closed	1.20	—	

[a]Time-weighted average (TWA) of acetone, 250 ppm. TWA = average concentration to which worker may be exposed continuously for 8 h without damage to health (National Institute for Occupational Safety and Health, 1971).

TABLE 2-9 Measured Concentrations of Various Toxic Agents in Rooms Polluted with ETS

Pollutant	Location	Concentration	Nonsmoke Control Concentration	References
Benzene	Public places	20–317 $\mu g/m^3$	—	Badre et al., 1978
N-Nitrosodimethylamine	Restaurant, public places	0.01–0.24 $\mu g/m^3$	0.005 $\mu g/m^3$ (inside)	Brunnemann et al., 1977; Stehlik et al., 1982
N-Nitrosodiethylamine	Restaurant, public places	<0.01–0.2 $\mu g/m^3$	—	Stehlik et al., 1982
Anthanthrene	Coffee houses	4.1–9.4 ng/m^3	2.8–7.0 ng/m^3 (outdoors)	Just et al., 1972
Benzo[*a*]fluorene	Indoors	39 ng/m^3	—	Grimmer et al., 1977
Benzo[*a*]pyrene	Restaurant, public	2.8–760 ng/m^3	4.0–9.3 ng/m^3 (outdoors)	Galuskinova, 1964; Just et al., 1972; Perry, 1973; Grimmer et al., 1977
Benzo[-]pyrene	Coffee houses	3.3–23.4 ng/m^3	3.0–5.1 ng/m^3 (outdoors)	Just et al., 1972
Coronene	Coffee houses	0.5–1.2 ng/m^3	1.0–2.8 ng/m^3 (outdoors)	Just et al., 1972
Perylene	Coffee houses	0.7–1.3 ng/m^3	0.1–1.7 ng/m^3 (outdoors)	Just et al., 1972
Pyrene	Coffee houses	4.1–9.4 ng/m^3	0.1–1.7 ng/m^3 (outdoors)	Just et al., 1972
Phenols (volatile)	Coffee houses	7.4–11.5 ng/m^3	—	Just et al., 1972

Hunt, 1964; Martell, 1975; Hill, 1982), are present in tobacco and therefore appear in tobacco smoke. Furthermore, when radon is present in the air, aerosol particles, including those of tobacco smoke, tend to adsorb the earlier decay products of radon, namely the so-called short-lived daughters (Po-218, Pb-214, Bi-214, and Po-214), i.e, those preceding the long-lived daughters in the decay chain (Raabe, 1969; Kruger and Nöthing, 1979; Bergman and Axelson, 1983).

The presence of Pb-210 and subsequent decay products in tobacco might derive from uptake of Pb-210 from the soil, especially if radium-rich phosphate fertilizers have been used (Tso et al., 1966). It may also result from adsorption of short-lived radon daughters on the leaves of the tobacco plant when phosphate fertilizers are used and the leakage of radon from the ground is therefore increased. This adsorption applies to short-lived daughters, which then decay to the long-lived Pb-210, and subsequent nuclides found in the tobacco when phosphate fertilizers, containing radium-226, are used (Fleischer and Parungo, 1974; Martell, 1975). The origin of these decay products could also be due to the general occurrence of radon in the atmosphere (Hill, 1982).

In recent years, relatively high concentrations of radon and short-lived radon daughters have been found in indoor air in homes in several countries (Nero et al., 1985). In clean air, the short-lived radon daughters tend to be more unattached to aerosol particles and therefore are more easily deposited on walls, furniture, etc., especially through electrostatic forces. In the presence of an aerosol like tobacco smoke, some of the short-lived radon daughters are attached to particles, and therefore remain available for inhalation to a much greater extent than would otherwise be the case. Indoor radon-daughter concentration can more than double in the presence of tobacco smoke (Bergman and Axelson, 1983). Since radon daughter exposure is a well-known cause of lung cancer in miners, the described attachment of radon daughters to cigarette smoke would contribute to the carcinogenic potential of ETS (Little et al., 1965; Rajewsky and Stahlhofen, 1966; Radford and Martell, 1978). Given the presence of appreciable amounts of radon in indoor air, irradiation of the bronchial tract from radon daughters attached to smoke aerosol could be more important than the irradiation from the long-lived daughters in the tobacco itself. This subject needs further research, especially in light of recent reports on the widespread prevalence of indoor radon throughout the world.

TOXIC AND CARCINOGENIC AGENTS IN TOBACCO SMOKE

Combustion products of cigarettes are the main contributors of ETS. Therefore, comparisons of concentrations of specific toxins and carcinogens in ETS (Tables 2-4 through 2-9) with corresponding concentrations in MS are relevant.

However, comparisons of MS and ETS can be appropriate only if one considers the important differences in chemical composition (including pH) and physicochemical nature (e.g., particle size, air dilution factors, and distribution of agents between vapor and particulate phases) between the two aerosols. Furthermore, ETS in indoor environments is often accompanied by pollutants in the work environment or derived from other sources, such as cooking stoves and space heaters. There are also important differences between inhaling ambient air and inhaling a concentrated smoke aerosol during puff-drawing. Finally, chemical and physicochemical characteristics based on analysis of smoke generated by machine smoking are not fully comparable with those of compounds generated when a smoker inhales cigarette smoke. Especially in the case of low-yield cigarettes, the yields of constituents appear to be different between machine smoking and human smoking (Herning et al., 1981).

Table 2-10 compares concentrations of some smoke constituents in the MS generated in the laboratory from one cigarette to those inhaled by a nonsmoker exposed to ETS for 1 hour.* The physical and chemical changes that occur in reactive smoke constituents during aging of the compounds after their emission into the environment must also be considered. For example, nitric oxide is generated in a cigarette during smoking and is chemically

---

* The computations for exposures to nonsmokers for 1 hour in Table 2-10 are made using the equation:

$$mg/h = mg/m^3 \times 10^{-3} m^3/L \times 600 L/h,$$

assuming an average respiratory rate of 10 L/minute. To convert from ppm (or ppb) to mg/m^3, the following equation is used:

$$mg/m^3 = \frac{ppm \times \text{molecular weight}}{RT},$$

where RT at 20°C is 24.45.

intact when it leaves the cigarette in MS about 2 seconds later. However, once emitted into SS and diluted to become an ETS component, nitric oxide is partially oxidized to nitrogen dioxide and progressively more oxidized as more time elapses, producing a potent hydrophilic nitrosating agent.

SUMMARY AND RECOMMENDATIONS

The smoldering of tobacco between puffs generates SS. Undiluted SS contains some toxic compounds in much higher concentrations than MS, especially ammonia, volatile amines, volatile nitrosamines, some nicotine decomposition products, and aromatic amines. Furthermore, decay products of radon from the tobacco and from other sources adsorbed on some particles in indoor air might contribute to the carcinogenic potential of ETS.

SS is a major contributor to ETS. Respiratory environments that are polluted with SS contain measurable amounts of nicotine and other toxic agents, including carcinogens. We lack data on the presence and concentrations of many of the known SS components in polluted, enclosed environments. The concentrations of toxic agents of ETS are governed primarily by the amount of tobacco smoked, the degree of ventilation, and the volatility of the agents. Future studies should concentrate on the analysis of toxic and carcinogenic agents in smoke-polluted environments.

What Is Known

1. SS is the aerosol that is freely emitted into the air from the smoldering tobacco products between puffs.

2. ETS consists of diluted SS, exhaled MS, smoke that escapes from the burning cone during puff-drawing, and vapor-phase components (such as carbon monoxide) that diffuse through cigarette paper into the environment. However, secondary reactions can occur before a nonsmoker inhales ETS, such as aging, volatilization of nicotine, and adsorption of radon daughters on particles.

3. Undiluted SS contains higher concentrations of some toxic compounds than undiluted MS, including ammonia, volatile amines, volatile nitrosamines, nicotine decomposition products, and aromatic amines.

4. Conventional cigarette filter tips primarily influence the yield of MS, but have little impact on the yield of SS. Highly

TABLE 2-10 Concentrations of Toxic and Carcinogenic Agents in Cigarette Mainstream Smoke and ETS in Indoor Environments[a]

	Mainstream Smoke from Nonfilter Cigarette		Inhaled as ETS Constituent During 1 Hour: Range		Exceptionally High Values[b]	
Agent[c]	Weight	Concentration	Weight	Concentration	Weight	Concentration
CO	10–23 mg	24,900–57,400 ppm	0.6–13 mg	1–18.5 ppm	22 mg	32 ppm
NO	100–600 μg	230,000–1,380,000 ppb	7–88 μg	9–120 ppb	144 μg	195 ppb
NO_2	<5 μg	<7,600 ppb	24–86 μg	21–76 ppb	119 μg	105 ppb
Acrolein	60–100 μg	75,000–125,000 ppb	8–69 μg	6–50 ppb	110 μg	80 ppb
Acetone	100–250 μg	120,000–300,000 ppb	210–710 μg	150–500 ppb	3,400 μg	2,400 ppb
Benzene[d]	12–48 μg	11,000–43,000 ppb	12–190 μg	6–98 ppb	190 μg	98 ppb
NDMA[e]	10–40 ng	9–38 ppb	6–140 ng	0.003–0.077 ppb	140 ng	0.072 ppb
NDEA[e]	4–25 ng	3–17 ppb	<6–120 ng	<0.002–0.05 ppb	120 ng	0.05 ppb
Nicotine	1,000–2,500 μg	430,000–1,080,000 ppb	0.6–30 μg	0.15–7.5 ppb	300 μg	75 ppb
BaP[f]	20–40 ng	5–11 ppb	1.7–460 ng	0.00027–0.074 ppb	460 ng	0.074 ppb

[a]Values for inhaled ETS components calculated from values in Tables 2-4 through 2-9 and respiratory rate of 10 L/min. Data from unventilated interiors of automobiles excluded (Badre et al., 1978). Concentrations for MS are calculated by diluting weights given in volume of 350 ml, that is 10 puffs at 35 ml/puff.

[b]Chosen to classify reported data that require confirmation.

[c]NDMA = *N*-nitrosodimethylamine; NDEA = *N*-nitrosodiethylamine; B*a*P = benzo[*a*]pyrene.

[d]Human carcinogen, according to International Agency for Research on Cancer (Vainio et al., 1985); suspected carcinogen, according to American Conference of Governmental Industrial Hygienists (1985).

[e]Animal carcinogen according to the International Agency for Research on Cancer (Vainio et al., 1985).

[f]Suspected human carcinogen according to the International Agency for Research on Cancer (Vainio et al., 1985) and according to the American Conference of Governmental Industrial Hygienists (1985).

active filter tips, especially perforated ones, also affect the yield of components in SS.

5. Radioactive decay products in tobacco itself, for instance, Pb-210 and Po-210, and short-lived radon daughters adsorbed on smoke particles in indoor air can contribute to the carcinogenic potential of ETS.

6. ETS in indoor environments is accompanied by pollutants, such as nitrogen oxides and carbon monoxide, derived from other sources, including cooking stoves and space heaters. ETS contains measurable amounts of nicotine and other toxic agents, including carcinogens. The concentrations of toxic agents of ETS are governed primarily by the amount of tobacco smoked, the degree of ventilation, and the volatility of the agents.

7. Nicotine, found in MS primarily in the particulate phase, occurs in ETS primarily in the vapor phase. Therefore, filters designed to reduce particles in the air will not substantially alter the nicotine concentration.

What Scientific Information Is Missing

1. We lack data on the presence and concentrations of toxic and carcinogenic components in tobacco-smoke-polluted enclosed environments.

2. The distributions of various agents in vapor and particulate phases of ETS are not well characterized. Further, the effect of air-cleaning systems on these distributions has not been studied. Distributions are important with respect to the carcinogenic potential of ETS.

3. We need to examine the importance of the abundant release of amines into ETS. We lack analytic data on secondary reactions of amines in polluted air, such as *N*-nitrosation and condensation with other ETS components.

4. The transfer of constituents other than nicotine from the particulate phase of SS to the vapor phase of ETS could be important with respect to the retention of ETS in the respiratory tract of nonsmokers.

5. We do not know the extent to which nitrogen dioxide can contribute to endogenous nitrosation in nonsmokers as a constituent of the respiratory environment. Endogenous nitrosation leads to nitrosamines in exposed subjects.

6. We need studies to determine the extent to which ETS differs from MS in ways related to health and their relative toxicities.

7. We should analyze toxic and carcinogenic agents in smoke-polluted environments, especially enclosed natural environments, and their uptake by nonsmokers.

8. Research should be conducted on interactions between ETS and radon daughters, especially as radon daughters can adhere to RSP, and can thereby enter the lung.

REFERENCES

Adams, J.D., K.J. O'Mara-Adams, and D. Hoffmann. On the mainstream-sidestream distribution of cigarette smoke components. Presented at the 39th Tobacco Chemists' Research Conference, Montreal, Canada, Oct. 2-5, 1985.

American Conference of Governmental Industrial Hygienists (ACGIH). TLV Threshold Limit Values and Biological and Experimental Indices of 1985-1986. Cincinnati, Ohio: ACGIH, 1985. 114 pp.

Armitage, A.K., and D.M. Turner. Absorption of nicotine in cigarette and cigar smoke through the oral musco. Nature 226:1231-1232, 1970.

Badre, R., R. Guillerme, N. Abram, M. Bourdin, and C. Dumas. Pollution atmospherique par la fumée de tabac. Ann. Pharm. Fr. 36:443-452, 1978.

Baker, R.R. The effect of ventilation on cigarette combustion mechanisms. Recent Adv. Tob. Sci. 10:88-150, 1984.

Bergman, H., and O. Axelson. Passive smoking and indoor radon daughter concentrations. Lancet 2:1308-1309, 1983.

Brunnemann, K.D., and D. Hoffmann. The pH of tobacco smoke. Food Cosmet. Toxicol. 12:115-124, 1974.

Brunnemann, K.D., and D. Hoffmann. Pyrolytic origins of major gas phase constituents of cigarette smoke. Recent Adv. Tob. Sci. 8:103-140, 1982.

Brunnemann, K.D., D. Hoffmann, E.L. Wynder, and G.B. Gori. Determination of tar, nicotine, and carbon monoxide in cigarette smoke. A comparison of international smoking conditions. XXXVII of Chemical Studies on Tobacco Smoke, pp. 441-449. In E.L. Wynder, D. Hoffmann, and G.B. Gori, Eds. Smoking and Health I. Modifying the Risk for the Smoker. Proceedings of the 3rd World Conference on Smoking and Health. NIH Publ. No. 76-1221. Bethesda, Maryland: U.S. Department of Health, Education, and Welfare, Public Health Service, National Cancer Institute, 1976.

Brunnemann, K.D., L. Yu, and D. Hoffmann. Assessment of carcinogenic volatile N-nitrosamines in tobacco and in mainstream and sidestream smoke from cigarettes. Cancer Res. 37:3218-3222, 1977.

Brunnemann, K.D., W. Fink, and F. Moser. Analysis of volatile N-nitrosamines in mainstream and sidestream smoke from cigarettes by GLC-TEA. Oncology 37:217-222, 1980.

Brunnemann, K.D., J.C. Scott, N.J. Haley, and D. Hoffmann. Endogeneous formation of N-nitrosoproline upon cigarette smoke inhalation. IARC Sci. Publ. 57:819-828, 1984.

Cano, J.P., J. Catalin, R. Badre, C. Dumas, A. Viala, and R. Guillerme. Determination de la nicotine par chromatographie en phase gazeuse. II. Applications. Ann. Pharm. Fr. 28:633-640, 1970.

Carter, W.L., and I. Hasegawa. Fixation of tobacco smoke aerosols for size distribution studies. J. Colloid Interface Sci. 53:134-141, 1975.

Chappell, S.B., and R.J. Parker. Smoking and carbon monoxide levels in enclosed public places in New Brunswick. Can. J. Public. Health 68:159-161, 1977.

Coburn, R.F., R.E. Forster, and P.B. Kane. Considerations on the physiological variables that determine the blood carboxyhemoglobin concentrations in man. J. Clin. Invest. 44:1899-1910, 1965.

Cuddeback, J.E., J.R. Donovan, and W.R. Burg. Occupational aspects of passive smoking. Am. Ind. Hyg. Assoc. J. 37:263-267, 1976.

Dalham, T., M.-L. Edfors, and R. Rylander. Mouth absorption of various compounds in cigarette smoke. Arch. Environ. Health 16:831-835, 1968a.

Dalham, T., M.-L. Edfors, and R. Rylander. Retention of cigarette smoke components in human lungs. Arch. Environ. Health 17:746-748, 1968b.

Dube, M.F., and C.R. Green. Methods of collection of smoke for analytical purposes. Recent Adv. Tob. Sci. 8:42-102, 1982.

Elliot, L.P., and D.R. Rowe. Air quality during public gatherings. J. Air Pollut. Control Assoc. 25:635-636, 1975.

Eudy, L.W., F.A. Thome, D.L. Heavner, C.R. Green, and B.J. Ingebrethsen. Studies on the vapor-particulate phase distribution on environmental nicotine by selected trapping and detection methods. Presented at the 39th Tobacco Chemists' Research Conference, Montreal, Canada, Oct. 2-5, 1985.

Fischer, T., A. Weber, and E. Grandjean. Air pollution due to tobacco smoke in restaurants. Int. Arch. Occup. Environ. Health 41:267-280, 1978.

Fleischer, R.L., and F.P. Parungo. Aerosol particles on tobacco trichomes. Nature 250:158-159, 1974.

Galuskinova, V. 3,4-Benzpyrene determination in the smoky atmosphere of social meeting rooms and restaurants: A contribution to the problem of the noxiousness of so-called passive smoking. Neoplasm 11:465-468, 1964.

Godin, G., G. Wright, and R.J. Shephard. Urban exposure to carbon monoxide. Arch. Environ. Health 25:305-313, 1972.

Goldsmith, J.R., and L.I. Friberg. Effects of air pollution on human health, pp. 458-610. In A.C. Stern, Ed. Air Pollution, Vol. II, 3rd ed. New York: Academic, 1977.

Grabowski, J., and C.S. Bell, Eds. Measurement in the Analysis and Treatment of Smoking Behavior. Publ. No. DHHS/PUB/ADM-83-1285. Rockville, Maryland: U.S. Department of Health and Human Services, National Institute on Drug Abuse, 1983. 132 pp.

Grimmer, G., H. Böhnke, and H.P. Harke. Passive smoking: Intake of polycyclic aromatic hydrocarbons by breathing of cigarette smoke containing air. Int. Arch. Occup. Environ. Health 40:93-99, 1977.

Harke, H.-P. Zum Problem des Passivrauchens. I. Über den Einfluss des Rauchens auf die CO-Konzentration in Büroräumen. Int. Arch. Arbeitsmed. 33:199-206, 1974.

Harke, H.-P., and H. Peters. Zum Problem des Passivrauchens. III. Über den Einfluss des Rauchens auf die CO-Konzentration im Kraftfahrzeug bei Fahrten im Stadtgebiet. Int. Arch. Arbeitsmed. 33:221-229, 1974.

Harmsen, H., and E. Effenberger. Tabakrauch in Verkehrsmitteln, Wohn- und Arbeitsräumen. Arch. Hyg. Bakteriol. 141:383-400, 1957.

Herning, R.I., R.T. Jones, J. Bachman, and A. Mines. Puff volume increases when low-nicotine cigarettes are smoked. Br. Med. J. 283:187-189, 1981.

Hill, C.R. Radioactivity in cigarette smoke. N. Engl. J. Med. 307:311, 1982.

Hill, P., and H. Marquardt. Plasma and urine changes after smoking different brands of cigarettes. Clin. Pharmacol. Ther. 27:652-658, 1980.

Hiller, F.C. Deposition of sidestream smoke in the human respiratory tract. Prev. Med. 13:602-607, 1984.

Hiller, F.C., K.T. McCusker, M.K. Mazumder, J.D. Wilson, and R.C. Bone. Deposition of sidestream cigarette smoke in the human respiratory tract. Am. Rev. Resp. Dis. 125:406-408, 1982.

Hinds, W.C., and M.W. First. Concentrations of nicotine and tobacco smoke in public places. N. Engl. J. Med. 292:844-845, 1975.

Hoffmann, D., and K.D. Brunnemann. Endogeneous formation of N-nitrosoproline in cigarette smokers. Cancer Res. 43:5570-5574, 1983.

Hoffmann, D., and S.S. Hecht. Nicotine-derived N-nitrosamines and tobacco-related cancer: Current status and future directions. Cancer Res. 45:935-944, 1985.

Hoffmann, D., N.J. Haley, K.D. Brunnemann, J.D. Adams, and E.L. Wynder. Cigarette sidestream smoke: Formation, analysis and model studies on the uptake by nonsmokers. U.S.-Japan Meeting, "New Etiology of Lung Cancer," Honolulu, Hawaii, Mar. 21-23, 1983.

Hoffmann, D., K.D. Brunnemann, J.D. Adams, and N.J. Haley. Indoor air pollution by tobacco smoke: Model studies on the uptake by nonsmokers, pp. 313-318. In B. Berglund, T. Lindvall, and J. Sundell, Eds. Indoor Air, Vol. 2. Radon, Passive Smoking, Particulates, and Housing Epidemiology. Stockholm, Sweden: Swedish Council for Building Research, 1984a.

Hoffmann, D., N.J. Haley, J.D. Adams, and K.D. Brunnemann. Tobacco sidestream smoke: Uptake by nonsmokers. Prev. Med. 13:608-617, 1984b.

Ingebrethsen, B.J., and S.B. Sears. Particle size distribution measurements of sidestream cigarette smoke. Presented at the 39th Tobacco Chemists' Research Conference, Montreal, Canada, Oct. 2-5, 1985.

International Committee for Cigar Smoke Study. Machine smoking of cigars. Coresta Inform. Bull. 1:31-34, 1974.

Johnson, W.R., and J.C. Karg. Mechanisms of hydrogen cyanide formation from the pyrolysis of amino acids and related compounds. J. Org. Chem. 36:189-192, 1971.

Johnson, W.R., R.W. Hale, J.W. Nedlock, H.J. Grubbs, and D.H. Powell. The distribution of products between mainstream and sidestream smoke. Tob. Sci. 17:141-144, 1973a.

Johnson, W.R., R.W. Hale, S.C. Cough, and P.H. Chen. Chemistry of the conversion of nitrate nitrogen to smoke products. Nature 243:223-225, 1973b.

Just, J., M. Borkowska, and S. Maziarka. Zanieczyszczenie dymem tytoniowym powietrza kawiarn warszawskich. (Tobacco smoke in the air of Warsaw coffee rooms.) Rocz. Panestw. Zakh. Hyg. 23:129-135, 1972.

Keith, C.H., and J.C. Derrick. Measurement of the particle size distribution and concentration of cigarette smoke by the "conifuge." J. Colloid Sci. 15:340-356, 1960.

Klus, H., and H. Kuhn. Distribution of various tobacco smoke constituents in main and sidestream smoke. A review. Beitr. Tabakforsch. Int. 11:229-265, 1982.

Krasnegor, N.A., Ed. Cigarette Smoking as a Dependence Process. Publ. No. DHEW/PUB/ADM-79/800. Rockville, Maryland: U.S. Department of Health and Human Services, National Institute on Drug Abuse, 1979. 92 pp.

Kruger, J., and J.F. Nöthling. A comparison of the attachment of the decay products of radon-220 and radon-222 to monodispersed aerosols. J. Aerosol. Sci. 10:571-579, 1979.

Ladd, K.F., H.L. Newmark, and M.C. Archer. N-nitrosation of proline in smokers and nonsmokers. J. Natl. Cancer Inst. 73:83-87, 1984.

Little, J.B., E.P. Radford, and H.L. McComb. Distribution of polonium-210 in pulmonary tissue of cigarette smokers. N. Engl. J. Med. 273:1343-1351, 1965.

Lu, P.H., Y.Z. Hong, N.G. Shi, W.D. Zhang, C.S. Dai, J.W. Huang, X.X. Qin, M.Z. Kiu, and D.H. Tong. Radiographic findings in cotton textile workers and the relationship to cigarette smoking. Regul. Toxicol. Pharmacol. 6:60-65, 1986.

Martell, E.A. Tobacco radioactivity and cancer in smokers. Am. Sci. 63:404-412, 1975.

Miller, J.E. Determination of the components of pipe tobacco and cigar smoke by means of a new smoking machine, pp. 584-595. Proceedings of the Third World Tobacco Scientific Congress, University College of Rhodesia and Nyasaland, Salisbury, Southern Rhodesia, Feb. 18-26, 1963. Salisbury: Salisbury Printers, Ltd., 1964.

National Institute for Occupational Safety and Health. Health Aspects of Smoking in Transport Aircraft. Publ. No. NIDA/RD-79/028, Research Monograph Series No. 23. Rockville, Maryland: National Institute for Occupational Safety and Health and Federal Aviation Administration, Washington, D.C., 1971. 92 pp.

National Research Council, Committee on Indoor Pollutants. Tobacco smoke, pp. 149-168. In Indoor Pollutants. Washington, D.C.: National Academy Press, 1981.

Nero, A.V., R.G. Sextro, S.M. Doyle, B.A. Moed, W.W. Nazaroff, K.L. Revzan, and M.B. Schwehr. Characterizing the sources, range and environmental influence of radon-222 and its decay products. Sci. Total Environ. 45:233-244, 1985.

Neurath, G., and H. Ehmke. Apparatur zur Untersuchung des Nebenstromrauches. Beitr. Tabakforsch. 2:117-121, 1964.

Neurath, G., and H. Horstmann. Einfluss des Feuchtigkeits gehaltes von Cigaretten auf die Zusammnensetzung des Rauches und die Glutzonentemperaturen. Beitr. Tabakforsch. Int. 2:93-100, 1973.

Perry, J. Fasten your seatbelts: Non smoking. B.C. Med. J. 15:304-305, 1973.

Pillsbury, H.C., C.C. Bright, K.J. O'Connor, and F.W. Irish. Tar and nicotine in cigarette smoke. J. Assoc. Off. Anal. Chem. 52:458-462, 1969.

Porthein, F. Zum Problem des "Passiv-Rauchens." Münch. Med. Wochenschr. 118:707-709, 1971.

Raabe, O.G. Concerning the interactions that occur between radon decay products and aerosols. Health Phys. 17:177-185, 1969.

Radford, E.P., Jr., and V.R. Hunt. Polonium-210: A volatile radioelement in cigarettes. Science 143:247-249, 1964.

Radford, E.P., and E.A. Martell. Polonium-210: Lead-210 ratios as an index of residence times of insoluble particles from cigarette smoke in bronchial epithelium, pp. 567-581. In W.H. Walton and B. McGovern, Eds. Inhaled Particles IV, Part 2. New York: Pergamon, 1978.

Rajewsky, B., and W. Stahlhofen. Polonium-210 activity in the lungs of cigarette smokers. Nature 209:1312-1313, 1966.

Rühl, C., J.D. Adams, and D. Hoffmann. Chemical studies on tobacco smoke. LXVI. Comparative assessment of volatile and tobacco-specific N-nitrosamines in the smoke of selected cigarettes from the USA, West Germany and France. J. Anal. Toxicol. 4:255-259, 1980.

Sakuma, H., M. Kusama, S. Munakata, T. Ohsumi, and S. Sugawara. The distribution of cigarette smoke components between mainstream and sidestream smoke. I. Acidic components. Beitr. Tabakforsch. Int. 12:63-71, 1983.

Sakuma, H., M. Kusama, K. Yamaguchi, T. Matsuki, and S. Sugawara. The distribution of cigarette smoke components between mainstream and sidestream smoke. II. Bases. Beitr. Tabakforsch. Int. 12:199-209, 1984a.

Sakuma, H., M. Kusama, K. Yamaguchi, and S. Sugawara. The distribution of cigarette smoke components between mainstream and sidestream smoke. III. Middle and higher boiling components. Beitr. Tabakforsch. Int. 12:251-258, 1984b.

Scassellati-Sforzolini, G., and A. Savino. Evaluation of a rapid index of ambient contamination by cigarette smoke in relation to the composition of gas phases of the smoke. Riv. Ital. Ig. 28:43-55, 1968.

Schmeltz, I., A. Wenger, D. Hoffmann, and T.C. Tso. Chemical studies on tobacco smoke. 63. On the fate of nicotine during pyrolysis and in a burning cigarette. J. Agric. Food Chem. 27:602-608, 1979.

Sebben, J., P. Pimm, and R.J. Shephard. Cigarette smoke in enclosed public facilities. Arch. Environ. Health 32:53-58, 1977.

Seiff, H.E. Carbon Monoxide as an Indicator of Cigarette-Caused Pollution Levels in Intercity Buses. Publ. No. BMCS-IHS-73-1. Washington, D.C.: U.S. Department of Transportation, Bureau of Motor Carrier Safety, 1973. 13 pp.

Slavin, R.G., and M. Hertz. Indoor air pollution: A study of the thirtieth annual meeting of the American Academy of Allergy. 30th Annual Meeting Am. Acad. Allergy, San Diego, Feb. 15-19, 1975.

Stehlik, G., O. Richter, and H. Altmann. Concentration of dimethylnitrosamine in the air of smoke-filled rooms. Ecotoxicol. Environ. Saf. 6:495-500, 1982.

Szadkowski, D., H.-P. Harke, and J. Angerer. Kohlenmonoxidbelastung durch Passivrauchen in Büraoräumen. Zentralbl. Prak. Inn. Med. 3:310-313, 1976.

Tso, T.C., N. Harley, and L.T. Alexander. Source of lead-210 and polonium-210 in tobacco. Science 153:880-882, 1966.

Tsuda, M., J. Niitusuma, S. Sato, T. Hirayama, T. Kakizoe, and T. Sugimura. Increase in the levels of N-nitrosoproline, N-nitrothioproline, and N-nitro-z-methylthioproline in human urine by cigarette smoking. Cancer Lett. 30:117-124, 1986.

U.S. Department of Health and Human Services. Third Annual Report on Carcinogens. National Toxicology Program. Research Triangle Park, North Carolina: U.S. Department of Health and Human Services, 1983. 137 pp.

U.S. Department of Transportation and U.S. Department of Health, Education, and Welfare. Health Aspects of Smoking in Transport Aircraft. U.S. Department of Transportation, Federal Aviation Administration, and U.S. Department of Health, Education, and Welfare, Washington, D.C.: NIOSH, 1971. 85 pp.

U.S. Public Health Service. Smoking and Health. A Report of the Surgeon General. DHEW Publ. No. (PHS) 79-50066. Washington, D.C.: U.S. Department of Health, Education, and Welfare, Public Health Service, 1979.

Vainio, H., K. Hemminki, and J. Wilbourn. Data on the carcinogenicity of chemicals in the IARC Monographs programme. Carcinogenesis (Lond.) 6:1653-1665, 1985.

Vilcins, G., and J.O. Lephardt. Aging process of cigarette smoke: Formation of methyl nitrite. Chem. Ind. (Lond.) 22:974-975, 1975.

Wartman, W.B., Jr., E.C. Cogbill, and E.S. Harlow. Determination of particulate matter in concentrated aerosols. Application to analysis of cigarette smoke. Anal. Chem. 31:1705-1709, 1959.

Weber, A. Annoyance and irritation by passive smoking. Prev. Med. 13:618-625, 1984.

Weber, A., and T. Fischer. Passive smoking at work. Int. Arch. Occup. Environ. Health 47:209-221, 1980.

Weber, A., C. Jermini, and E. Grandjean. Irritating effects on man of air pollution due to cigarette smoke. Am. J. Public Health 66:672-676, 1976.

Weber, A., T. Fischer, and E. Grandjean. Passive smoking: Irritating effects of the total smoke and gas phase. Int. Arch. Occup. Environ. Health 43:183-193, 1979.

Wynder, E.L., and D. Hoffmann. Tobacco and Tobacco Smoke: Studies in Experimental Carcinogenesis. New York: Academic Press, 1967. 730 pp.

3
In Vivo and In Vitro Assays to Assess the Health Effects of Environmental Tobacco Smoke

INTRODUCTION

Suitable methods for assessing the potential for adverse health effects resulting from exposure to environmental tobacco smoke (ETS) are limited by the complexity of the composition of the mixture. In vivo and in vitro assays are commonly used to establish carcinogenicity and in some cases to extrapolate risks to humans. For complex mixtures such as ETS, these assays may be done on the mixture itself or on individual chemical constituents. Many properties of ETS change as the smoke "ages" after its initial generation. Aging probably affects the bioavailability, as well as physicochemical characteristics, of the smoke.

As inhalation is the primary route by which humans are exposed to tobacco smoke, it is obviously the preferred method of administration in animal models for evaluating the toxicological properties of both cigarette smoke and ETS. While extensive inhalation studies have been performed on the toxicological properties of mainstream cigarette smoke (MS), far fewer studies have been performed on sidestream smoke (SS) and ETS. The selection of appropriate animal models requires familiarity with exposure systems, as well as with basic anatomical differences between the model and human respiratory tracts.

Methods other than inhalation, such as in vitro assays, have been developed for the evaluation of MS. A few of these methods have been applied to the assessment of the relative toxicological properties of SS versus MS. These methods are frequently criticized because of differences in the way the smoke constituents are presented to the test system as compared with that which occurs in the human situation. Despite these limitations, the use of cigarette smoke condensate (CSC) from MS has provided insight into the relative carcinogenic potential of various constituents in the MS of cigarettes. Similar studies using suitable condensates from SS and aged ETS could provide additional data on the effects of ETS.

IN VIVO ASSAYS ON ENVIRONMENTAL TOBACCO SMOKE

Exposure Methods in Laboratory Research

Several methods are available to evaluate the potential health effects of inhaled pollutants. Some common ones are whole-body exposure, head-only exposure, nose- or mouth-only exposure, lung-only exposure, or partial-lung exposure. Since the primary objective of an inhalation experiment is to determine the effects of the test substances or mixture on the respiratory system, it is preferable to eliminate or limit exposure through the skin or through ingestion (such as through contact with materials deposited on the fur or contaminated food and water).

Three methods have been used to determine the amount of material deposited in the respiratory tract (Phalen, 1984): direct measurement, calculations using airborne concentrations and uptake models, and calibration of the exposure apparatus using tracer substances. Direct measurement requires analysis of major components and their metabolites in tissues as well as in urine and feces or measurement of the amounts of material in the inspired and expired air. Aside from calculating dose based upon particle aerodynamic size and physiological data on lung function of experimental animals, tracers can provide reasonable estimates of exposure.

Inhalation exposure chambers are used for those studies in which whole-body exposure is desired. The ability to expose a large number of animals at one time and the absence of a need to restrain or anesthetize the animals are among the advantages in using this approach. There are, however, several major disadvantages. The animals are exposed through skin absorption and mouth ingestion and, in prolonged instances, by food and possibly water contamination. Animals tend to avoid exposure in such chambers by huddling together or covering their noses with their own fur. Losses of particulate aerosols to the interior walls of the chambers are also frequently a problem.

Head-only exposure systems eliminate many of these problems. The disadvantages of these systems are that the animal must be restrained and is stressed or anesthetized, and there is difficulty in forming an adequate seal.

Nose- or mouth-only exposure systems further limit exposure to the oral cavity and the respiratory tract. Masks or the use of catheters in the nose are generally used with larger animals. Lung and partial-lung-only exposure systems such as endotracheal tubes are employed to bypass the upper respiratory tract and to directly expose the lung. Most of these methods require that the animal be anesthetized, which may alter normal respiration. Other disadvantages include disruption of normal airflow by the presence of tubes in the airways and the loss of normal humidification and thermal regulation of the inspired air caused by bypassing the upper respiratory tract.

Intratracheal instillation is an alternative to inhalation for evaluating the effects of individual compounds on the respiratory system. While there are several advantages in employing this bioassay technique, it is also known that the distribution of test material to respiratory tissue may differ from that which would be obtained by actual inhalation exposures. Instillation of an aqueous suspension of radiolabeled particles resulted in a less uniform deposition than inhalation (Brain et al., 1976).

Animal Models in Inhalation Studies

The selection of an appropriate animal model for inhalation studies with potentially toxic agents is compounded by the fact that one of the major functions of the mammalian sensory apparatus is to limit the exposure to toxic agents either by altering breathing or by producing avoidance behavior (Alarie, 1973; Wood, 1978). Also, the selection of animal species and strains for inhalation exposure studies requires thorough evaluation. The use of several (at least three) animal species, several dose levels, and animals that metabolize the suspect toxin in a similar manner to humans is recommended for those studies that attempt to evaluate human hazards (Stuart, 1976). The appropriate animal model should have (1) a similarity to the human respiratory tract with respect to anatomy, physiology, and susceptibility; (2) a life span appropriate for the proposed study; (3) a sensitivity to certain classes of toxic agents; (4) anatomical or physiological properties that could lead to increased precision in empirical measurements; (5) an existing data base; (6) a documented history of appropriate procedures; and (7) an adaptability for generating data that might be used for mathematically modeling the animal system and its responses to airborne particulates.

Results of Inhalation Studies

Inhalation studies on the carcinogenicity of MS have been performed on a variety of laboratory animals. The early studies with rodents have been previously reviewed (Wynder and Hoffmann, 1967; Mohr and Resnik, 1978). More recent studies verify these findings for several animal species exposed to whole smoke or MS. A few studies have exposed mice to the vapor phase of fresh MS, and one (see below) exposed mice to the vapor phase of flue-cured MS. Because commonly utilized filter systems do not remove many of the vapor-phase constituents, studies contrasting the effects of exposure to whole smoke with the effects of exposure to the gas phase should throw some light on the possible health effects of ETS.

Male and female C57Bl mice (100 in each group) were exposed nose only for 12 minutes daily to the gas phase of smoke of cigarettes prepared from flue-cured tobaccos (Harris et al., 1974). The treated mice had lung tumors and emphysema, independent of the tumors, which were not found in control mice.

A total of 219 C57Bl and 186 BLH mice were exposed to the gas phase of cigarette MS. The particulate matter was removed by passing the smoke through a Cambridge filter. The animals were exposed to the gas phase of 12 cigarettes for 90 minutes daily over 27 months. The percentages of mice with lung adenomas were 5.5% and 32% in the smoke-exposed C57Bl and BLH mice, as compared with 3.4% and 22% for their respective controls (Otto and Elmenhorst, 1967). Therefore, it appears that there are carcinogenic constituents in the vapor phase of the smoke.

Using Snell's mice, similar studies evaluated the toxicological properties of whole MS and the gas phase of MS. In these studies, the animals were housed in individual chambers during the exposure (Leuchtenberger and Leuchtenberger, 1970). There was a significant difference ($p < 0.1$) in the incidence of pulmonary tumors between the animals exposed to whole smoke and control animals. The difference was greater ($p = 0.005$) for animals exposed to only the gas phase of cigarette smoke as compared with the same controls, so that the rate of tumors among the gas-phase-exposed animals was greater than among the whole-smoke exposed animals.

In Vivo Bioassays Other Than Inhalation

Alternative methods have been used to assess the relative chronic toxicity of cigarette MS in an attempt to reduce the cost and technical difficulties associated with inhalation experiments. The most common approach has been to use the CSC in bioassay procedures. In preparing the condensate, many of the volatile and semivolatile components are lost. In addition, it is not known how the aging of the CSC may affect chemical composition and biological activity.

To date, only one study has examined the carcinogenic potential of the condensate of SS of cigarettes (Wynder and Hoffmann, 1967; International Agency for Research on Cancer, 1986). Cigarette "tar" from the SS of nonfilter cigarettes, which had settled on the funnel covering a multiple-unit smoking machine, was suspended in acetone and applied to mouse skin for 15 months. Fourteen of 30 Swiss-ICR mice developed benign skin tumors, and 3 had carcinomas. In a parallel assay of MS from the same source, a 50% CSC:acetone suspension applied to deliver a comparable dose of CSC to 100 Swiss-ICR female mice led to benign skin tumors in 24 mice and malignant skin tumors in 6. This indicates that the smoke condensate of SS has greater tumorigenicity per equivalent dose on mouse skin than MS "tar" ($p < 0.05$; Wynder and Hoffmann, 1967).

IN VITRO ASSAYS ON ENVIRONMENTAL TOBACCO SMOKE

Several short-term bioassays have been performed to evaluate the genotoxicity of cigarette MS. These studies have been the subject of two recent reviews (DeMarini, 1981; Obe et al., 1984). While most of them have evaluated the effects of CSC, some have attempted to evaluate either the gas phase or the whole smoke.

The most commonly employed assay for mutagenic activity employs various strains of *Salmonella typhimurium*. Whole smoke as well as CSC from four types of tobacco were found to be mutagenic in *S. typhimurium* TA1538 (Basrur et al., 1977). Recent studies have shown that SS is also mutagenic in a system where the smoke was tested directly on the bacterial plates (Ong et al., 1984). They support extensive assays performed on CSC that indicate that tobacco smoke has significant mutagenic potential and show that the particulate matter of SS is likely to be a significant contributor to the mutagenic activity of indoor air particulate matter (Bos et al., 1983; Lofröth et al., 1983). Thus, similar mutagenic activity for the CSC of SS would be expected.

In another study (Lewtas et al., in press), condensate from air polluted with ETS for 10 hours was used in an assay employing *S. typhimurium*. The average indoor air mutagenicity per cubic meter was significantly correlated with the number of cigarettes smoked.

Another in vitro assay measures the number of sister-chromatid exchanges (SCEs) in human lymphocytes. Valadand-Barrieu and Izard (1979) used a solution of the gas phase from cigarette MS. They showed that this solution induced a significant dose-related increase in SCEs.

SUMMARY AND RECOMMENDATIONS

Sufficient data are not available to assess the relative genotoxicity and toxicity of whole ETS. A few isolated reports have dealt with the genotoxicity of SS and ETS, and the relative toxicity of MS and SS. In order to evaluate ETS, it is suggested that in vitro genotoxicity assays in at least two systems should be done with ETS per se as well as with its particulate matter. These assays under controlled and, subsequently, under field conditions should not be limited to freshly generated ETS, but should also attempt to determine effects of various degrees of air dilution and aging. In a comprehensive analytical approach, data should be generated to determine systematically the concentrations of toxic and tumorigenic agents in various milieus with ETS. At the same time, it may be useful to examine the uptake of tobacco-specific agents as well as the mutagenicity of the urine of nonsmokers exposed to ETS. All of these measures should be considered in the context of detailed exposure histories.

What Is Known

1. The lungs of various species have different physiological properties, making each of them the experimental species of choice only for certain situations, depending on the objective of the research study.

2. ETS and SS have been shown to be mutagenic in a system where the smoke was tested directly on bacterial plates.

3. The extensive studies of MS can serve as a guideline for the evaluation of ETS. Many of the constituents in the smokes are similar. Despite the limitations of extrapolating from various bioassays to man, the use of CSC from MS has provided insight as to the contribution of various components to the carcinogenic potential of MS from cigarettes.

4. In the only study reported to date using SS condensate, SS condensate was shown to be more carcinogenic than MS condensate.

What Scientific Information Is Missing

1. Only a few laboratory methods have been applied toward the assessment of the relative toxicological and genotoxic properties of SS generated from cigarettes and, more importantly, of ETS. Research is needed to clarify the appropriate methods for estimating genotoxicity and to isolate and identify the active agents in body fluids of ETS-exposed nonsmokers.

2. Comparative inhalation studies with MS, SS, and ETS are still needed. Such assays, while not duplicating human exposure patterns, would provide more definitive information about the relative carcinogenic potential of SS in comparison to the MS of the same cigarettes.

3. The aging of the atmosphere in which ETS occurs can have a profound effect on its chemical composition, physical characteristics, and overall biological effects. Therefore, studies of aged ETS are needed.

4. Where exposure histories can be specified clearly, validation and quantitative determination of genotoxic markers for substances in ETS that also occur in the environment would be of value for measuring dose of ETS.

5. In examining the effects of MS, many research workers have used condensates of the smoke painted on the shaved skin of mice.

Similar work with skin painting has not been done with ETS and would be of value for assessing the differential toxicity of ETS and MS.

6. In vitro assays are needed for estimation of the tumor promotion and cocarcinogenic effect of ETS. In vitro tests are quicker than in vivo tests, and enough material can not be collected to do in vivo tests.

REFERENCES

Alarie, Y. Sensory irritation by airborne chemicals. CRC Crit. Rev. Toxicol. 2:299-363, 1973.

Basrur, P.K., S. McClure, and B. Zilkey. A comparison of short term bioassay results with carcinogenicity of experimental cigarettes, pp. 2041-2048. In H.E. Nieburgs, Ed. Prevention and Detection of Cancer, Vol. 1. New York: Marcel Dekker, 1977.

Bos, R.P., J.L.G. Theuws, and P.Th. Henderson. Excretion of mutagens in human urine after passive smoking. Cancer Lett. 19:85-90, 1983.

Brain, J.D., D.E. Kundson, S.P. Sorokin, and M.A. Davis. Pulmonary distribution of particles given by intratracheal instillation or by aerosol inhalation. Environ. Res. 11:13-33, 1976.

DeMarini, D.M. Mutagenicity of fractions of cigarette smoke condensate in *Neurospora crassa* and *Salmonella typhimurium.* Mutat. Res. 88:363-374, 1981.

Harris, R.J., G. Negroni, S. Ludgate, C.R. Pick, F.C. Chesterman, and B.J. Maidment. The incidence of lung tumours in c5761 mice exposed to cigarette smoke: Air mixtures for prolonged periods. Int. J. Cancer 14:130-136, 1974.

International Agency for Research on Cancer (IARC) Monographs: Evaluation of Carcinogenic Risk of Chemicals to Humans, Vol. 38, pp. 163-314. Tobacco Smoking. Lyons: IARC, 1986. 421 pp.

Leuchtenberger, C., and R. Leuchtenberger. Effects of chronic inhalation of whole fresh cigarette smoke and of its gas phase on pulmonary tumorigenesis in Snell's mice, pp. 329-346. In P. Nettesheim, M.G. Hanna, Jr., and J.W. Deatherage, Jr., Eds. Morphology of Experimental Respiratory Carcinogenesis. Proceedings of a Biology Division, Oak Ridge National Laboratory, Conference, Gatlinburg, Tenn., May 13-16, 1970. Washington, D.C.: U.S. Atomic Energy Commission, 1970.

Lewtas, J., S. Goto, K. Williams, J.C. Chuang, B.A. Petersen, and N.K. Wilson. The mutagenecity of indoor air particles in a residential pilot field study. Atmos. Environ., in press.

Lofröth, G., L. Nilsson, and I. Alfheim. Passive smoking and urban air pollution: Salmonella/microsome mutagenicity assay of simultaneously collected indoor and outdoor particulate matter, pp. 515-525. In M.D. Waters, S.S. Sandhu, J. Lewtas, L. Claxton, N. Chernoff, and S. Nesnow, Eds. Short-Term Bioassays in the Analysis of Complex Environmental Mixtures. III. New York: Plenum, 1983.

Mohr, U., and G. Resnick. Tobacco carcinogenesis, pp. 263-367. In C.C. Harris, Ed. Pathogenesis and Therapy of Lung Cancer. New York: Marcel Dekker, 1978.

Obe, G., W.-D. Heller, and H.-J. Vogt. Mutagenic activity of cigarette smoke, pp. 223-246. In G. Obe, Ed. Mutations in Man. Berlin: Springer-Verlag, 1984.

Ong, T., J. Stewart, and W.Z. Whong. A simple in situ mutagenicity test system for detection of mutagenic air pollutants. Mutat. Res. 139:177-181, 1984.

Otto, H., and H. Elmenhorst. Experimentelle Untersuchungen zur Tumorinduktion mit der Gasphase des Zigarettenrauchs. Z. Krebsforsch. 70:45-47, 1967.

Phalen, R.F. Inhalation Studies: Foundations and Techniques. Boca Raton, Florida: CRC Press, 1984.

Stuart, B.O. Selection of animal models for evaluation of inhalation hazards in man, pp. 268-288. In E.F. Aharonsen, S. Ben-David, and M.A. Klingberg, Eds. Air Pollution and the Lung. New York: John Wiley & Sons, 1976.

Valadaud-Barrieu, D., and C. Izard. Action de la phase gazeuse de fumée de cigarette sur le taux d'echanges des chromatides-soeurs du lymphocyte humain in vitro. C.R. Acad. Sci. (Paris) 288:899-901, 1979.

Wood, R.W. Stimulus properties of inhaled substances. Environ. Health Perspect. 26:69-76, 1978.

Wynder, E.L., and D. Hoffmann. Tobacco and Tobacco Smoke: Studies in Experimental Carcinogenesis. New York: Academic Press, 1967. 730 pp.

II
ASSESSING EXPOSURES TO ENVIRONMENTAL TOBACCO SMOKE

4
Introduction

Exposure to a variety of air contaminants has been shown to produce adverse health and discomfort responses in humans. In another report from the National Academy of Sciences (NRC, 1985), the methodological issues of studying exposures to air pollutants and subsequent health effects are discussed in detail. This part of the report considers issues relevant to assessing exposure to ETS. Ideally, evidence for health effects in humans should be demonstrated in epidemiologic studies that are consistent with a plausible hypothesis across a range of exposures or doses. However, many epidemiologic studies have substantial uncertainties associated with exposure variables. A framework for assessing exposures to environmental tobacco smoke (ETS) is discussed below. A variety of approaches to current and historic exposures to ETS, such as personal monitoring, locational monitoring, questionnaires, and biologic monitoring, are presented.

Concentrations of air contaminants exhibit pronounced spatial and temporal variations, regardless of the microenvironments in which they are found (outdoors, residential, industrial, etc.). Ideally, identifying the air contaminant or class of contaminants implicated in producing adverse health or comfort effects is essential in designing an air-monitoring program. In practice, however, it is often necessary to monitor a class of contaminants (for instance, total mass of respirable particles) or a proxy contaminant (for instance, nicotine), when the specific air contaminant producing the adverse impact can not be identified or easily measured. The air contaminants associated with ETS are comprised of a broad range of many vapor- and particle-phase inorganic and organic chemicals noted in Chapter 2, some of which can undergo pronounced physicochemical changes. Assessing impact on human health and comfort requires the identification of proxy air contaminants for ETS that will permit a determination of exposure in a background of contaminants from other sources (see Chapter 5).

In epidemiologic studies of air contaminants, it is important to specify exposure to specific particulates or gases on a time scale corresponding to the health or comfort effect sought. The impact of exposure to an air contaminant should, ideally, be evaluated in terms of the biologic dose of the contaminant or its metabolites received by the target tissue. In most cases, this is not practical. The uptake, distribution, metabolism, and site and mode of action of the contaminant in humans is neither well understood nor easily measured. Moreover, dose cannot be directly assessed. Factors affecting the uptake of air contaminants include physical characteristics of the contaminant, as well as physiological characteristics and activity levels of the exposed person (see Chapter 7). In the absence of an ability to measure or specify the *dose* of a contaminant received, *exposures* to air contaminant(s) are assessed by either using biological markers, measured in the subject population, or by measuring the air-contaminant concentrations in the physical environment (Figure 4-1).

Exposures to airborne contaminants can be assessed by three basic approaches (Figure 4-1):

- personal air-contaminant monitoring,
- modeling, based on air sampling, time-activity patterns, and questionnaires, and
- biological markers.

Personal monitoring employs samplers (worn by subjects) that record the integrated concentration individuals are exposed to in the course of their normal activity for time periods of several hours to several days (see Chapter 5).

The modeling approach employs the use of stationary monitors to measure the air-contaminant concentrations in a number of microenvironments. These measured concentrations are combined with time activity patterns (time budgets) to determine the average exposure of an individual as the sum of the concentrations in each environment weighed by the time spent in that environment.

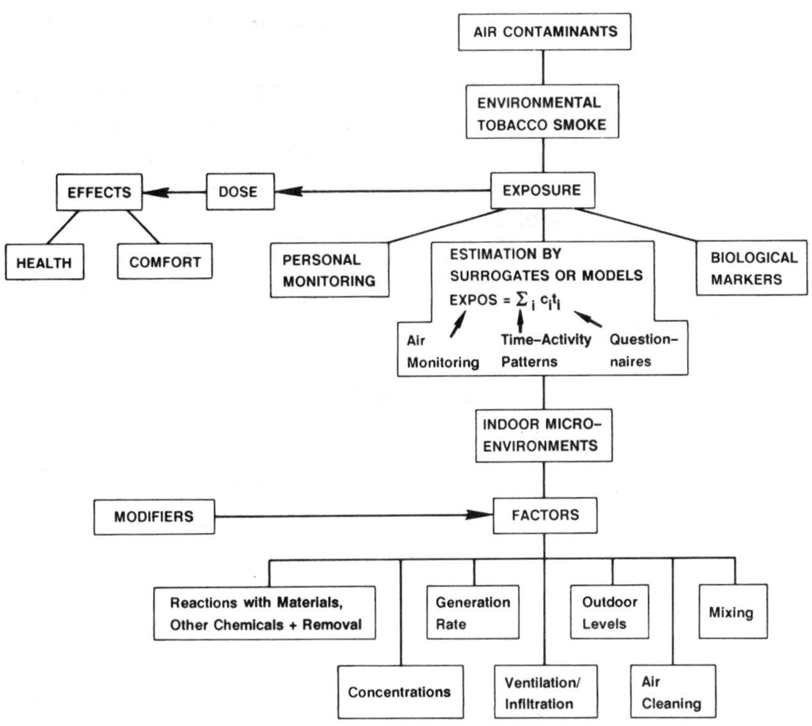

FIGURE 4-1 Flow diagram of components for assessing human exposures to air contaminants from environmental tobacco smoke.

Questionnaires are employed in two capacities: (1) to provide information on the physical properties of each environment, including source use parameters, in order to model the concentration of air contaminants in the microenvironment, thus permitting a prediction of air-contaminant concentrations in spaces not monitored; and (2) to provide a simple categorization of exposure levels, such as exposed versus unexposed or none versus low versus high.

Questionnaires have been used to categorize subjects' exposure to ETS in all studies of risk of chronic lung disease reported to date. Chapter 6 discusses the use of questionnaires to categorize ETS exposures.

Chapter 7 reviews assumptions required to estimate exposure-dose relationships for ETS and gives an approximation to the dose received under a specific situation.

Chapter 8 examines the use of biological markers, such as urinary cotinine, as indices of exposure to ETS.

There are several factors (Figure 4-1) that determine the composition and level of ETS air contaminants in the indoor environments. Determining the range of values for each of these factors will lead to an understanding of their impact on ETS exposures. Efforts to modify or eliminate exposures to ETS must focus on the factors that control the concentrations in the physical environment, since these factors result in the exposure that relates to the adverse health or comfort effect.

REFERENCE

National Research Council, Committee on the Epidemiology of Air Pollutants. Epidemiology and Air Pollution. Washington, D.C.: National Academy Press, 1985. 224 pp.

5
Assessing Exposures to Environmental Tobacco Smoke in the External Environment

Environmental tobacco smoke (ETS) is composed of more than 3,800 compounds. The emitted compounds are found in vapor or particulate phases, or in some cases both. Volatile material may evaporate from particles within seconds to minutes after emission (e.g., nicotine, see Chapter 2). ETS has not yet been adequately characterized such that its chemical and physical nature can be clearly defined. The concentration of any individual or group of ETS constituents in an enclosed space is a function of: (a) the generation rate of the contaminant(s) from the tobacco, (b) the source consumption rate, (c) the ventilation or infiltration rate, (d) the concentration of the contaminant(s) of interest in the ventilation or infiltration air, (e) the degree to which the air is mixed, (f) the removal of the contaminant(s) by surfaces or chemical transformations, and (g) the effectiveness of any air-cleaning devices that may be in use. Exposure to ETS takes place in many settings—such as public, industrial, nonindustrial occupational, and residential buildings—and is a function of the time an individual spends in a microenvironment and the concentration of the ETS constituents in that environment. ETS exposures can be determined either by extrapolation from fixed-location monitoring survey instruments that are portable or by direct personal monitoring, using lightweight pumps and filters worn by subjects.

This chapter will consider the methodology and data available for assessing human exposures to ETS in the physical (external) environment, including the suitability of proposed tracers or proxy air contaminants that would be representative of ETS, available data on ETS exposure from personal monitoring and monitoring of indoor environments, and the application of modeling to assessing ETS exposures.

TRACERS FOR ENVIRONMENTAL TOBACCO SMOKE

It is difficult to assess the ETS contribution to exposures because it usually exists in a complex mix of air contaminants from other sources. It is not practical, or possible, to monitor the full range of air contaminants associated with ETS, even under laboratory conditions. Chamber and field studies of ETS have monitored proxy contaminants as indicators of ETS. Most studies to date have been less than ideal because the component that was measured did not meet all the following criteria for an ETS tracer. A marker or tracer for quantifying ETS concentrations should be:

- unique or nearly unique to the tobacco smoke so that other sources are minor in comparison,
- a constituent of the tobacco smoke present in sufficient quantity such that concentrations of it can be easily detected in air, even at low smoking rates,
- similar in emission rates for a variety of tobacco products, and
- in a fairly consistent ratio to the individual contaminant of interest or category of contaminants of interest (e.g., suspended particulates) under a range of environmental conditions encountered and for a variety of tobacco products.

While a variety of measures have been used as proxies or tracers of ETS, no single measure has met all the criteria outlined above, nor has any measure been universally accepted or recognized as representing ETS exposure.

Carbon monoxide (CO) has been measured extensively both in chamber studies (Bridge and Corn, 1972; Hoegg, 1972; Penkala and De Oliveira, 1975; Weber et al., 1976, 1979a,b; Weber and Fisher 1980; Weber, 1984; Muramatsu et al., 1983; Leaderer et al., 1984; Winneke et al., 1984; Clausen, et al., 1985) and in occupied public and nonindustrial occupational indoor spaces (see Table 2-4) to represent ETS levels. Under steady-state conditions in chamber studies, where outdoor CO levels are known and the tobacco brands and smoking protocols constant, CO can be a reasonably reproducible indicator of ETS exposure. The variability of CO production from tobacco combustion is not well known and may vary considerably as a function of a number of variables (puff volume, puff duration, temperature, etc.). The ratio of CO, a nonreactive contaminant, to the more reactive gas-phase contaminants in ETS and to reactive suspended particulate mass is not well established, particularly in the dynamic phase of smoking, that is, the non-steady-state phase. Chamber and field studies have indicated that, under realistic smoking conditions that would be encountered in residences or offices, the typical smoking and ventilation rates would produce CO levels well within the levels observed in the outdoor air or in the indoor air generated from the indoor sources, such as kerosene heater, gas stove, etc. Consequently, it is difficult to factor out the contribution of CO from ETS in any specific, uncontrolled situation. In areas where heavy smoking is experienced, and where other sources of CO do not exist, CO may provide a rough measure of ETS exposure because the CO produced by the tobacco combustion will dominate.

Both chamber and field studies (Table 5-1) have demonstrated that tobacco combustion has a major impact on the mass of suspended particulate matter in occupied spaces in the size range $<2.5\ \mu m$, defined in this report as respirable suspended particulates (RSP). Suspended particulate mass is a major component of environmentally emitted tobacco smoke. Even under conditions of low smoking rates, easily measurable increases in RSP have been recorded above background levels (Table 5-1). The term RSP, however, encompasses a broad range of particulates of varying chemical composition and size emanating from a number of sources (outdoors, cooking indoors, etc).

Smoking is not the only source of particulate matter suspended in the indoor air. The apportionment of the measured RSP to tobacco combustion in an occupied space will not be accurate unless the RSP emission rates for a variety of brands of tobacco are similar under a variety of conditions and source use information is obtained. The variability of RSP emissions into the environment for a variety of brands of tobacco needs to be investigated, as does the relationship between the vapor and particulate phases of tobacco-combustion emissions under a variety of environmental conditions, such as different humidities, and under a variety of smoking conditions, such as subject smokers versus smoking machines.

TABLE 5-1 Particulate Levels Measured in Indoor Environments, Including Smoking and Nonsmoking Occupancy

Study	Type of Premise	Occupancy	Volume, m^3	Ventilation Type/Rate	Monitoring Type/Time	Concentrations Mean (range), $\mu g/m^3$	Comments
Brunekreef and Boleij, 1982	4 residences	NS	—	N/—	G/2 mo	55 (20–90)	TSP, repeat measures 0.2 mg
	7 residences	S = 1	—	N/—	G/2 mo	125 (60–250)	TSP sensitivity
	14 residences	S = 2	—	N/—	G/2 mo	152 (60–340)	TSP sensitivity
	1 residence	S = 3	—	N/—	G/2 mo	335 (—)	TSP sensitivity
	Outdoors	—	—	—	G/2 mo	— (41–73)	
Cuddeback et al., 1976	2 taverns	S = 5–40 NS = 5–260 T = 10–300	—	N,M/1–6 ach	G/9 h	446 (233–986)	TSP ventilation estimated
Elliot and Rowe, 1975	3 arenas	NS	—	—	G/24 h	55 (42–92)	TSP
	3 arenas	S T = 2,000–14,277	—	M/—	G/0.3 h	350 (148–620)	TSP
First, 1984	1 school	NS	—	M/—	P/—	20 (—)	TSP
	8 public buildings	S	—	N,M/—	P/—	260 (40–660)	TSP
Hawthorne et al., 1984	11 residences	NS	150–674	M/0.18–0.96	QCMI/5–15 min (over 6 h)	9–40 (—)	RSP, winter/summer—no sources
	8 residences	NS	150–674	M/0.26–1.98	QCMI/5–15 min (over 6 h)	12–46	RSP, winter/summer—sources[e]
	2 residences	S	150–674	M/0.27–1.47	QCMI/5–15 min (over 6 h)	96–106	RSP, winter/summer—sources[e] + cig.
Leaderer et al., personal communication	3 public buildings	NS	163–1,326	M/0.37–5.6[d]	G/4–21 h	17.8 (9.1–32.2)	TSP, repeat measures, all var.
	7 public buildings	1.7–4.57[b] T = 2–6	168–600	M/0.77–7.53[d]	G/2–24 h	205.1 (58–452)	Measured (160.0 peak)

Moschandreas et al., 1981	Outdoors	—	—	—	G/24 h	17.0 (—)	RSP, TSP also measured
	2 offices	—	—	—	G/24 h	16.8–20.2 (53 peak)	RSP, TSP also measured
	5 residences	NS T = 2–6	—	N/0.5–1.3 ach	G/24 h	19.4–4.01 (118.9 peak)	RSP, TSP also measured
	5 residences	S	—	N/0.5–1.3 ach	G/24 h	36.9–99.9	RSP, TSP also measured
Nitschke et al., 1985	Outdoors	—	—	—	G/168 h	11.3 ± 6.0 (1–28)	RSP
	19 residences	NS	315–1,021	N/—	G/168 h	26.0 ± 22.6 (6–88)	RSP, repeat measures, source mix[e]
	11 residences	S	290–800	N/—	G/168 h	59.2 ± 38.8 (10–144)	RSP, repeat measures, source mix[e]
Parker et al., 1984	1 residence	NS T = 3	—	N/0.2–1.9 ach	0/24 h	< 10 (—)	TSP
	2 residences	S = 1–2 T = 3–4	—	N/0.2–0.7 ach	0/24 h	10–46 (—)	TSP
Repace and Lowrey, 1980, 1982	Outdoors	—	—	—	P/2 min	42.9 (22–63)	RSP, average of 2-min samples
	27 Public buildings	0.13–3.54[f]	—	M/—	P/2 min	278 (86–1,140)	RSP, average of 2-min samples
Sexton et al., 1984	Outdoors 19 homes	—	—	—	G/24 h	17.0 ± 1.6 (6–23)	RSP, repeat samples
	24 residences	NS[c]	—	N/—	G/24 h	25.0 ± 1.0 (13–63)	Used fireplaces
Spengler et al., 1981	Outdoors	—	—	—	G/24 h	21.1 ± 11.9 (—)	RSP, repeat measures
	35 residences	NS	—	N/—	G/24 h	24.1 ± 11.6 (—)	RSP, repeat measures
	15 residences	S = 1	—	N/—	G/24 h	36.5 ± 14.5 (—)	RSP, repeat measures
	5 residences	S = 2	—	N/—	G/24 h	70.4 ± 42.9 (—)	RSP, repeat measures
Spengler et al., 1985	Outdoors	—	—	N/—	G/24 h	18 ± 2.1 (—)	RSP, repeat measures
	73 residences	NS	—	—	G/24 h	28 ± 1.1 (—)	RSP, repeat measures
	28 residences	S	—	—	G/24 h	74 ± 6.6 (—)	RSP, repeat measures
Sterling and Sterling, 1983	1 office	S restr.	—	—	G(?)/—	25.5 (15–36)	TSP
	22 offices	S	—	—	G(?)/—	31.7 (—)	TSP

TABLE 5-1 *Continued*

Study	Type of Premise	Occupancy	Volume, m^3	Ventilation Type/Rate	Monitoring Type/Time	Concentrations Mean (range), $\mu g/m^3$	Comments
U.S. Department of Transportation, 1971	8 domestic planes	S T = 27-110	—	M/—	G/1-1/4, 2-1/2 h	Not given (—)	TSP
	20 military planes	S T = 165-219	—	M/—	G/6-7 h	<10-120 (—)	TSP
Weber and Fischer, 1980	44 offices	S	—	N,M/—	P/2 min (30 ea)	133 ± 130 (962 peak)	RSP, minus background level

[a]Active smokers per 100 m^3.

[b]Grams of tobacco consumed.

[c]Some smoking was reported during 9 of the 280 samples.

[d]Measured during 24-h periods by the perfluorocarbon tracer technique.

[e]Some residences had combinations of sources (kerosene heaters, wood stoves, etc.) and no cigarettes.

[f]Active smokers density per 100 m^3.

ABBREVIATIONS:

ach = Air changes per hour
G = Gravimetric
M = Mechanical ventilation
N = Natural ventilation
NS = No smokers
O = Optical monitor
P = Piezoelectric balance
QCMI = Quality Crystal Microbalance Cosade Impactor
RSP = Respirable suspended particles
S = Smokers
T = Total occupants
TSP = Total suspended particles
restr. = building with smoking restrictions

Nicotine exhibits many of the properties necessary to serve as a potential marker for ETS. It is unique to tobacco smoke, is a major constituent of the smoke, and occurs in environmental concentrations that are easily measurable. It has been used as a marker for ETS in several studies (Table 2-5). The major problems with using nicotine are: (a) the ratio of nicotine [recently found to be in vapor phase in ETS (Eudy et al., 1985)] to other ETS constituents (RSP, in particular) for a variety of brands of tobacco is not known, (b) the reactivity rate (removal rate) of nicotine relative to other ETS constituents is not known, (c) particulate- or vapor-phase nicotine once deposited on surfaces may be re-emitted, and (d) until recently sampling methods for nicotine have not been efficient in collecting total nicotine (both vapor and particulate phase). Two new air-sampling methods for nicotine (Muramatsu et al., 1984; Hammond et al., in press) hold promise for obtaining total nicotine concentrations with the sensitivity and accuracy required for environmental air monitoring.

A number of aromatic hydrocarbons (benzene, toluene, benzo-[*a*]pyrene, pyrene, etc.) have been measured in field studies (Galuskinova, 1964; Just et al., 1972; Perry, 1973; Elliot and Rowe, 1975; Badre et al., 1978) investigating the impact of smoking on indoor air quality. Many of these air contaminants have other important sources, indoors and outdoors, that make measured levels difficult to interpret. Therefore, the aromatic hydrocarbons generally are poor indicators of ETS alone. Controlled chamber studies that elevate the variability of emission of the compounds from a variety of brands of tobacco have not been carried out, and the ratios of these compounds to categories of ETS contaminants (for instance, RSP) have not been established.

Tobacco-specific nitrosamines and nitrogen oxides (Tables 2-6 and 2-9), acrolein and acetone (Tables 2-7 and 2-8), and polonium-210 have been measured as indicators of ETS. The low environmental concentrations, existence of other sources, reactivity of the tracer contaminants, and lack of data on the ratios of these contaminants to ETS contaminants for a variety of brands of tobacco limit their usefulness as indicators of ETS in indoor spaces.

Research efforts need to be directed toward identifying a tracer or proxy air contaminant for ETS that meets the four criteria outlined above. At present, RSP is widely used as a general measure of ETS exposure indoors, particularly if the measurements are limited to locations where the levels of RSP from other sources are known and present at a low background concentration. The variability of RSP emissions for a number of brands of cigarettes, however, has yet to be evaluated.

PERSONAL MONITORING

Measurements of concentrations of air contaminants in the immediate breathing zone of an individual provide information on personal exposure. Personal monitoring can be accomplished with active samplers that integrate concentrations across a variety of locations or conditions using filters or vapor traps with subsequent laboratory analysis. Continuous portable monitoring instruments are available but have not been widely used. Particles are measured by light-scattering principles or frequency change as mass is deposited on a vibrating quartz crystal. For the most part, gases are measured using IR absorption or electrochemical reactions. Continuous-recording instruments have been utilized more for characterizing microenvironments than for direct measurements of personal exposures. Passive personal monitoring utilizes diffusion and permeation to concentrate gases on a collection medium for subsequent laboratory analysis. Both active and passive monitors have been employed in assessing an individual's total exposure to individual or general categories of air contaminants. A discussion of the type, application, and usefulness of passive monitors to assess air contaminant exposures can be found in Elliott and Rowe (1975) and Wallace and Ott (1982).

A relatively small number of studies have utilized personal monitors to determine total exposures to ETS (Muramatsu et al., 1984; Schenker et al., 1984; Sexton et al., 1984; Spengler et al., 1985; Hammond et al., in press). In one study (Spengler et al., 1985) indoor (residential), outdoor, and personal 24-hour concentrations of RSP (measured in this study as particles with a 50% cut point of 3.5 μm) were obtained for a sample of 101 nonsmoking individuals living in Roane County, Tennessee. In the sample, 28 of those monitored reported some exposure to ETS in either the home or workplace (nonindustrial), while 73 reported no such exposure. Each participant was sampled on 3 nonconsecutive days. Personal exposures to respirable particles for the subgroup exposed to ETS and the subgroup not exposed to ETS are shown in Figure 5-1. Personal exposures to RSP were dominated by indoor levels of ETS. Those reporting passive smoke exposure had

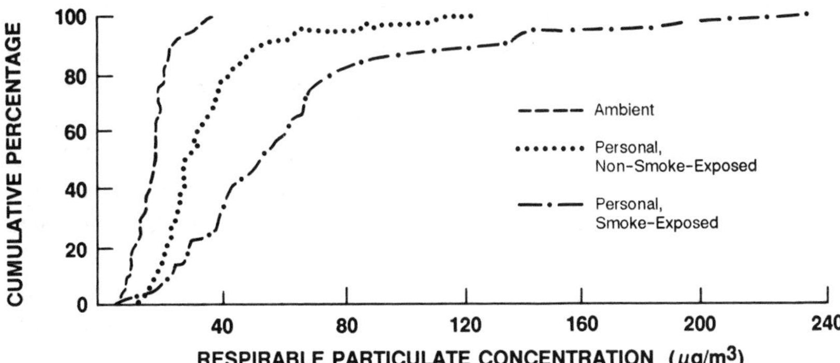

FIGURE 5-1 Cumulative frequency distributions of RSP concentrations from central site ambient and personal monitoring of smoke-exposed and nonsmoke-exposed individuals. Reprinted with permission from Spengler et al. (1985).

mean personal respirable particulate levels 28 $\mu g/m^3$ higher than those without passive smoke exposure. Particulate levels for those exposed to ETS showed a large variation, with approximately 25% of the personal samples having RSP levels in excess of the EPA ambient standard for outdoor total suspended particles. The EPA standard, however, includes particles up to approximately 50 μm and does not specify chemical composition. A direct comparison with the EPA standard requires a consideration of average time exposed as well as concentration.

Sexton et al. (1984) conducted 24-hour personal monitoring for RSP for 48 nonsmoking individuals for 24 different residences. Samples were collected every other day, for a 2-week period, during a heating season in Vermont. Those individuals reporting exposure to ETS for more than 2 hours per day had RSP levels 18.4 $\mu g/m^3$ higher than those who reported no exposure (50.1 $\mu g/m^3$ versus 31.7$\mu g/m^3$).

In demonstrating a new method for the collection and analysis of nicotine in air, one study (Muramatsu et al., 1984) obtained personal-monitoring samples of nicotine for one nonsmoker in 53 nonindustrial indoor microenvironments, including offices, houses, restaurants, cars, buses, etc. The samples were collected over a 1-hour to 8-hour time period in each space and were specific for nicotine. A wide range of nicotine concentrations were reported, from 1.76 $\mu g/m^3$ in a laboratory to 83.13 $\mu g/m^3$ in a car. It is difficult to interpret these results in terms of an integrated exposure for a large segment of the population, since the sampling scheme did not explicitly provide population estimates of exposure—that is, personal samples were obtained on a microenvironment basis for only one individual. Lacking good data for the ratio of total nicotine to RSP in ETS, it is difficult to estimate the RSP exposure levels. The data, however, do demonstrate that the variability of nicotine concentrations and the occurrence of high concentrations of other ETS components can be found in various microenvironments.

In an epidemiologic study of the health effects of diesel exhaust on railroad workers (Schenker et al., 1984), which included a control group of railroad office workers who were not exposed to diesel exhaust but were exposed to ETS, ETS was recognized as an important component of the respirable particulate exposures. Hammond et al. (in press) used a newly developed air-sampling and analytical method for measuring total nicotine in collected RSP personal samples to determine the contribution of ETS to the RSP levels measured. Their results indicated that the major portion of the office workers' RSP exposure is due to ETS. Ratios of nicotine to RSP for a variety of brands of tobacco need to be established before absolute ETS exposures can be assessed.

Personal monitoring can provide a useful measure of an individual's exposure to an air contaminant or class of contaminants over a period of several hours to several days. The usefulness of personal monitors for assessing ETS exposure would be greatly enhanced if the personal monitor were passive in nature and inexpensive. Personal and portable monitors, however, need to be evaluated to determine their usefulness in establishing ETS exposures associated with long-term adverse health outcomes, such as cancer. They may be useful in establishing ETS exposures, in a background of confounding air contaminants, associated with short-term effects.

A variety of sample collection and analysis methods has been used to monitor individual constituents and categories of contaminants found in ETS for both personal monitoring and air monitoring of spaces. While this report does not offer a review and evaluation of the monitoring methods that have been employed and are available, it should be clearly noted that the specificity and sensitivity of the measurement method must be evaluated to assess the uncertainties in the measured concentrations. The constituents of ETS will exhibit a pronounced spatial and temporal distribution in an indoor space and among indoor environments, due to variations in smoking rates and building characteristics. In interpreting measured concentrations of ETS constituents, one must recognize the potential for pronounced spatial and temporal variations.

CONCENTRATIONS OF ENVIRONMENTAL TOBACCO SMOKE IN INDOOR ENVIRONMENTS

Various Environmental Tobacco Smoke Constituents

There is a sizable body of literature reporting on measurements of various constituents (acrolein, aromatic hydrocarbons, carbon monoxide, nicotine, etc.) of ETS in a variety of microenvironments. These studies have reported a wide range of concentrations of ETS-related air contaminants under conditions of normal space use (Tables 2-4 to 2-9). However, the majority of the measurements are of very limited use in assessing actual human exposures to ETS for a large segment of the population for the following reasons:

- the representativeness of the air contaminant measured to the total ETS in the space is unknown;
- the proxy air contaminant measured may have a variety of other potential sources that were not accounted or controlled for;
- data were not collected on smoking rates or numbers of smokers; and
- important building characteristics such as infiltration or volume were not recorded.

While these studies have indicated the range of concentrations of several ETS-related air contaminants that can be found indoors, they do not provide a sufficient basis on which ETS indoor exposure estimates can be made.

Particulate Levels and Smoking Occupancy

The most extensive and suitable data base for modeling ETS is the RSP (<2.5 μm) associated with ETS. This RSP comprises

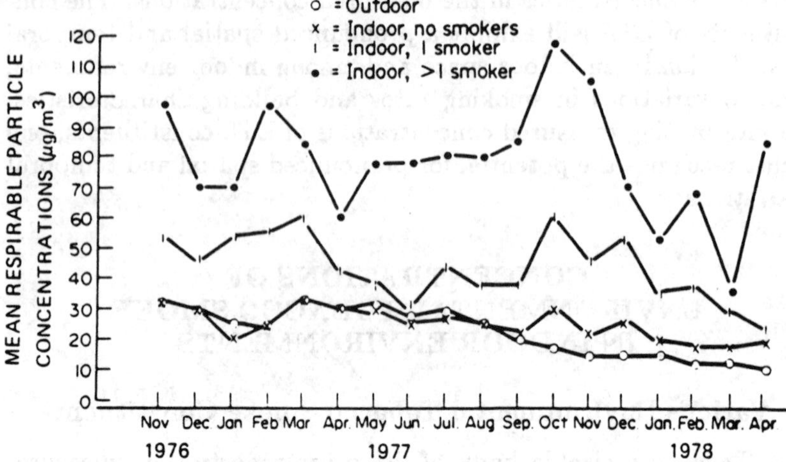

FIGURE 5-2 Monthly mean RSP concentrations in six U.S. cities. Reprinted with permission from Spengler (1981).

a major general category of ETS contaminants and is produced in concentrations that are easily measured in occupied spaces where smoking occurs.

In a survey of more than 80 homes in six U.S. cities (Spengler et al., 1981), 24-hour gravimetric samples of RSP were collected every sixth day for up to 2 years in stationary samplers in each home and outdoors. The resulting data (monthly RSP means) aggregated by the number of smokers are shown in Table 5-1 and Figure 5-2. Homes without smokers exhibited RSP levels roughly equal to outdoor levels and followed outdoor trends. The presence of just one smoker in a home had a pronounced impact on RSP levels. Using regression analysis, the authors estimated that the impact on overall average RSP levels in a residence of a pack-per-day smoker was approximately 20 $\mu g/m^3$. The impact of smoking in a home with central air conditioning was effectively doubled, presumably due to reduced air exchange.

Table 5-1 presents the range of RSP levels measured in a variety of indoor microenvironments for smoking and nonsmoking occupancies. It also indicates whether direct measures of the variables necessary for the model outlined in Equation 5-1 below, or necessary to explain the RSP levels measured, were recorded. These variables include, among others, ventilation, mixing, removal by surfaces, and smoking occupancy. Outdoor levels of

RSP or total suspended particulates are generally lower than or equal to indoor levels in homes without smoking.

Smoking occupancy is strongly associated with elevated levels of RSP in a variety of indoor microenvironments at levels well above outdoor concentrations and indoor concentrations where there is nonsmoking occupancy. However, few studies have directly recorded the data on the parameters that are necessary to validate models for predicting RSP levels due to smoking occupancy (see section below). Even so, using a number of assumptions, data in Table 5-1 have been used for model validation by some studies (Repace and Lowrey, 1980, 1982).

MODELING

The process of assessing exposure and attributing it to various microenvironments requires knowledge of the time individuals spend in such microenvironments and the typical air-contaminant levels (average and peak) occurring in them. The nature of the health or comfort effect under study determines the time-average concentration of concern. A number of microenvironments have been identified (Moschandreas, 1981), and time-budget surveys have shown that most individuals spend more than 90% of their time indoors, that is, in residential, industrial, and nonindustrial occupational environments (Szalai, 1972). The indoor residential and nonindustrial occupational environments represent the major microenvironments in which exposure to ETS takes place.

Tobacco combustion is a major source category that affects the quality of the air indoors. The air-contaminant concentrations in an enclosed space resulting from tobacco combustion, and hence human exposures, are the result of a complex interaction of several interrelated variables (Figure 4-1), including source air-contaminant emission characteristics and source use, building characteristics, infiltration or ventilation rates, air mixing, loss terms (removal by surfaces or chemical transformations), and the efficiency of air-cleaning equipment. The interaction of these variables in determining the resultant indoor concentrations of ETS has typically been evaluated in both controlled laboratory (chamber and test house) studies and field studies within the theoretical framework of the general mass-balance equation (Turk, 1963; Shair and Heitner, 1974; Esmen, 1978; Ishizu, 1980; Repace and Lowrey, 1980; Leaderer et al., 1984).

The mass-balance equation may be applied to tobacco smoke as either an equilibrium model (time-independent) or a dynamic model (time-dependent). Equilibrium models rely on the assumption that many of the input parameters—such as source rates, removal or loss rates, and ventilation rates—are constant, even though these parameters in actuality may vary considerably in time. These models are useful in developing air-contaminant emission factors for ETS in controlled laboratory studies and in assessing long-term average exposures in given indoor microenvironments. Dynamic models are usually more flexible than equilibrium models and can provide information on short-term concentrations. They may be used to compare the sensitivity of results to variations of input parameters. Equilibrium models, when applied to field studies of ETS, require average information on the impact variables, while dynamic models require a great amount of detailed information obtained as a function of time. Dynamic and equilibrium models are useful in laboratory studies; equilibrium models are best suited to evaluating and predicting ETS concentrations in field studies, particularly when average concentrations over a period of days or longer are of interest.

Equilibrium Models for RSP

Laboratory and field studies typically utilize some form of a single-compartment equilibrium model to evaluate the input parameters to the mass-balance equation, to evaluate field-study data, and to project RSP concentrations from ETS indoors. These studies have reduced the general single-compartment mass-balance equation to the following simplified form.

$$C_{eq} = \frac{G}{m(n_v + n_s)V}, \tag{5-1}$$

where C_{eq} is the equilibrium concentration of RSP in a space expressed as micrograms per cubic meter (μg/m^3) due to ETS, G is the RSP generation rate from tobacco combustion into the space in micrograms per hour (μg/hour), n_v is the ventilation or filtration rate in air changes per hour (ach), n_s is the loss rate of RSP due to surface removal in a space in air changes per hour, V is the volume of the space in cubic meters (m^3), and m is the mixing rate expressed as a fraction. The above model assumes no air-cleaning devices, either in the space or recirculated air.

Under laboratory conditions, the input parameters can be controlled and evaluated. In conducting field studies or in estimating past RSP levels indoors, the values on the right side of Equation 5-2 have to be determined from available data. It should be emphasized that this equation assumes equilibrium conditions, and, to the extent that any of the generation or removal terms are intermittent (e.g., smoking rate) or variable (e.g., ventilation rate), errors are introduced.

Generation Rate

The generation rate of RSP for ETS is a function of the number of cigarettes smoked and the emission rate of RSP per cigarette. Few studies have investigated the RSP emission rate for SS plus exhaled MS, i.e., contributions to ETS. One recent study (Rickert et al., 1984) examined sidestream and mainstream emissions of tar, nicotine, and carbon monoxide in 15 brands of Canadian cigarettes with a range of advertised mainstream tar deliveries (0.7 to 17.0 mg tar/cigarette). The experiments utilized a single-port smoking machine and collected mainstream emissions and sidestream emissions, from a small chamber, onto Cambridge filters. The subsequently measured sidestream emissions of tar were found to average 24.1 mg/cigarette with a range of 15.8 to 36.0 mg/cigarette. These emissions were independent of mainstream emissions, which averaged 11.4 mg of tar per cigarette with a range of 2.5 to 19.4 mg/cigarette. Sidestream emissions were higher for ventilated brands.

RSP emission rates were developed for 10 brands of U.S. cigarettes with rated tar deliveries from 1.0 to 23.0 mg and for one standard cigarette (University of Kentucky #1R3F). The study (B.P. Leaderer, S.K. Hammond, and T. Tosun, personal communication) utilized a 34-m^3 chamber in which the cigarettes were smoked by occupants at a prescribed rate in an effort to create realistic environmental conditions. RSP measurements were made over a 4-hour period during equilibrium conditions via collection of well-mixed room air on filters with subsequent gravimetric analysis. RSP emission levels were found to range from 18.0 to 35.4 mg/cigarette, with an average of 26.9 ± 4.8 mg/cigarette.

Three brands of British cigarettes (very low tar, 1.5 mg; low tar, 12 mg; and medium tar, 18 mg) were evaluated for both mainstream and sidestream emissions of tar (U.K. Government,

1980). The average RSP sidestream emission rate measured was 24.5 mg/cigarette, with a range of 23.0 to 26.4 mg. This study utilized a small test chamber and a smoking machine. The emission by-products were collected onto Cambridge filters.

Only one study (Hoegg, 1972) reports mainstream and sidestream RSP levels for cigarettes prior to 1970. This test chamber study reported a sidestream particle emission rate of 25.8 mg/cigarette and mainstream particle emission rate of 36.2 mg/cigarette for one brand of cigarette.

Current data would suggest an overall RSP emission rate from ETS in the range of approximately 20 to 36 mg tar/cigarette. An accurate estimate of an average emission rate for modeling purposes requires the weighing of the above emission data by the sales-weighted average cigarette brand sold. Data are not available to estimate the historical trend, if any, in the RSP emissions for ETS.

Equation 5-1 assumes a constant, or near constant, source emitting over a sufficiently long time period to reach and maintain equilibrium conditions. In controlled experiments a constant rate of tobacco combustion is easily obtained. In practice, however, tobacco combustion rates in terms of numbers of cigarettes consumed over some period of time in different indoor environments is variable. In the absence of detailed data on cigarette consumption in a space, such as number of cigarettes smoked, time smoked, total weight of tobacco consumed, etc., estimates are required. For example, one smoker in a household smoking at a national average rate of two cigarettes/hour and 10 minutes/cigarette constitutes an intermittent source $[G(t)dt]$. A continuous source would be the smoking of six cigarettes/hour. Using a 26-mg/cigarette emission rate, the estimated total RSP emissions from the intermittent source, i.e., 52 mg/hour, would be represented as being emitted uniformly over a 1-hour period for the full averaging time considered. In large occupied spaces where smoking is permitted, such as nonindustrial occupational environments, estimates (Bridge and Corn, 1972; Jaffe, 1978; Repace and Lowrey, 1980) would indicate that, at any given time, 11% of the population would be smoking (one-third of the U.S. population are smokers, who are smoking at the rate of two cigarettes/hour and 10 minutes/cigarette). This would constitute a continous source. In practice, the smoking rate is probably highly variable in time. The RSP emissions from this example would also be averaged over time to produce uniform average emission rates per hour. For the estimation of equilibrium conditions in Equation 5-1, $G = NE$, where N is equal to the number of cigarettes consumed per hour in a space and E is the number of milligrams of RSP emitted into the environment per cigarette. The assumption of a continuous source introduces errors in the estimated RSP concentration.

It is also important to note that the equilibrium model assumes that the source will be emitting contaminants over a sufficiently long period of time to achieve balance with the removal mechanisms (ventilation, removal by surfaces, and air cleaning). If C_t is the concentration at time t (in hours) then:

$$C_t = C_{eq}(1 - e^{-tN}), \qquad (5\text{-}2)$$

where C_{eq} is the equilibrium concentration and N is the effective removal rate ($N = n_v + n_s$). If the total impact of the removal rate, i.e., ventilation plus loss to surfaces, is equivalent to one *ach*, 85% of the equilibrium concentration would be obtained in 2 hours. Thus, to the extent that the source emissions do not combine over long periods of time, the equilibrium concentration will not be reached and maintained, introducing errors into the estimated or modeled RSP.

Ventilation/Infiltration

The supply of fresh air to a space by ventilation (air supplied by mechanical systems) or by infiltration (uncontrolled movement of air through cracks and unintentional openings in the building envelope) serves to reduce the levels of air contaminants generated by an indoor source.

Building codes adopted and enforced by local, state, and federal government agencies generally specify minimal acceptable ventilation criteria to be maintained in buildings. These codes are usually derived from standards that have been promulgated by authoritative bodies (American National Standards Institute, American Society of Heating, Refrigerating and Air-Conditioning Engineers, etc.). These standards are usually developed by consensus and are generally voluntary until adopted by municipal or state governments. The studies of Yaglou et al. (1936) formed the basis of minimum required ventilation rates that persisted until 1979. These studies reported ventilation rates (fresh odor-free air) in cubic feet per minute per person (cfm/person) necessary to provide an acceptable odor environment. They found that, as occupant density increased, so did the required cfm/person ventilation rate. Because of the odor level, smoking occupancy required significantly more ventilation air. A minimum ventilation rate of approximately 10 cfm/person for nonsmoking occupancy and an occupant density of 400 ft^3/person was recommended. Prior to 1936, minimum recommended ventilation rates were as high as 30 cfm/person.

In 1973, the American Society of Heating, Refrigerating and Air-Conditioning Engineers (ASHRAE) adopted and published Standard 62-73 (Standards for Natural and Mechanical Ventilation). This standard recommended ventilation rates for various residential and commercial spaces on an occupancy-density basis. In 1981, ASHRAE adopted Standard 62-81 (Ventilation for Acceptable Indoor Air Quality), which also recommended ventilation rates for various residential and commercial spaces on an occupancy-density basis but distinguished between smoking and nonsmoking occupancy. Modal ventilation rates in this standard equaled 35 cfm/occupant for smoking occupancy and 7 cfm/occupant for nonsmoking occupancy.

As noted in Equation 5-1, ventilation rates are incorporated as *ach*. ASHRAE 62-73 recommended from 15 to 25 cfm/person for general office space with an estimated 10 persons/1,000 ft^2 density, while ASHRAE 62-81 recommended 20 cfm/person when smoking is permitted and a 5-cfm/person minimum for nonsmoking occupancy with an estimated 7 persons/1,000 ft^2 density occupancy. Assuming full occupancy and an 8-ft ceiling, ASHRAE 62-73 ventilation rate ranges are 1.13 and 1.9 *ach*, while ASHRAE 62-81 recommends a rate of 1.3 *ach* for smoking occupancy and 0.26 *ach* for nonsmoking occupancy. When considered on a space-by-space basis for commercial or residential environments as recommended by either ASHRAE 62-73 or ASHRAE 62-81, the *ach* rates vary considerably, depending on the use of the space and whether smoking is permitted.

In estimating *ach*'s for inputs into Equation 5-1, to assess either current or past RSP concentrations in occupied space due to ETS, the following points should be kept in mind:

- There are no data to indicate the current or past distribution of *ach*'s currently are or have been in a variety of commercial spaces in which smoking is or has been permitted.
- Air-exchange rates are calculated from cfm/person rates specified in the standards for full occupancy. To the extent that occupancy is less than or greater than the designed figure, the cfm/person could be significantly different.
- Ventilation codes are equivalent to design standards. In actual practice, the heating, ventilation, and air-conditioning (HVAC) system may not operate as designed. Interior alterations, modifications in occupancy, maintenance, and repair of equipment, and operator practice can significantly affect the performance of the HVAC system.

Air-infiltration values in housing are induced by differences in pressure across the structure envelope. Limited data exist to indicate what the current or past distribution of air-exchange rates in houses in the United States are or what the intra- or interseasonal variations are. One study of seasonal infiltration rates of 312 houses in North America (Grimrsud et al., 1982; Figure 5-3) found a median value of 0.5 *ach*. This study was based on new energy-efficient houses. Another study (Grot and Clark, 1979; Figure 5-3) of 266 low-income houses in North America found the median seasonal air-exchange rate to be 0.9 *ach*. Air-infiltration rates for both studies were taken without occupants in the houses. Normal activities of occupants would add an average 0.10 to 0.15 *ach* to the values reported in these two studies.

Ventilation or infiltration rates in commercial and residential buildings can vary by an order of magnitude among and within buildings, season to season and within a season. Unfortunately, there are few data available that would allow for an accurate estimate of the distribution of air-exchange rates in commercial and residential spaces currently or over the past several years. A range of 0.4 to 1.5 *ach* would seem reasonable.

Removal by Surfaces

Next to ventilation, the major mechanism for removal of suspended particulate matter is surface deposition. Surface deposition of particles indoors is a function of several variables, including particle size and composition, temperature, humidity, type and quantity of surface material in a room, surface-to-volume rates,

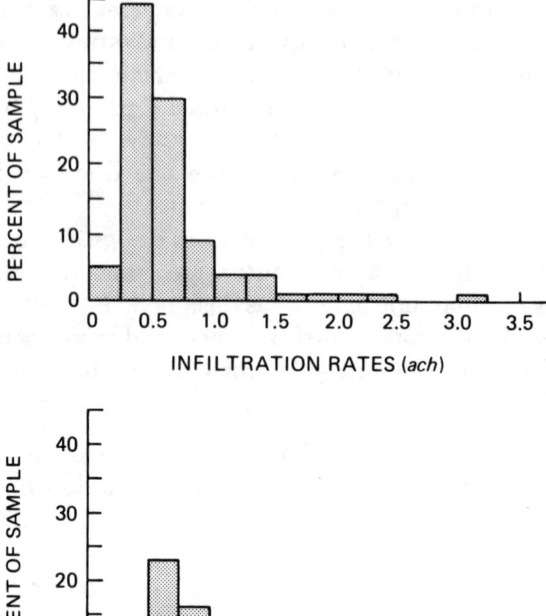

FIGURE 5-3 Histograms of infiltration values in two different samples of North American housing. (a) Average seasonal infilitration of 312 recently constructed houses; the median value is 0.5 air changes per hour (*ach*). Reprinted with permission from Grimsrud et al. (1982). (b) Average seasonal infiltration of 266 older low-income houses; the median is 0.9 *ach*. Reprinted with permission of Grot and Clark (1979).

and turbulence. In laboratory studies under conditions of ideal mixing, surface-deposition rates (h^{-1}) for ETS were found to vary from an equivalent 0.1 h^{-1} to 1.8 h^{-1} (Leaderer et al., 1986). The greater the degree of turbulence introduced into the chamber and the higher the surface-to-volume ratio, the higher the surface deposition.

One recent chamber study evaluated the importance of materials (rugs, wall paper, and painted wall board), surface area of materials, temperature, humidity, and turbulence on the deposition rate of RSP generated by tobacco combustion under conditions of ideal mixing (Leaderer et al., 1986). In these experiments, the deposition rate of RSP was determined by monitoring the decay of RSP and carbon dioxide (injected into the chamber) under the experimental conditions examined. The difference between the RSP and carbon dioxide (nonreactive tracer gas) represented the RSP deposition rate. This study found the most pronounced impact on deposition in this chamber to be the air-recirculation rate (fresh-air-ventilation rate held constant) or turbulence. The type and quantity of material, temperature, and humidity were also found to impact particle deposition in a significant way. The results of this study indicate that a particle deposition rate of 0.2 to 0.8 h^{-1} for ideal mixing might typically be encountered in occupied spaces.

Mixing

Once released into an enclosed space, air contaminants move through it by dispersion. Dispersion determines where the high and low concentrations of the contaminant will occur. Dispersion is controlled by diffusion, which is the movement from areas of high to low concentrations, and by mixing, which is the movement of air in the space. When ideal mixing occurs in a space, i.e., $m = 1$ in Equation 5-1, no spatial gradient of an air contaminant like RSP exists, and the full effectiveness of ventilation and sink rates in removing the contaminant is seen. In controlled laboratory studies, ideal mixing is easily obtained through the use of mixing fans or the rapid recirculation of the air. In occupied spaces, however, ideal mixing is hardly ever obtained unless a great deal of turbulence is introduced to the space and the supply- and exhaust-air system is carefully designed. Less than ideal mixing can result in a pronounced concentration gradient of a contaminant in the space. The ventilation rates and removal by surfaces under those conditions are not as effective in lowering air-contaminant levels. The mixing term is usually defined as the ratio of effective ventilation to theoretical ventilation.

In an occupied space, the value of the mixing factor is affected by the source and its use, room geometry, air supply and exhaust design, air-flow rates, obstacles in a room, and activity of the occupants. In addition, the mixing factor is specific for a precise location. No data exist that would indicate the distribution of the values for the mixing factor in occupied spaces. A limited number of studies show a range of mixing factors from 0.1 to near 1.0 (Brief, 1960; Kasuda, 1976).

Volume

The volume of the space in which smoking occurs is highly variable. It can range from a few cubic meters in a car to several thousand cubic meters in large auditoriums or sports arenas. The highest RSP levels from ETS will tend to occur in smaller spaces with high smoking rates.

Predicting Environmental Tobacco Smoke Exposures from Tobacco Combustion

Utilizing Equation 5-1, expected RSP concentrations indoors from ETS can be estimated for a range of the input parameters that realistically can be expected under normal smoking occupancy. Figures 5-4 and 5-5 allow for the easy calculation of RSP levels due to ETS as a function of smoking rate, ventilation, sink rate, mixing, and volume of the space (see the example outlined in the legends of these figures). The calculations treat the spaces of concern (e.g., multiroom home or a single room in a house) as a single compartment with no air-cleaning devices. The total amount of RSP (in milligrams) from ETS can be determined in Figure 5-5 as a function of the smoking rate and effective removal rate (N). The removal rate is equal to the sum of ventilation plus removal by surfaces times the mixing factor. The total amount of RSP calculated from Figure 5-4 is then entered into Figure 5-5 to determine the RSP concentrations (in micrograms per cubic meter) expected for a given volume of space. The calculations used to generate these figures assume that:

- an average total RSP emission rate is 26 mg/cigarette,
- the emissions are nearly consistent and averaged over a 1-h period,
- near steady-state or equilibrium conditions are reached quickly,
- no air-cleaning devices are in use,
- background levels of RSP in a space are zero, and

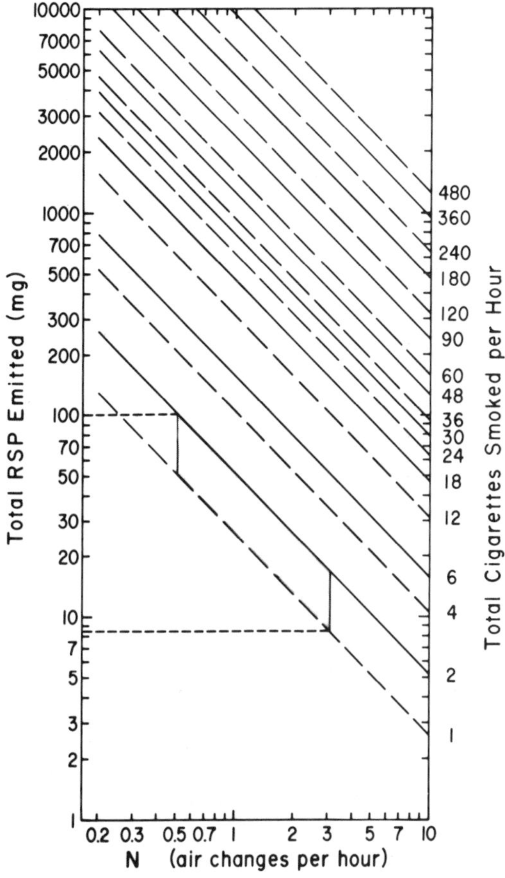

FIGURE 5-4 Diagram for calculating the RPS mass from ETS emitted into any occupied space as a function of the smoking rate and removal rate (N). The removal rate is equal to the sum of the ventilation or infiltration rate (n_v) and removal rate by surfaces (n_s) times the mixing factor m. The calculated ETS RSP mass determined from this figure serves as an input to Figure 5-5 to determine the ETS respirable suspended particulate mass concentration in any space in $\mu g/m^3$. Smoking rates (diagonal lines) are given as cigarettes smoked per hour. Mixing is determined as a fraction and n_v and n_s are in air changes per hour (*ach*). All three parameters have to be estimated or measured. Calculations were made using the equilibrium form of the mass-balance equation (Equation 5-3) and assume a fixed emission rate of 26 mg/cigarette of RSP.

Shaded area shows the range of RSP emissions that could be expected for a residence with one smoker smoking at a rate of either 1 or 2 cigarettes per hour for the range of mixing, ventilation, and removal rates occurring in residences under steady-state conditions.

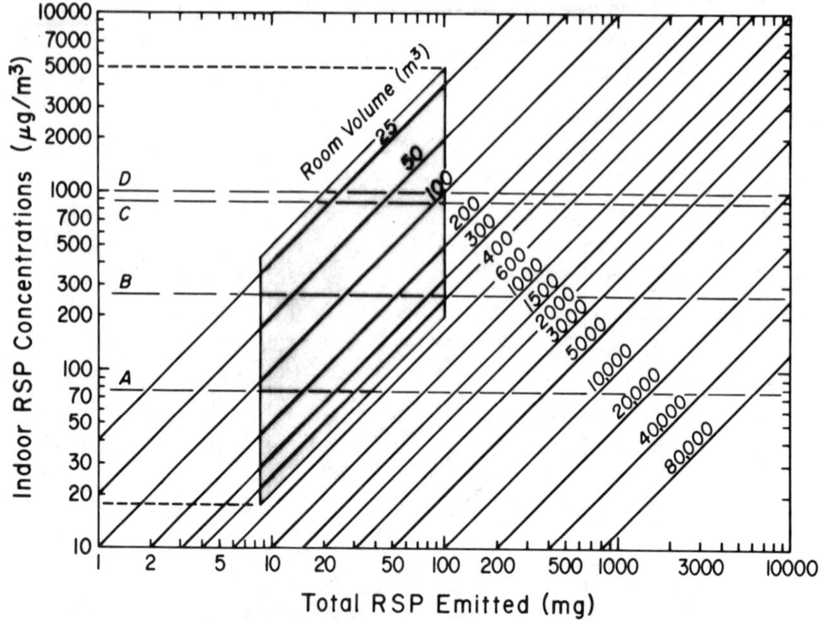

FIGURE 5-5 Diagram to calculate the ETS RSP concentration in a space as a function of the total mass of ETS RSP emitted (determined from Figure 5-4) and the volume of a space (diagonal lines). The concentrations shown assume a background level in the space of zero. The particulate concentrations shown are estimates during smoking occupancy. The dashed horizontal lines (*A*, *B*, *C*, and *D*) refer to National Ambient Air Quality Standards (health-related) for total suspended particulates established by the U.S. Environmental Protection Agency. *A* is the annual geometric mean. *B* is the 24-hour value not to be exceeded more than once a year. *C* is the 24-hour air pollution emergency level. *D* is the 24-hour significant harm level. Shaded area shows the range of concentrations expected (from Figure 5-4) for a range of typical volumes of U.S. residences and rooms in these residences.

- a one-chamber model is appropriate.

In these figures, the RSP-emission rate is assumed constant. If, in fact, this rate is variable, then the predicted RSP level will also vary. As already discussed, the input parameters to Equation 5-1 are known to vary greatly under realistic occupancy conditions, with few or no data available on the distribution of the values of those input parameters. Figures 5-4 and 5-5 highlight the large effect that small variations in the input parameters can have on the predicted RSP concentration.

For example, for a range of conditions that can be expected to be encountered in private residences with one smoker (shaded areas in Figures 5-4 and 5-5), RSP levels in residences or public places during smoking occupancy can vary by more than two orders of magnitude from approximately 17 to 5,000 $\mu g/m^3$. This example assumes one smoking resident smoking at a rate of either one or two cigarettes/hour. Relatively easy-to-obtain information on some of the input parameters, such as building volume or typical smoking densities, obtained through questionnaires or observation, can serve to significantly reduce the range of estimated exposures. It is also clear from Figures 5-4 and 5-5 that, for the vast majority of conditions, RSP levels due solely to ETS can be expected to equal or exceed levels specified in National Ambient Air Quality Standards for the total suspended particulates (Code of Federal Regulations, 1985). These standards are health-based and reflect different averaging times as well as levels of exposure. Direct comparison of exposures with the standards requires consideration of particle size, concentration, and time. The physical and chemical nature of the particulate matter resulting from tobacco smoke is different from particulate matter observed outdoors in ambient air. These different particulate matters no doubt have different biological effects. Therefore, direct comparisons of exposures to outdoor standards should be made with caution.

Application of Respirable Suspended Particulates Model

The most extensive use of the mass-balance equation for assessing RSP levels due to ETS in occupied spaces has been by Repace and Lowrey (1980). Drawing upon the best available data from several sources, including both measured and estimated parameters, they proposed and applied in field observations a condensed version of the mass-balance equation for estimating RSP exposures due to ETS in a variety of indoor microenvironments. Their model is

$$C_{eq} = 650 D_s / n_v, \qquad (5\text{-}3)$$

where C_{eq} is the equilibrium of concentration of RSP due to ETS expressed in micrograms per cubic meter, D_s is the density of active smokers expressed as units of burning cigarettes observed in a space per 100 m^3 over the sampling time frames, and n_v is the ventilation or infiltration rate in *ach*. The constant term (650) is calculated from a standard set of assumed conditions for smoking rates, RSP emission rates, mixing factors, ventilation rates, and sink rates. These standard sets of conditions are derived largely from experimental data and building standards.

Although many of the input parameters were estimated from the literature, which is based on limited experimental data, Repace and Lowrey (1980, 1982) applied Equation 5-3, or similar equations, to a variety of situations and found that they produced reasonably accurate estimates in a limited number of occupied spaces with smoking occupancy. Apparently, easy-to-obtain data on building volumes, design occupancy, smoking occupancy, type of ventilation systems, and building standards can improve the prediction of RSP concentrations. In using Equation 5-3, the major assumptions deal with mixing, ventilation rates, and sink rates. Additional field testing of the Repace and Lowrey model, as well as a better understanding of the variability of the input parameters, either estimated or measured for use in Equation 5-3, is needed.

SUMMARY AND RECOMMENDATIONS

In investigating the adverse health and comfort impact of air contaminants, it is important to specify the exposure to a specific air contaminant or a class of air contaminants on the time scale corresponding to the health or comfort effect being evaluated. Accurate data on exposure is essential to minimize misclassification of exposure in epidemiologic studies of air contaminants. In the absence of an indicator of the dose of the contaminant, target tissue exposures may be estimated by use of biological markers, by personal monitors, or by the air monitoring of microenvironments in which people spend time combined with time activity patterns.

ETS is comprised of several thousand chemicals in both the gas and particulate phases. While several individual constituents of ETS have been measured in a number of microenvironments as a proxy for ETS (nicotine, CO, acrolein, etc.), none have met all of the criteria necessary for a suitable proxy, nor has an individual contaminant been uniformly accepted or recognized as representing ETS exposure. New methods of measuring nicotine in air hold promise for using nicotine as a suitable proxy for ETS, but considerable development and testing need to be done. The single largest component of ETS by weight is the RSP, which refers to particles less than 2.5 μm and is highly variable in chemical composition. The RSP fraction of ETS is currently the best and most-utilized general category of air contaminants to represent ETS exposure.

A limited number of studies that employed personal monitors to measure total RSP found that individuals who reported being exposed to ETS were exposed to RSP concentrations consistently greater than those who reported no exposure. Furthermore, the distribution of RSP concentrations varied widely (from 10 $\mu g/m^3$ to more than 200 $\mu g/m^3$). The limited number of samples, lack of data on the environments where the exposure took place, and lack of a specific proxy for ETS do not permit accurate estimation of the ETS exposure or extension of the data to a larger population. They do indicate, however, that individuals who report exposure to ETS will have greater RSP exposures than those who do not.

Measurements of RSP levels in various indoor environments (residences, offices, restaurants, bars, bowling alleys, airplanes, arenas, etc.) have clearly shown that RSP levels will be considerably above background levels (outdoor levels or nonsmoking levels) when smoking is reported in the space.

Modeling of RSP concentrations due to ETS in any indoor environment usually utilizes a simplified form of the mass-balance equation. These models are typically single-chamber models that assume steady-state or equilibrium conditions to estimate RSP levels and require as input parameters an RSP-emission rate for tobacco combustion, number of cigarettes consumed, ventilation or infiltration rates, removal rates by surfaces, air mixing in the space, and volume of the space. Information on the current or past distribution of these input parameters in the range of microenvironments in which individuals spend the majority of their time (residences, offices, etc.) is not available. The variability of one or more of the input parameters can make a difference of as much as an order of magnitude in the estimated RSP concentration. Additional variability in the estimated RSP levels is introduced to the extent that the equilibrium assumptions do not hold (i.e., an intermittent rather than continuous source).

Gathering data on easily measured input parameters such as smoking rates or volume can substantially reduce the variability of the estimated RSP levels. Limited field tests of the general equilibrium model, in which some of the input parameters were measured and others were estimated either from chamber studies or building codes, have predicted RSP levels reasonably well over a wide range of values of input parameters. While the predicted level of RSP exposure due to ETS may be highly variable using models, it is clear from the models that, even using the most conservative estimates for the input parameters, RSP levels when smoking is allowed will result in substantial increases over nonsmoking occupancy RSP levels. This is consistent with the concentrations measured through personal monitoring or area monitors in various microenvironments.

What Is Known

1. Various individual chemical constituents of ETS have been measured in indoor spaces as proxies for ETS, but their suitability as proxies for ETS exposures has not been well established.

2. The total RSP, measured by personal monitors, has been found to be elevated for individuals who reported being exposed to ETS as compared with those who reported no exposure.

3. The distributions of RSP measured by personal monitors and by portable monitors vary widely. However, levels of RSP measured in various indoor environments have clearly shown that RSP levels will be considerably above background levels when smoking is reported in the space.

4. Limited field tests of the mass-balance, general-equilibrium model in which some of the input parameters are measured and others are estimated have predicted RSP levels reasonably well over a wide range of values of input parameters.

What Scientific Information Is Missing

1. There is a lack of data on the environments where measurements have been taken. Consequently, an accurate estimate of the ETS exposure or extension of the data to a large population based upon present data may not be possible.

2. A suitable proxy or tracer air contaminant is not available for total ETS exposure. Nicotine may be a good indicator for exposure to the vapor phase. However, the relative proportions of various constituents of ETS in the particulate and vapor phases need further study to determine the extent to which a tracer for one phase can be used to infer exposure to the other phase.

3. Information on current or past distributions of the input parameters for the mass-balance models of RSP concentrations is

not available for a range of microenvironments in which individuals spend the majority of their time.

4. When levels of various constituents of ETS are measured in field situations, data should be gathered on input parameters such as smoking rates or volume so that a detailed field evaluation of the equilibrium model can be made.

5. ETS exposure in epidemiologic studies needs to be improved. Questionnaires must be validated. Personal and microenvironmental monitoring studies should be conducted to determine the predictive value of various exposure assessment methodologies. This might be achieved as part of a nested design in a larger epidemiologic study.

6. The variability of RSP emissions into the environment and the relationship between vapor and particulate phases need to be investigated for a variety of brands of tobacco.

REFERENCES

ASHRAE Standards 62-1973. Standards for Natural and Mechanical Ventilation. Atlanta: ASHRAE, 1973.

ASHRAE Standards 69-1981. Ventilation for Acceptable Indoor Air Quality. Atlanta: ASHRAE, 1981. 19 pp.

Badre, R., R. Guillerme, N. Abram, M. Bourdin, and C. Dumas. Pollution atmospherique par la fumée de tabac. Ann. Pharm. Fr. 36:443-452, 1978.

Brief, R.S. Simple way to determine air contaminants. Air Eng. 2:39-44, 1960.

Bridge, D.P., and M. Corn. Contribution to the assessment of nonsmokers to air pollution from cigarette and cigar smoke in occupied spaces. Environ. Res. 5:192-209, 1972.

Brunekreef, B., and J.S.M. Boleij. Long-term average suspended particulate concentrations in smokers' homes. Int. Arch. Occup. Environ. Health 50:299-302, 1982.

Clausen, G., W.S. Cain, P.O. Fanger, and B.P. Leaderer. The influence of aging, particle filtration and humidity on tobacco smoke odor, pp. 345-350. In P.O. Fanger, Ed. CLIMA 2000, Vol. 4. Indoor Climate. Copenhagen: VVS Kongress-VVS Messe, 1985.

Code of Federal Regulations (CFR). National primary and secondary ambient air quality standards. Code Fed. Regul. 40(PT50):500-573, 1985.

Cuddeback, J.E., J.R. Donovan, and W.R. Burg. Occupational aspects of passive smoking. Am. Ind. Hyg. Assoc. J. 37:263-267, 1976.

Elliot, L.P., and D.R. Rowe. Air quality during public gatherings. J. Air Pollut. Control Assoc. 25:635-636, 1975.

Esmen, N.A. Characterization of contaminant concentrations in enclosed spaces. Environ. Sci. Technol. 12:337-339, 1978.

Eudy, L.W., F.A. Thorne, D.L. Heavner, C.R. Green, and B.J. Ingebrethsen. Studies on the vapor-particulate phase distribution of environmental nicotine by selected trapping and detection methods. Presented at the 39th Tobacco Chemists' Research Conference, Montreal, Canada, Oct. 2-5, 1985.

First, M.W. Environmental tobacco smoke measurement: Restrospect and prospect. Eur. J. Respir. Dis. 5(Suppl.):9-16, 1984.

Galuskinova, V. 3,4-Benzpyrene determination in the smoky atmosphere of social meeting rooms and restaurants. A contribution to the problem of the noxiousness of so-called passive smoking. Neoplasma 11:465-468, 1964.

Grimsrud, D.T., M.H. Sherman, and R.C. Sonderegger. Calculating infiltration: Implications for a construction quality standard, pp. 422-452. Proceedings of the ASHRAE-DOE Conference on the Thermal Performance of the Exterior Envelope of Buildings II, held in Las Vegas, Nev., Dec. 1982. New York: ASHRAE. 442 pp.

Grot, R.A., and R.E. Clark. Air leakage characteristics and weatherization techniques for low-income housing, pp. 178-194. Proceedings of the ASHRAE-DOE Conference on the Thermal Performance of the Exterior Envelope of Buildings, held in Orlando, Fla., Dec. New York: ASHRAE, 1979.

Hammond, S.K., B.P. Leaderer, and A. Roche. Collection and analysis of nicotine as a marker for environmental tobacco smoke in personal samples. Atmos. Environ., in press.

Hawthorne, A.R., D. Gammage, C.S. Dudney, B.E. Hingerty, D.D. Schuresko, D.C. Parzyek, D.R. Womack, S.A. Morris, R.R. Westeley, D.A. White, and J.M. Schrimscher. Air Indoor Quality Study of Forty East Tennessee Homes. ORNL 5965. Oak Ridge, Tennessee: Oak Ridge National Laboratory, 1984. 134 pp.

Hoegg, U.R. Cigarette smoke in closed spaces. Environ. Health Perspect. 2:117-128, 1972.

Ishizu, Y. General equation for the estimation of indoor pollution. Environ. Sci. Technol. 14:1254-1257, 1980.

Jaffe, J.H. Behavioral pharmacology of tobacco use. Life Sci. Res. Rep. 8:175-198, 1978.

Just, J., M. Borkowska, and S. Maziarka. Zanieczyszczenie dymen tytoniowym powietrza kawiarn Warszawskich. (Tobacco smoke in the air of Warsaw coffee house.) Rocz. Panstw. Zakl. Hig. 23:129-135, 1972.

Kusada, T. Control of ventilation to conserve energy while maintaining acceptable indoor air quality. ASHRAE Trans. 82:1169, 1976.

Leaderer, B.P., W.S. Cain, and R. Isseroff, and L.G. Berglund. Ventilation requirements in buildings. II. Particulate matter and carbon monoxide from cigarette smoking. Atmos. Environ. 18:99-106, 1984.

Leaderer, B.P., S. Renes, P. Bluyssen, and H. Van De Loo. Chamber studies of NO_2, SO_2 and RSP deposition rates indoors. Proceedings of the 79th Annual Meeting of Air Pollution Control Association, Minneapolis, Minn., June 23-27, 1986. APCA No. 86-38.3, 1986.

Moschandreas, D.J., D.J. Pelton, and J. Zabransky. Comparison of indoor and outdoor air quality. EPRI EA-1733. Electric Power Research Institute, 1981.

Moschandreas, D.J. Exposure to pollutants and daily time budgets of people. Bull. N.Y. Acad. Med. 57:845-859, 1981.

Muramatsu, M., S. Umemura, T. Okada, and H. Tomita. Estimation of personal exposure to tobacco smoke with a newly developed nicotine personal monitor. Environ. Res. 35:218-227, 1984.

Muramatsu, T., A. Weber, S. Muramatsu, and F. Ackermann. An experimental study on irritation and annoyance due to passive smoking. Int. Arch. Occup. Environ. Health. 51:305-317, 1983.

Nitschke, I.A., W.A. Clarke, M.E. Clarkin, G.W. Traynor, and J.B. Wadach. Indoor air quality, infiltration and ventilation in residential buildings. NYSERDA #85-10. Albany: New York State Energy Research and Development Authority, 1985.

Parker, G.B., G.L. Wilfert, and G.W. Dennis. Indoor Air Quality and Infiltration in Multifamily Naval Housing, pp. 1-14. Annual PNWIS/APCA Meeting, held in Portland, Oreg., Nov. 12-14, 1984.

Penkala, S.J. and G. De Oliveira. The simultaneous analysis of carbon monoxide and suspended particulate matter produced by cigarette smoking. Environ. Res. 9:99-114, 1975.

Perry, J. Fasten your seatbelts: No smoking. B.C. Med. J. 15:304-305, 1973.

Repace, J.L., and A.H. Lowrey. Indoor air pollution, tobacco smoke, and public health. Science 208:464-472, 1980.

Repace, J.L., and A.H. Lowrey. Tobacco smoke, ventilation, and indoor air quality. ASHRAE Trans. 88:894-914, 1982.

Rickert, W.S., J.C. Robinson, and N. Collishaw. Yields of tar, nicotine and carbon monoxide in the sidestream smoke from 15 brands of Candian cigarettes. Am. J. Public Health 74:228-231, 1984.

Schenker, M.B., T. Smith, A. Munoz, S. Woskie, and F.E. Speizer. Diesel exposure and mortality among railway workers: Results of a pilot study. Br. J. Ind. Med. 41:320-327, 1984.

Sexton, K., J.D. Spengler, and R.D. Treitman. Personal exposure to respirable particulates: A case-study in Waterbury, Vermont. Atmos. Environ. 18:1385-1398, 1984.

Shair, F.H., and Heitner, K.L. Theoretical model for relating indoor pollutant concentrations to those outside. Environ. Sci. Tech. 8:444-451, 1974.

Spengler, J.D., D.W. Dockery, W.A. Turner, J.M. Wolfson, and B.J. Ferris, Jr. Long-term measurements of respirable sulphates and particles inside and outside homes. Atmos. Environ. 15:23-30, 1981.

Spengler, J.D., R.D. Treitman, T.D. Tosteson, D.T. Mage and M.L. Soczek. Personal exposures to respirable particulates and implications for air pollution epidemiology. Environ. Sci. Technol. 19:700-707, 1985.

Sterling, T.D., and E.M. Sterling. Investigations on the effect of regulating smoking on levels of indoor pollution and on the perception of health on comfort of office workers. Eur. J. Respir. Dis. 65(Suppl. 133):17-32, 1983.

Szalai, A, Ed. The Use of Time. Daily Activities of Urban and Suburban Populations. The Hague: Mouton, 1972. 868 pp.

Turk, A. Measurements of odorous vapors in test chamber: Theoretical. ASHRAE 9(5):55-8, 1963.

U.S. Department of Transportation and U.S. Department of Health, Education, and Welfare. Health aspects of smoking in transport aircraft. Washington, D.C.: U.S. Department of Transportation, Federal Aviation Administration, and U.S. Department of Health, Education, and Welfare, National Institute of for Occupational Safety and Health, 1971. 85 pp.

U.K. Government. Smoking and health, p. 83. In U.K. Government. London Laboratory of the Government Chemist Report 1979. Annual Report. London: U.K. Government, 1980. 197 pp.

Wallace, L.A., and W.R. Ott. Personal monitors: A state-of-the-art survey. J. Air Pollut. Control Assoc. 32:601-610, 1982.

Weber, A. Acute effects of environmental tobacco smoke. Eur. J. Respir. Dis. 68(Suppl. 133):98-108, 1984.

Weber, A., and T. Fischer. Passive smoking at work. Int. Arch. Occup. Environ. Health 47:209-221, 1980.

Weber, A., C. Jermini, and E. Grandjean. Irritating effects on man of air pollution due to cigarette smoke. Am. J. Public Health 66:672-676, 1976.

Weber, A., T. Fischer, and E. Grandjean. Passive smoking in experimental and field conditions. Environ. Res. 20:205-216, 1979a.

Weber, A., T. Fischer, and E. Grandjean. Passive smoking: Irritating effects of the total smoke and the gas phase. Int. Arch. Occup. Environ. Health 43:183-193, 1979b.

Winneke, G., K. Plischke, A. Roscovanu, and H.-W. Schlipkoeter. Patterns and determinants of reaction to tobacco smoke in an experimental exposure setting, pp. 351-356. In B. Berglund, T. Lindvall, and J. Sundell, Eds. Indoor Air, Vol. 2. Radon, Passive Smoking, Particulates, and Housing Epidemiology. Stockholm, Sweden: Stockholm Swedish Council for Building Research, 1984.

Yaglou, C.P., E.C. Riley, and D.I. Coggins. Ventilation requirements. ASHRAE Trans. 42:133-162, 1936.

6
Assessing Exposures to Environmental Tobacco Smoke Using Questionnaires

The active component(s) of environmental tobacco smoke (ETS) associated with various health effects may be different for acute and chronic outcomes. Also, the mechanisms of action differ. Furthermore, as discussed in Chapter 2, the relative concentrations of various components of ETS change over time, i.e., as the smoke ages. Therefore, the use of a single proxy pollutant, such as respirable particulates, or an indirect measure of ETS limits the ability to assess responses to ETS exposure. For some investigations, indirect assessment is probably not adequate to evaluate health effects for at least two reasons. First, the tobacco smoke components that affect the health outcome may not be related to the indirect assessment in a simple way, e.g., vapor-phase-component concentrations cannot be adequately measured by particulate-phase components. Secondly, a variety of host factors affect the actual dose received so that assessment of exposure does not accurately (or completely) represent dose (see Chapter 7).

A variety of methods is used to estimate individual exposures associated with human health effects in industrial and nonindustrial settings. These exposure indicators may be direct—such as the use of personal-monitoring data or biochemical measures obtained by testing body fluids for the compound or its metabolites—or indirect—such as the use of data from interview responses of family members regarding activities of the subject and modeling based on environmental monitoring of the ambient or industrial setting. The resulting data from direct and indirect indicators of exposure can be expressed in quantitative or qualitative terms.

The advantages and disadvantages of the various exposure measures used in industrial and nonindustrial settings are summarized in Table 6-1. The issues raised in this table are directly relevant to assessing ETS exposure. The use of surrogate measures derived from questionnaire responses and the issues resulting from use of these measures are discussed in this chapter.

EXPOSURE HISTORIES DERIVED FROM QUESTIONNAIRES

Questionnaire responses of study subjects or family/household members are used for two purposes. First, questionnaires are used to obtain data on the physical characteristics of each environment and the time-activity patterns of the individual in each environment. These data can be used with individual monitoring data to estimate (usually by modeling) the air-contaminant levels in the microenvironment and to estimate time-weighted, integrated individual exposures. Second, questionnaire responses provide a basis for classification of individuals into broad categories of exposure based on self (or proxy) reports of exposure to individuals who smoke. Questionnaires of the latter type have provided the bases for associating ETS to the increased risk of nonmalignant and malignant disease.

There are several major issues in epidemiologic studies of health effects of exposure to ETS that rely on indirect measures of exposure as derived from questionnaire data.

First, the assessment of ETS exposures associated with acute health effects requires a different approach than that for chronic health effects. Acute health effects, such as respiratory infections, are manifested shortly after exposure and are of short duration. By inference, these health outcomes depend only on exposures in the recent past. In contrast, chronic health effects are conditions that are associated with long-term exposure to ETS, that is, they are manifested after some prolonged period of time and are of long duration. In evaluating the association of ETS with chronic diseases, knowledge about the duration of exposure and the duration of time from initial exposure to disease onset is more important than the duration of the disease.

Second, quality of information obtained by interview or self-administered questionnaires may vary among studies and may vary for different disease outcomes. For example, the assessment

TABLE 6-1 Indicators of Individual Exposure in Industrial and Nonindustrial Settings—Advantages and Disadvantages

Indicator	Advantages	Disadvantages
1. DIRECT		
A. Biologic monitoring of body fluids for the compound and/or its metabolites—*quantitative* (e.g., blood level)	1. Identifies exposed individuals 2. Provides measure of body burden for some agents (e.g., metals) 3. Measures absorption of compound from all routes of entry—respiratory, cutaneous, and oral 4. Gives information about prior exposure	1. Many methods still in developmental stages and lack validation 2. May be expensive due to need for specially trained personnel and sophisticated equipment 3. May require concurrent air sampling if exposures are not constant 4. Interpretation may be influenced by variation in uptake with physical exertion and interference from diet and drugs 5. Requires careful timing of specimen collection, especially for blood samples 6. Subject consent required to obtain specimens 7. Lack of population reference values
B. Personal industrial hygiene or ambient monitoring, single and multiple—*quantitative*	1. Estimates exposure for individual employees 2. Can be performed easily by the employer 3. Exposure to multiple compounds can be assessed simultaneously	1. Requires cooperation of worker or study subjects to wear monitoring equipment 2. Does not measure body burden 3. Limited ability to assess multiple routes of exposure 4. Gives no information about prior exposures 5. May not correspond with results of area sampling 6. Samples may not reflect "average" work day; taking of measurements should consider shifts, production, seasons, etc.

TABLE 6-1 *Continued*

Indicator	Advantages	Disadvantages
C. Employer or other reports of exposure to compound—*qualitative*	1. Provides details of accidental releases 2. Can indicate safety procedures/protective measures	1. Data may be incomplete (unreported) 2. Exposure quantified subjectively 3. Episodic measurement of unusual occurrences rather than "average" workday exposure
D. Self-reports of exposure to compound—*qualitative*	1. Provides details of accidental releases 2. Can indicate personal hygiene and safety habits 3. Can obtain chronology of work experience with multiple agent exposures	1. Potential for recall bias 2. Employees may be unaware of exposure 3. Potential for falsification of exposure for personal gain 4. Potential for lost to follow-up (missing information) in retrospective studies
2. INDIRECT		
A. Biological monitoring		
(1) with chromosome studies—*quantitative* or *qualitative*	1. Identified changes in the genetic material 2. Indicates systemic exposure to a mutagen	1. Expensive, due to need for specially trained personnel and sophisticated equipment 2. Relationship between changes in mutation rates and reproductive outcomes is unknown 3. Results may be confounded by smoking and environmental factors (e.g., effect of smoking on sister chromatid exchanges in lymphocytes; radiation effects) 4. Individual variability in baseline rates 5. Most chromosomal aberrations are nonspecific
(2) by measuring changes in biochemical responses (e.g., elevated rate of thiocyanate production in	1. Identifies alterations in normal constituents of body fluids and changes in rate of normal biochemical processes	1. Does not quantify body burden 2. Results may be confounded by drugs, nutrition, and disease

response to cyanide exposure)—*quantitative* or *qualitative*		3. Requires understanding of compound's metabolism in body
B. Area industrial hygiene or ambient monitoring—*quantitative*	1. Documents concentration of agent in work environment 2. Variety of measurement techniques available 3. Can be performed easily by the employer	1. May not correspond with results of personal sampling 2. Measurements have multiple sources of variation 3. Does not indicate specific exposure level for individual employees 4. No information about previous exposures 5. Type of sample taken may be inappropriate for health effects being studied
C. Employer work area assignment records (work histories)—*qualitative* (specific estimates may be made using job-exposure linkage) or *quantitative* (may be developed by using duration of time spent in different environments)	1. Can provide chronologic work experience for duration of exposure 2. Can indicate exposure to multiple agents 3. May provide supplementary information	1. May be incomplete or may be unavailable 2. Records not designed for research purposes 3. Presumed exposure by work assignment may be based on subjective criteria 4. Record review is time-consuming
Activity diaries of study subjects, recording time spent in different microenvironments		
D. Surrogate (next of kin) interview responses regarding work history and activity history of study subject—*qualitative* (specific estimates made using a job-exposure linkage) or *quantitative* (estimates developed using duration of time spent in environments)	1. Can obtain information about confounding factors 2. Identifies major agents to which exposed 3. May provide supplementary demographic information about employees	1. Limited by knowledge of employee's work 2. May produce overestimate or underestimate of exposure 3. Time-consuming to locate and interview 4. Lack of validation of data 5. Differential quality of information by degree of kinship

of maternal smoking during the first year of life of a child may be a much more accurate measure of exposure to ETS related to respiratory illness than a summary history of ETS exposure related to lung cancer. Data quality for ETS exposures can be affected in major ways by differential and nondifferential misclassification of exposure. In Chapter 12, the impact of misclassifying exposed subjects as nonsmokers, when they are in fact current smokers or exsmokers, is discussed. Therefore, it is important to determine whether nonsmoking subjects are, in fact, never smokers or currently nonsmokers, i.e., exsmokers. Another source of bias is the misclassification of exposure among nonsmokers. That is, nonsmokers who say they have not been exposed may in fact have had significant exposures. In both cases, detailed probes are needed.

Third, the role of major confounding exposures needs to be assessed. For instance, occupational exposures to other air contaminants may cause pulmonary disorders.

Fourth, the evaluation of ETS exposures should attempt to assess all such exposures rather than focus solely on exposures from smoking by family members (spouse, mother, or father) or focus solely on the home environment. An adequate assessment of total ETS exposure will necessitate a consideration of exposure levels in specific microenvironments—such as home, school, work, vehicle, and recreation—and the duration of time an individual is exposed in these environments. Developing such a measure is complex even for relatively acute health outcomes, such as acute cardiovascular, respiratory, or neurotoxic symptoms, for which it may be sufficient to estimate recent exposures. Developing a comprehensive measure to ETS exposures is far more complex for diseases with long induction times, such as cancer and chronic obstructive pulmonary disease. The data required for modeling a long-term integrated ETS exposure may be far more detailed than are available or can be reliably obtained. Further, when a surrogate informant is used, that person most likely will be able to report on exposures in only some of the microenvironments. In this case, it may be impossible to develop a comprehensive index.

ENVIRONMENTAL TOBACCO SMOKE EXPOSURE DATA FOR STUDIES OF ACUTE AND CHRONIC HEALTH EFFECTS

The acute health effects of ETS in children, such as respiratory illnesses, have been assessed in the National Health Interview Survey (NHIS) by determining smoking status of one or both parents or smoking status of adults in the household (Bonham and Wilson, 1981). In this national probability sample of households, parental smoking histories and reports of respiratory illness among children were obtained at one point in time. By contrast, in the Harvard Air Pollution Respiratory Health Study (Six Cities Study), information on current smoking habits for parents and all household members who smoke regularly in the home is obtained annually to determine amount of cigarette smoking in the home environment to which the children aged 6-13 years are exposed (Ware et al., 1984). (In Chapter 11 the assessment of exposure to parental smoking in studies of respiratory illness in children is discussed in more detail.)

In studies of chronic health effects in adults, such as cancer, exposure of nonsmokers to ETS has been largely determined by smoking status of the spouse. Most studies of lung cancer among nonsmoking women have relied solely or principally on information regarding smoking status of the spouse to assess ETS exposures, with little attempt to corroborate self-reports of exposure to ETS.

The difficulties in assessing ETS exposure are similar to difficulties of assessing occupational exposures (Axelson, 1985). Both exposures are complex and variable. The problem of obtaining adequate information about ETS exposure might be overcome by obtaining data from multiple respondents and by using corroborating procedures. However, the conceptual difficulty concerning the determination of exposure is unresolved or unaddressed in most studies. Exposure to a substance involves a varying intensity over some period of time prior to the development of disease. These factors may influence the absorption and distribution of an agent in the body as well as the biotransformation and excretion of the agent. Therefore, these factors probably influence the risk of the health outcome of interest. For exposures extending over long periods of time, a simple "cumulative dose" usually is calculated by a time integration of the intensity. The estimate of exposure over long periods of time is expressed as average number of cigarettes per day or the calculation of "pack years." This type of measure does not provide for an independent consideration of latency, does not consider variability in exposure over the time period, and represents two components of exposure, one of which may be more precisely measured (duration) than the other (intensity) (Doll and Peto, 1978). Axelson (1985) describes some sophisticated adjustments that have been proposed for weighting time periods of exposure to estimate cumulative-dose measures.

These proposed methods have not been widely adopted, probably due to both the complexity of the method as well as the recognized limitations of exposure data typically available. The more common, simplified procedure is to apply an appropriate induction/latency period in the analysis of studies of cancer or other chronic diseases. This practice suggests, however, that more attention be given to identifying the separate effects of late (recent) exposures versus early (remote) exposures on development of various diseases. These effects may also be mediated by the age at which the exposures occurred.

The proposal described by Johnson and Letzel (1984) advocates a method of assessing exposures to ETS experienced over an entire lifetime. The major limitation of this approach is that it has not been validated. Johnson and Letzel (1984) argue that since no objective criteria for lifetime exposure to ETS exists, a direct validation of an instrument to assess lifelong ETS exposure cannot be obtained. They propose that the instrument be validated on a recent time frame, such as 24-hour data. From these data the investigators argue by analogy that the method, when expanded to a longer time frame, can be regarded as valid. While this approach may seem less than ideal, the constraints due to data availability and quality emphasize the importance of the type of methods development and corroboration illustrated by the work of Johnson and Letzel (1984).

DATA QUALITY

Misclassification of individual ETS exposure may be differential (biased) or nondifferential (random). Differential misclassification would result in a distortion of the estimate of risk in either direction, depending on the direction of the misclassification. Nondifferential misclassification would result in a reduction of power in a study, thus making it more difficult to detect a true association of exposure with risk of disease.

One form of differential misclassification that is a major concern in studies of ETS exposures is the active smoking status of study subjects. This misclassification may be considered differential because spouses and children of smokers are more likely to be smokers (or have smoked) themselves, even though they are reported as "nonsmokers." The effects of this differential misclassification are discussed in Chapters 11 and 12. One way to minimize this problem is to have multiple questions that probe for previous cigarette usage, even if the subject has defined himself or herself as a nonsmoker.

Another form of differential misclassification is that resulting from the biased reporting of exposure to ETS by individuals with existing respiratory diseases, such as asthma or chronic bronchitis. One might conjecture that individuals with existing respiratory diseases may be more or may be less likely to report exposure to ETS than individuals without such existing conditions.

In studies of ETS exposures, information about the smoking habits of the subject, family, and household members is obtained by interviews with the study subject when available, or by interview with a family member when the study subject is deceased or unavailable. That is, surrogate respondents may be used to collect information regarding personal exposures of the study subject.

The validity of surrogate information in most studies is uncertain, and the direction of any potential bias is rarely known (Gordis, 1982). The feasibility of this approach for a variety of exposures and habits has been examined (Pickle et al., 1983). Also, several studies have assessed the reliability and validity of surrogate respondents for various kinds of exposures (Rogot and Reid, 1975; Kolonel et al., 1977; Marshall et al., 1980; Baumgarten et al., 1983; Humble et al., 1984; Greenberg et al., 1985; Herrmann, 1985; Lerchen and Samet, 1986). In all of these studies, agreement between self and surrogate responses improves when the amount of detail required for the response is decreased. This observation was first reported by Rogot and Reid (1975) and subsequently observed in studies comparing self versus spouse/surrogate responses.

Lerchen and Samet (1986) reported perfect agreement of cigarette-smoking status (ever/never) as reported by lung cancer cases and their wives, but only 66 (86%) of the 77 wives married to smokers were able to supply complete details about their husbands' cigarette-smoking habits. In this study, agreement (expressed as correlation coefficients) was quite good for all smoking-related variables, such as age at which the subject started to smoke (0.48), total years of smoking (0.91), and average number of cigarettes smoked per day (0.44). The mean values reported by cases and their wives were not significantly different for any variable. Overall, the agreement observed for self- and surrogate-reported smoking-related information was better than the agreement for education, occupation, and dietary information.

Pershagen and Axelson (1982) also reported perfect agreement for smoking status information obtained by interview with a close relative (parent, wife, or child) for 14 lung cancer cases when information was compared with that obtained previously by the plant physician. Their inquiry was limited to smoker/nonsmoker status. Damber (1986) and Pershagen (1984) reported 99% agreement between reports of close relatives and hospital records for ever/never smoking studies in a sample of 86 patients admitted for respiratory disease. The agreement for number of years smoked (±5 years) was 74%.

Other studies have noted additional features of the responses from surrogates. The report by Pickle et al. (1983) indicates that respondents other than spouse and direct next-of-kin (siblings, parents, and children) are more likely to not know relevant information. Marshall et al. (1980) demonstrated the increase in sensitivity obtained by combining information from two or more surrogate respondents, and Herrmann (1985) showed that husbands reported data for wives as reliably as wives reported exposures of husbands.

Recent data from the NCHS Epidemiologic Followup Study (NHEFS) in 1982-1984 of participants in the National Health and Nutrition Examination Survey (NHANES I) in 1971-1975 provides a strong confirmation of these earlier reports (S.R. Machlin, J.C. Kleinman, J.H. Madans, National Center for Health Statistics, personal communication). This analysis is based on a subsample of 5,669 individuals with data regarding baseline smoking status available from both NHANES I and NHEFS. Agreement rates between NHANES I and NHEFS for the 5,029 subject responses versus the 640 proxy responses at follow-up are compared (Tables 6-2 and 6-3). When smoking status is broadly defined as ever/never, the 91% agreement rate for proxy responses compares quite favorably with the 95% agreement rate of subject responses

(Table 6-2). Similar high agreement is observed for proxy and subject responses at follow-up when smoking status is considered as current/not current (Table 6-3). Additional analyses of these data to assess the factors associated with agreement between baseline and follow-up responses considered age, race, gender of subject, type of respondent at follow-up, and smoking status at baseline. Estimates of the relative odds of disagreement indicated that only the effect of race did not interact with any of the other variables included in the multiple logistic model. Significant two-way interactions were observed for type of informant and age of subject, baseline smoking status and gender of subject, and baseline smoking status and age of subject. These results suggested that proxy respondents were more than twice as likely to misclassify smoking status for subjects less than 65 years of age, but not for subjects age 65 years and over. When amount smoked (current amount at baseline versus usual amount at follow-up) is compared for smokers only, the agreement rates are substantially affected by type of respondent; 55% agreement for subject responses versus 35% agreement for proxy responses. When this comparison is made with nonsmokers included, a much higher rate of agreement for both subject (80%) and proxy (74%) responses is observed. This comparison is strongly influenced by the substantial proportion of nonsmokers (over 60%). Of concern, however, is the high proportion of self-reported current and former smokers at baseline who are reported as never smokers at follow-up; 5.6% by self respondents and 12.9% by proxy respondents. These results are discussed later in the section concerned with confounding.

Another large cohort study in England and Wales provides information regarding the proportion of people who say that they have never smoked but, in fact, have done so in the past (N. Britten, University of Bristol, England, personal communication). A large longitudinal study of children born in 1 week in England and Wales in 1946 has included several follow-up visits, the most recent of which was done in 1982 when the subjects were 36 years of age. Table 6-4 presents some results. A portion (4.9%) of the subjects said they had never smoked as much as one cigarette a day in 1982 when in fact they had previously reported that they smoked. These subjects had reported smoking at a rate of about half the current smokers. Nearly all of exsmokers (93%) had smoked 10 or more years earlier.

TABLE 6-2 Percent Distribution of Smoking Status at Baseline Exam (NHANES I, 1971–75), According to Smoking Status at Follow-up (NHEFS, 1982–84) by Type of Respondent at Follow-up

	Smoking Status Reported at Follow-up				
Baseline Smoking Status (NHANES I)	Ever No.	Percent	Never No.	Percent	Total No.
		Type of Follow-up Respondent: Self			
Ever	2,675	95.6	125	5.6	2,800
Never	122	4.6	2,107	94.4	2,229
Total	2,797	100.0	2,232	100.0	5,029
		Type of Follow-up Respondent: Proxy			
Ever	329	95.1	38	12.9	367
Never	17	4.9	256	87.1	273
Total	346	100.0	294	100.0	640

SOURCE: Information obtained from National Center for Health Statistics (S. R. Machlin, J. C. Kleinman, J. H. Madans, personal communications).

TABLE 6-3 Percent Distribution of Smoking Status at Baseline Exam (NHANES I, 1971–75), According to Smoking Status at Follow-up (NHEFS, 1982–84) by Type of Respondent at Follow-up

	Smoking Status Reported at Follow-up				
Baseline Smoking Status (NHANES I)	Current No.	Percent	Not Current No.	Percent	Total No.
		Type of Follow-up Respondent: Self			
Current	1,722	89.5	124	4.0	1,846
Not Current	202	10.5	2,981	96.0	3,183
Total	1,924	100.0	3,105	100.0	5,029
		Type of Follow-up Respondent: Proxy			
Current	186	83.4	24	5.8	210
Not Current	37	16.6	393	94.2	430
Total	223	100.0	417	100.0	640

SOURCE: Information obtained from National Center for Health Statistics (S. R. Machlin, J. C. Kleinman, and J. H. Madans, personal communication).

TABLE 6-4 Smoking Habits of Cohort Members at Age 36 Who Previously Reported That They Had Smoked at Least One Cigarette a Day

Smoking Status Reported in 1982	Most Recent Age at Which Smoking Was Reported	Number of Subjects	Percentage of All Reported Ever-Smokers (No. = 2,080)	Mean No., cig./day	Interval Between Age Started Smoking and Age 36
Nonsmokers who had previously reported smoking (No. = 102)	31 yr (1977)	7	0.34	12.7	—
	25 yr (1971)	18	0.87	5.1	9.5
	20 yr (1966)	49	2.36	4.2	5.4
	<20 yr (before 1966)	28	1.35	5.8	1.8
	Total	102	4.90		
			Percent of Current Smokers (No. = 1,127)		
Current smokers who had previously reported smoking (No. = 1,048)	31 yr (1977)	819	72.67	20.6	
	25 yr (1971)	136	12.07	12.7	
	20 yr (1966)	84	7.45	11.4	
	<20 yr (before 1966)	9	0.80	16.1	

SOURCE: Based on data from the MRC National Survey of Health and Development (N. Britten, personal communication, University of Bristol, England).

Therefore, both longitudinal studies indicate that about 5% of self-reported lifelong nonsmokers may, in fact, have smoked. Rogot and Reid (1975) observed that there was a tendency of surrogate informants to report a higher tobacco consumption than previously reported by the study subjects. However, Lerchen and Samet (1986) observed no such differential in the reporting by wives of amount smoked by their husbands as compared with that reported by husbands.

The body of evidence on surrogate responses to questions about smoking status suggests that the validity of such data may be limited and that spouses and, perhaps, other close family members can provide an accurate, but simple, smoking history (ever/never, smoker/nonsmoker). However, detailed information about amount and number of years smoked may be inaccurate and may result in substantial misclassification of study subjects by exposure status. These findings, although from a limited number of studies, have direct implications for the studies of ETS exposures where ETS exposure information is derived from surrogate reports. It should be noted that in the special instance where the spouse surrogate is reporting on his personal smoking history, the information regarding ETS exposure of the nonsmoking study subject may be more accurate with regard to home exposures than the report by the study subject.

Cotinine, the major metabolite of nicotine, can be detected in blood, urine, and saliva of active cigarette smokers and of those passively exposed to ETS. Coultas et al. (1986) demonstrated that nonsmokers exposed to cigarette smoke in their homes have detectable levels of salivary cotinine that increase as the number of smokers in the home increases from 1 to 2 or more (Table 6-5). Biochemical corroboration is not as promising for remote exposures to ETS. Corroboration of historical exposures, therefore, must rely on other methods, such as review of historical records. Results of recent biochemical measures may be used to corroborate self-reports of recent exposures for individuals for whom reports of both recent and remote exposures are available. The quality of historical data for an individual can be inferred from data using results from biochemical corroboration. This approach has been proposed by Johnson and Letzel (1984).

The true validity of retrospective ETS exposures is impossible to establish. Wherever possible, other methods to corroborate exposure estimates should be used to assess and confirm the quality

TABLE 6-5 Salivary Cotinine Concentration (ng/ml) in Nonsmokers by Age and Number of Active Smokers in Household

	Number of Household Smokers		
Age, yr	None	One	Two or More
Younger than 6	0;1.7;68[a]	3.8;4.1;41	5.4;5.6;21
6–17	0;1.3;200	1.8;2.4;96	5.3;5.6;25
Older than 17	0;1.5;316	0.65;2.8;60	0;3.7;12

[a]Median; mean; number of subjects.

SOURCE: Coultas et al. (1986).

of self- and proxy reports of ETS exposure as well as active smoking status of study subjects. Other methods currently available for comparison with questionnaire and interview responses include biochemical measures, environmental modeling, review of existing records, and reports of additional respondents.

OTHER VARIABLES

Confounding factors that should be considered in the design, collection, and use of questionnaire data are other risk factors associated with the disease that may or may not be correlated with exposures to ETS. In the case of lung cancer, such risk factors include, but are not limited to:

- occupation and industry of employment,
- exposure to specific respiratory carcinogens, such as asbestos, arsenic, radon, etc., in occupational or nonoccupational settings,
- dietary factors,
- family history of cancer (Ooi et al., 1986),
- residential history,
- housing characteristics,
- years of education, and
- socioeconomic status.

Confounding factors relevant to the assessment of pulmonary function and respiratory illness are listed in Table 11-1. In addition, exsmokers and current smokers have been (or are) exposed to active smoking for some period of time. Therefore, these individuals may have been exposed to higher concentrations and longer duration of ETS, due to their own smoking patterns. Thus, an evaluation of the increased risk associated with exposure to ETS for any disease that is strongly associated with active smoking will need to control for smoking status of the individual study subjects. The confounding effects of active smoking were not adequately controlled in several investigations of lung cancer (discussed in Chapter 12). This concern is particularly relevant in studies of acute respiratory illness in children and adolescents where the study subjects may be disinclined to report their smoking behavior accurately or the parents may be unaware of their child's active smoking (described in Chapter 11).

A history of exposure to all other known or suspected confounding factors should be obtained in a comparable manner for cases and comparison subjects by interview and corroborated whenever possible by comparison with existing records or self-reports obtained before development of the disease. The exposure data collected should strive to be as detailed as possible with respect to intensity, duration, and calendar time for all exposures, including ETS exposures. However, one should be cognizant of the limitations imposed on data quality, especially when the investigation relies on surrogate responses. Such quantification at best provides an approximation of exposure, whether the information is obtained from the individual himself or from a surrogate.

SUMMARY AND RECOMMENDATIONS

There are problems with self- and proxy reports of ETS exposure inferred from questionnaire responses that limit the utility of these data. The best method by which to estimate individual ETS exposures is not known, and this lack of information hampers all efforts at assessing data quality, including data validity. At present all methods used and proposed are indirect, although some provide quantitative measures and some qualitative measures (smoker/nonsmoker). However, information on exposure from monitoring and detailed environmental-modeling studies of RSP indicate that only 30-40% of the variation in exposure can be explained using this approach (see Chapter 5). Further, biochemical methods to assess ETS exposure are extremely limited in the assessment of historical exposures that are most important with regards to chronic health effects. Therefore, exposure data derived from questionnaire responses have an extremely important role in existing and future studies of ETS exposures.

What Is Known

1. Surrogate responses from spouses or close family members can provide data as accurate as self-reports for simple ever/never smoker status and current amount smoked. However, with such simple classifications, an error rate of about 5% is observed whereby ever smokers are misclassified as lifelong nonsmokers. This error is present for self-respondents as well as proxies.

What Scientific Information Is Missing

1. Differences in exposure levels between home and work environments have not been described in existing studies. In addition to the amount of time that an individual may spend in a work setting, the actual exposure may vary within the setting due to physical characteristics of the work environment as well as the number of active smokers present.

2. Future investigations should be concerned with detailed characterization of ETS that would provide a more precise estimation of individual exposures and include additional considerations of physical characteristics of the environment, activity patterns of the study subject, and ages at which exposures occurred. These data could be entered into a model, from which exposure estimates can be made.

3. Because of the importance of misclassification of active smoking status, repeated and complementary efforts to determine and corroborate smoking status should be made in the collection of exposure data. Specific probes regarding former smoking status might be included in the questionnaire, even if the study subject has defined himself or herself as a nonsmoker.

4. Confounding factors should be considered in the design, collection, and use of questionnaire data. These will vary with the health effect being assessed. The evaluation of ETS exposures should attempt to assess all such exposures, including both the home and work environment rather than focus solely on the smoking status of one family member, e.g., spouse.

5. The comparability of questionnaires used to assess ETS has not been established, and this would be desirable.

REFERENCES

Axelson, O. Dealing with the exposure variable in occupational and environmental epidemiology. Scand. J. Soc. Med. 13:147-152, 1985.

Baumgarten, M., J. Siemiatycki, and G.W. Gibbs. Validity of work histories obtained by interview for epidemiologic purposes. Am. J. Epidemiol. 118:583-591, 1983.

Bonham, G.S., and R.W. Wilson. Children's health in families with cigarette smokers. Am. J. Public Health 71:290-293, 1981.

Coultas, D.B., J.M. Samet, C.A. Howard, G.T. Peake, and B.J. Skipper. Salivary cotinine levels and passive tobacco smoke exposure in the home. Am. Rev. Respir. Dis. 133:A157, 1986.

Damber, L. Lung cancer in males: An epidemiological study in northern Sweden with special regard to smoking and occupation. Umeä University Medical Dissertations, Umeä, Sweden, 1986. 135 pp.

Doll, R., and R. Peto. Cigarette smoking and brochial carcinoma: Dose and time relationships among regular smokers and lifelong non-smokers. J. Epidemiol. Comm. Health 32:303-313, 1978.

Gordis, L. Should dead cases be matched to dead controls? Am. J. Epidemiol. 115:1-5, 1982.

Greenberg, E.R., B. Rosner, C.H. Hennekens, R. Rinsky, and T. Colton. An investigation of bias in a study of nuclear shipyard workers. Am. J. Epidemiol. 121:301-308, 1985.

Herrmann, N. Retrospective information from questionnaires. I. Comparability of primary respondents and their next-of-kin. Am. J. Epidemiol. 121:937-947, 1985.

Humble, C.G., J.M. Samet, and B.E. Skipper. Comparison of self- and surrogate-reported dietary information. Am. J. Epidemiol. 119:86-98, 1984.

Johnson, L.C., and H.W Letzel. Measuring passive smoking: Methods, problems and perspectives. Prev. Med. 13:705-716, 1984.

Kolonel, L.N., T. Hirohata, and A.M.Y. Nomura. Adequancy of survey data collected from substitute respondents. Am. J. Epidemiol. 106:476-484, 1977.

Lerchen, M.L, and J.M. Samet. An assessment of the validity of questionnaire responses provided by a surviving spouse. Am. J. Epidemiol. 123(3):481-489, 1986.

Marshall, J., R. Priore, B. Haughey, T. Rzepka, and S. Graham. Spouse-subject interviews and the reliability of diet studies. Am. J. Epidemiol. 112:675-683, 1980.

Ooi, W.L., R.C. Elston, V.W. Chen, J.E. Bailey-Wilson, and H. Rothschild. Increased familial risk for lung cancer. J. Natl. Cancer Inst. 72:217-222, 1986.

Pershagen, G. Validity of questionnaires data on smoking and other exposures, with special reference to environmental tobacco smoke. The Respir. Dis. 133(Suppl.):76-80, 1984.

Pershagen, G., and O. Axelson. A validation of questionnaire information on occupational exposure and smoking. Scand. J. Work Environ. Health 8:24-28, 1982.

Pickle, L.W., L.M. Brown, and W.J. Blot. Information available from surrogate respondents in case-control interview studies. Am. J. Epidemiol. 118:99-108, 1983.

Rogot, E., and D.D. Reid. The validity of data from next-of-kin in studies of mortality among immigrants. Int. J. Epidemiol. 4:51-54, 1975.

Ware, J.H., D.W. Dockery, A. Spiro III, F.E. Speizer, and B.G. Ferris, Jr. Passive smoking, gas cooking, and repiratory health of children living in six cities. Am. Rev. Respir. Dis. 129:366-374, 1984.

7
Exposure-Dose Relationships for Environmental Tobacco Smoke

ESTIMATING DOSE

When considering the risks of exposure to environmental tobacco smoke (ETS) by nonsmokers, it is not enough to evaluate exposure and response. The actual dose received should be considered. Typically, for smokers, the exposure is given in terms of number of cigarettes smoked per day or cumulative pack-years. For nonsmokers, the exposure is usually characterized in terms of particle or gas concentration in micrograms per cubic meter. But what is known about the total integrated dose to the respiratory tract resulting from exposure to ETS by nonsmokers? What fraction of inspired particles and gases is deposited and fails to exit with the expired air? Moreover, what is the fate of the deposited smoke?

Although highly variable in concentration, ETS includes many of the same constituents as the smoke entering the active smoker's lungs. Both particulate and gaseous phases are present, as described in Chapter 2. In principle, the retained dose for either inhaled particles or gases can be approximated in a straightforward manner:

$$\text{Dose} = \dot{V} \times [C] \times CE. \qquad (7\text{-}1)$$

The deposited dose, in micrograms per hour, equals the ventilation rate in cubic meters per hour ($\dot{V}$) times the concentration of particle or gas in the inspired air in milligrams per cubic meter ($[C]$), times the collection efficiency (CE). CE has no dimensions; it is the fraction of the inhaled particle or gas that deposits and thus fails to exit with the expired air. Thus, the dose is directly proportional to three variables: ventilation, pollutant concentration, and the fraction deposited.

First, consider ventilation ($\dot{V}$). The standard 70-kg adult at rest breathes about 7.5 L/min (International Commission on Radiological Protection, 1975). However, a value of 20 L/min would be more appropriate for adults in indoor environments who periodically stand, walk, type, or perform other modest tasks. During heavy exercise, ventilation can increase by a factor of as much as 10, to exceed 100 L/min (International Commission on Radiological Protection, 1975).

The concentration of various constituents in ETS ($[C]$) that might be encountered in various situations has been discussed in Chapters 2 and 5.

PARTICLE SIZE

For particles, collection efficiency (CE) is determined primarily by two factors: particle size and breathing pattern. If the geometric size, shape, and density of the individual particles or droplets are known, then the distribution of particle diameters can be described. Because it is a better predictor of the behavior of the particle in the respiratory tract, aerodynamic diameter rather than optical measurement is used to express the range of particle sizes. Aerodynamic diameter is defined as the diameter of a sphere of unit density that has the same settling velocity as the particle being measured. It may be expressed as the count median aerodynamic diameter (CMAD) or mass median aerodynamic diameter (MMAD). These are, respectively, the diameters for which half of the number (or mass) of the particles are less than that diameter and for which half exceed it.

The particles in mainstream cigarette smoke have been measured by several investigators using a variety of analytical devices. Because of the different apparatus and methods of smoke generation and dilution, results vary. However, to an order of magnitude, the findings are reasonably consistent. McCusker et al. (1983) used a device called the single particle aerodynamic relaxation time (SPART) analyzer to size mainstream particles from several brands of cigarettes, with and without filters. The MMAD for all brands averaged approximately 0.46 mm and was not markedly different when the filters were removed. Particulate concentrations per milliliter ranged from 0.3×10^9 to 3.3×10^9, depending on whether the cigarettes were rated ultralow, low, or medium in tar content.

Hinds (1978) compared the particulate size distribution in cigarette smoke using an aerosol centrifuge and a cascade impactor. Although these devices are based on different physical principles, the MMAD values were comparable to those measured by McCusker et al. (1983), ranging from 0.37 to 0.52 μm. Variations depend primarily on the dilution of the smoke. Keith and Derrick (1960) used a specially modified centrifuge, termed a conifuge, to analyze cigarette smoke and reported MMAD and concentration values similar to Hinds (1978) and McCusker et al. (1983). Particulate analysis by a light-scattering photometer yielded a MMAD of 0.29 μm and particulate concentrations of 3×10^{10}/ml.

Time and concentration can modify tobacco smoke. Cigarette smoke aerosols contain volatile components, and evaporation gradually reduces particle diameters. It is also true that when the particle concentrations are extremely high, like those encountered in mainstream smoke, the aerosol can agglomerate rapidly because nearby particles collide with each other and coalesce. If smoke is cooled (reducing the vapor pressure of volatile components) and diluted in room air (reducing the probability of particle collisions), the size of the particles will become more stable. Particle size may also change within the human respiratory tract. After air containing smoke is drawn into the mouth and upper respiratory tract, it becomes humidified. Smoke particles can grow in size because of their affinity for water, termed hygroscopicity (Hiller, 1982a).

BREATHING PATTERN

Particle size is a critical factor in determining the collection efficiency, but breathing pattern is also important For example, large slow tidal volumes will favor alveolar deposition, while high inspiratory flows will promote deposition at bifurcations in the airways. Breath-holding is also important. The greater the elapsed time before the next expiration, the higher the fraction of inspired particles deposited, since there is more time for particles to sediment or diffuse. Individual anatomic differences may influence the amount and distribution of deposited particles. The cross section of airways will influence the linear velocity of the inspired air.

Increasing alveolar size decreases alveolar deposition. Preexisting disease can also modify the deposition of smoke. For environmental tobacco smoke (diameters of particles ranging from 0.1 μm to 1 μm) the sedimentation and diffusion mechanisms will be the primary mechanisms of deposition.

Changes in the rate and pattern of breathing associated with exercise can also affect the total dose of cigarette particulates deposited in the lungs. Bennett et al. (1985) reported that exercise increased the percent deposition of experimentally generated aerosols (MMAD of 2.6 μm) in human subjects. The reason for this observation was that during exercise, breathing patterns change so that flow rates are increased. Increasing the flow rates also increases the inertial impaction. Also, exercise is frequently associated with a shift from nose to mouth breathing. Consequently, the filtration of large particles that takes place in the upper respiratory tract no longer occurs. Increased deposition was also measured in exercising hamsters that inhaled a radiolabelled aerosol (activity median diameter of 3 μm) (Harbison and Brain, 1983). These results are relevant to those who breathe air containing ETS when their minute ventilation is increased while working or during periods of exercise.

DEPOSITION OF CIGARETTE SMOKE PARTICLES

The factors discussed in the previous sections indicate that experimental measurements of the concentration of smoke aerosols in indoor environments, i.e., exposure concentrations, are insufficient for predictions of smoke deposition. ETS smoke is constantly changing, thereby complicating the collection of accurate and reproducible data regarding its particulate size. In addition, alterations in respiratory structure and respiratory rate can affect deposition of particulates. These complexities stress the importance of actual measurement of regional deposition of cigarette smoke particles in human lungs. However, little is published on this important area, despite the prevalence of passive smoking and concerns about its impact on human health. The majority of the available information on deposition of particles present in cigarette smoke is based on theoretical or physical models of the lungs and measurements of differences between the concentrations of tobacco smoke aerosol or model aerosols in inhaled and exhaled air.

A model to predict the percent of deposition of particles based on MMAD was developed by the Task Group on Lung Dynamics (1966) of the International Commission on Radiological Protection. The respiratory tract was divided into three main regions: nasopharynx, trachea and bronchi, and the alveolar. In conjunction with estimates of particle clearance, deposition calculations were made for these regions at three different inhalation volumes. This model suggests that about 30% of the particles within the size range present in cigarette smoke will deposit in the alveolar region and 5-10% in the tracheobronchial region. This model also emphasizes the impact of particle solubility on the total integrated dose with time. Brain and Valberg (1974) developed convenient nomograms and a computer program to calculate how particle solubility and particle size significantly affect the net amount of particulates retained in the lungs. Although the basic outline of the model is generally correct, more recent measurements suggest that values for alveolar deposition of particles 0.1-1.0 μm are too high by a factor of at least 2 (Heyder, 1982). The extent to which ETS particles are hygroscopic and increase in size within the respiratory tract is an important and unresolved issue that adds further uncertainty.

Aerosol deposition has also been studied in airway casts. Physical models of the upper airways of human lungs have been made by a double-casting technique to study particulate deposition at several airway generations (Schlesinger and Lippman 1972). Different flow rates and particle sizes were used to study deposition patterns. Schlesinger and Lippman (1978) reported a correlation between the deposition sites of test aerosols in their lung casts and the most common sites of origin of bronchogenic carcinoma in smoking humans. Both occurred preferentially at bifurcations. Martonen et al. (1983) added an oropharyngeal compartment and a replica cast of the larynx to the tracheobronchial casts in order to better simulate airflow patterns in the upper respiratory tract. They used these models to evaluate the amount of cigarette smoke condensate deposited in the airways at different flow rates. More condensate was present in areas where airways branched and especially at the bifurcation points, indicating increased levels of impaction. Aerosol was also deposited preferentially along posterior airway walls of the branching regions.

Hiller et al. (1982a) measured the collection efficiency in adults of an aerosol containing three different sizes of polystyrene latex spheres in nonsmoking humans. They measured a 10% deposition for 0.6-μm (MMAD) spheres, which is similar to the results of Davies et al. (1972) and Muir and Davies (1967) using 0.5-μm aerosols and Heyder (1982) using aerosols that were 0.2 to 1.0 μm in size. The size ranges of these aerosols are comparable to those experimentally measured in cigarette smoke, as previously discussed.

In contrast to passive smoking, the estimates of the collection efficiency of smoke particles during active smoking are substantially higher (about 70%) for at least two reasons (Hiller et al., 1982b). First, the much higher particulate concentrations in mainstream smoke may give rise to more agglomeration and greater hydroscopic growth in the respiratory tract. Both processes produce larger particles with higher collection efficiencies. Second, and more important, the breathing pattern used by the active smoker is markedly different than normal breathing. It is characterized by a slow deep inspiration followed by breath-holding. This increases the average residence time of the smoke particles and thus increases the fraction of inhaled particles that deposit in the lung.

To compare the amount of smoke deposited in the lungs of an active smoker with an individual exposed to ETS, first consider a pack-a-day smoker (about 20 cigarettes during an 8-hour period). The average tar rating in mainstream smoke (MS) over the past couple of decades has been about 14 mg/cigarette. Therefore, the total amount of tar inspired is 280 mg/8 h. Assuming a collection efficiency of 70%, the amount of tar deposited is 196 mg/8 h.

As pointed out in Chapter 5, smoke particles can range from 50 to 500 $\mu g/m^3$ in public places where smoking occurs and from 20 to 150 $\mu g/m^3$ in homes with smokers. Consider a nonsmoker who breathes at 10 L/min, or 4,800 L/8 h. With modest exercise, this could increase to 20 L/min, or 9,600 L/8 h. Based on estimates by Hiller et al. (1982a,b), the collection efficiency of particles in ETS is about 10%. Therefore, the total amount of smoke particles deposited in a nonsmoker in these environments for 8 h could range from approximately $0.0096 \text{ mg/8 h} = 20\ \mu g/m^3 \times 4.8\ m^3/8 \text{ h} \times 0.1$ to an extreme of $0.5 \text{ mg/8 h} = 500\ \mu g/m^3 \times 10\ m^3/8 \text{ h} \times 0.1$. This would be approximately 0.005% to 0.26% of that amount of tar deposited in the active smoker's lungs after smoking 20 cigarettes. The active smoker, of course, also breathes the ETS, so that the total dose received by the active smoker is the mainstream smoke plus a passive smoking dose equivalent to that received by the nonsmoker exposed to ETS. However, since the dose received due to breathing ETS-contaminated air is so small, this additional contribution to the total dose is negligible.

Benzo[*a*]pyrene (B*a*P) is one of the primary constituents of particles in mainstream smoke. From Table 2-10 one can estimate that a nonsmoker exposed to ETS receives a higher relative dose of B*a*P than of RSP. However, the ambient measurements, which are used to estimate the dose for the nonsmoker, may be elevated in view of the high outdoor concentrations that are reported in these studies. More data on the fate of B*a*P in ETS and on ambient concentrations are needed before estimates of the relative doses can be made meaningfully.

Although the amount of smoke deposited in the lungs of nonsmokers during exposure to ETS is small compared with that encountered by the active smoker regarding mainstream smoke, it may differ in composition and toxicity. For example, as discussed in Chapter 2, certain constituents are present in much higher concentrations in sidestream smoke as compared with mainstream smoke (Weiss et al., 1983). These possible differences in composition must be explored.

PARTICLE RETENTION IN THE LUNGS

The amount of particles present at different sites in the lungs is not only dependent on deposition. Retention of smoke depends on the balance between the amount of each constituent that deposits in the respiratory tract and the efficiency of the lung clearance mechanisms in the airways and alveoli. Clearance mechanisms are a dynamic component of normal lung function and operate to keep the lung clean and sterile. Particles depositing in the airways are entrained in the mucus layer that lines the airway. This layer is swept toward the mouth by the action of ciliated cells and eventually swallowed. Mucus transport is approximately 1-2 cm per minute in the trachea, but is slower in smaller airways. In addition, macrophages present in the airways may phagocytose deposited particulates and be carried towards the mouth by the mucociliary transport system. Particulates reaching the alveolar region—those that are usually less than several micrometers—are soon engulfed by alveolar macrophages. Some of these cells gradually migrate towards the airways and exit the lung via the mucociliary escalator. Dissolution of particles is an additional important clearance mechanism.

Lung disease and cigarette smoking itself can affect particle clearance and retention in smokers' lungs. Previous studies have shown that smokers have different aerosol deposition patterns and slower clearance rates than nonsmokers (Albert et al., 1969; Sanchis et al., 1971; Cohen et al., 1979). These alterations in clearance are, in part, caused by components within cigarette smoke that affect the quantity and rheological properties of the mucous. Components of cigarette smoke, also, can impair phagocytosis by alveolar macrophages (Ferin et al., 1965). Clearance mechanisms in smokers may be further compromised by lung diseases, such an emphysema and fibrosis, and by exposure to other air pollutants.

Measurements of the long-term retention of compounds associated with cigarette particulates in the lungs are difficult to estimate from data obtained with airway casts or from differences between inhaled and exhaled aerosol concentration, since these methods do not take into account clearance mechanisms. Unfortunately, few data are available regarding the actual retention and sites of deposition of cigarette smoke particles in either nonsmoking humans or animals exposed to ETS. The most accurate method that could be used is quantification of particulate deposits in individual pieces of tissue dissected from the lung. Impossible in living animals, this is a tedious procedure in animal lungs or human material obtained at surgery or autopsy and is especially difficult for large lungs. One can also attempt to quantify dose by examining saliva, serum, or urine. These possibilities are discussed in Chapter 8.

GASES IN ENVIRONMENTAL TOBACCO SMOKE

In addition to the particulate phase, we must also consider exposure-dose relationships for gases in ETS. As before, breathing pattern influences gas uptake. Of particular importance is the difference between oral and nasal breathing. Breathing by mouth increases the exposure of the airways, while breathing by nose (as would be true for nonsmokers exposed to ETS most of the time) offers some protection for the lower respiratory tract.

The most important variable determining the amount and site of uptake is the water solubility of the gas in question. Gases that are highly soluble in water, such as formaldehyde or acrolein, will be almost completely removed by the upper respiratory tract, especially during nasal breathing. The concentration of other gases, such as the oxides of nitrogen, which have an intermediate solubility, will decrease as the inspired bolus penetrates deeper and deeper into the lungs. There will be uptake of gas in the upper airways, but significant amounts will also penetrate to respiratory bronchioles and alveoli. Finally, there are gases of low solubility, such as carbon monoxide. No significant uptake of CO occurs in the upper airways, and it is only slowly absorbed across the air-blood barrier. In the absence of heavy exercise and very high ventilation rates, many hours are required to establish an equilibrium between inspired CO and carboxyhemoglobin in the blood.

As was true for particles, we can estimate the gas uptake for active smokers and for passive smokers. As reviewed in Chapter 2, CO from ETS can range from less than 1 to 8 ppm. If the background air has little or no CO, even the upper estimates of 8 ppm will have a negligible effect on carboxyhemoglobin levels. Almost 2 hours would be required to reach 1% carboxyhemoglobin (Peterson and Stewart, 1975). This is approximately the same as background levels of carboxyhemoglobin, which are associated with endogenous production of carbon monoxide. Even after 15 hours, when the equilibrium value of 1.7% COHb is finally reached, the effect should be insignificant. However, if air pollution from mobile and stationary sources produces higher background levels of CO, then an incremental exposure of 1 to 8 ppm could produce some added burden of carboxyhemoglobin.

Reactive or highly soluble gases such as formaldehyde, acrolein, or oxides of nitrogen present a different situation. Acrolein has a very high water solubility (40 g/100 ml). Because of this high solubility in the airway lining fluids, one would anticipate a collection efficiency approaching 100%. Moreover, this would occur rapidly, so that acrolein is classified as an upper respiratory tract irritant. According to Table 2-10, there are between 60 and 100 μg of acrolein generated per cigarette. Thus, from 20 cigarettes, 1.2 to 2.0 mg of acrolein would be deposited in the respiratory tract of the active smoker.

Chapter 2 suggests that levels of acrolein in public places where smoking is permitted could range from 10 to 50 $\mu g/m^3$. Using similar assumptions to that made for particles, we estimate that the nonsmoker would inhale 4.8 to 10 m^3 of air per 8 hours. Assuming a collection efficiency of 100%, the total amount of acrolein deposited in the passive smoker would be approximately 0.048 to 0.5 mg. We select 1.6 mg/8 hours as the mid-range dose for the active smokers, which assumes 20 cigarettes smoked per 8 hours with 80 μg acrolein per cigarette. Using this value, the nonsmoker exposed to ETS for 8 hours would then receive approximately 3 to 31% of that received by the active smoker. When the contribution of ETS is included for the active smoker, the nonsmoker exposed to ETS for 8 hours would receive between 5 and 24% of that of an active smoker. The relatively high dose of acrolein received by the nonsmoker reflects the high collection efficiency for this hydrophilic component and the persistence of vapor-phase components in the air even when filtration is used. Table 2-10 gives comparisons of the amount of other materials inspired for both active smokers and individuals exposed to ETS over shorter periods of time.

SUMMARY AND RECOMMENDATIONS

A number of studies have measured the levels of specific constituents of ETS under natural conditions (reviewed in Chapters 2 and 5). The extrapolation from relative exposures to relative doses received is difficult. Variation in the percent of time individuals spend in particular environments such as home, workplace, and so forth, and the variations in uptake and clearance, discussed in this chapter, will affect the actual dose received.

Using a simple, first-approximation model for exposure and retention, the relative daily dose received for a nonsmoker exposed to ETS can be compared with the dose received by an active smoker. For RSP, the estimates were up to 0.26%. For acrolein, a hydrophillic, vapor-phase constituent, the relative dose is estimated to be much higher, 3 to 31%, whether or not the ETS exposure of the active smoker is considered. Nicotine, another constituent that appears primarily in the vapor phase of ETS, has an estimated relative dose of up to 1% (see Chapter 8).

The extent to which these are indicative of the relative exposures to specific constituents that are important for particular health effects in active smokers or in nonsmokers exposed to ETS cannot be determined for any of the health effects reviewed later in this report. Nevertheless, the estimated relative exposures give some idea of the potential range of relative exposures, for constitutents that are found both in the vapor phase and in the particulate phase.

Because of the range of estimated relative doses, it would be ideal to make estimates of the relative dose based on the specific constituent(s) that are most relevant to the health effect being assessed. However, many of these specific constituents, for instance the carcinogenic constituents such as benzo[*a*]pyrene, *N*-nitrosodimethylamine, and *N*-nitrosodiethylamine, are difficult to measure; therefore, there are not enough data available to make meaningful estimates of the relative doses of these constituents. Also, biological markers might be potentially informative indicators of the relative doses. However, as reviewed in Chapter 8, to date only carbon monoxide, nicotine, and cotinine have been measured extensively in humans.

What Is Known

1. Particle size and breathing pattern are critical factors in the deposition of ETS in humans.
2. Theoretical models predict that 30 to 40% of the particles with the size range present in cigarette smoke will deposit in the alveolar region and 5 to 10% in the tracheobronchial region.
3. The collection efficiency of smoke particles during active smoking has been measured to be about 70%. On the other hand, the collection efficiency is estimated to be only 10% for nonsmokers exposed to ETS.

What Scientific Information Is Missing

1. Actual measurement of regional deposition of cigarette smoke particulates in human lungs is not available.
2. There are little data regarding the actual retention and sites of deposition of ETS particulates in either humans or animals.
3. The concentrations of various components in vapor and particulate phases of MS and ETS differ. Consequently, research is needed, particularly for vapor-phase components, to see how these differences affect dose.

REFERENCES

Albert, R.E., M. Lippmann, and W. Briscoe. The characteristics of bronchial clearance in humans and the effect of cigarette smoking. Arch. Environ. Health 18:738-755, 1969.

Bennett, W.D., M.S. Messina, and G.C. Smaldone. Effect of exercise on deposition and subsequent retention of inhaled particles. J. Appl. Physiol. 59:1046-1054, 1985.

Brain, J.D., and P.A. Valberg. Models of lung retention based on ICRP Task Group report. Arch. Environ. Health 28:1-11, 1974.

Cohen, D., S.F. Arai, and J.D. Brain. Smoking impairs long-term dust clearance from the lung. Science 204:514-517, 1979.

Davies, C.N., J. Heyder, and M.C. Subba Rama. The breathing of half-micron aerosols. I. Experimental. J. Appl. Physiol. 32:591-600, 1972.

Ferin, J., G. Urbankova, and A. Vlokova. Influence of tobacco smoke on the elimination of particles from the lungs. Nature 206:515-516, 1965.

Harbison, M.L., and J.D. Brain. Effects on exercise of particle deposition in Syrian golden hamsters. Am. Rev. Respir. Dis. 128:904-908, 1983.

Heyder, J. Particle transport onto human airway surfaces. Eur. J. Respir. Dis. 63(Suppl. 119):29-50, 1982.

Hiller, F.C., M.K. Mazumder, J.D. Wilson, P.C. McLeod, and R.C. Bone. Human respiratory tract deposition using multimodal aerosols. J. Aerosol. Sci. 13:337-343, 1982a.

Hiller, F.C., K.T. McCusker, M.K. Mazumder, J.D. Wilson, and R.C. Bone. Deposition of sidestream cigarette smoke in the human respiratory tract. Am. Rev. Respir. Dis. 125:406-408, 1982b.

Hinds, W.C. Size characteristics of cigarette smoke. Am. Ind. Hyg. Assoc. J. 39:48-54, 1978.

International Commission on Radiological Protection (ICRP), Task Group of Committee 2 of the International Commission on Radiological Protection. Physiological data for reference man, pp. 346-347. In ICRP. Report of the Task Group on Reference Man (ICRP 23). New York: Pergamon, 1975.

Keith, C.H., and J.C. Derrick. Measurement of the particle size distribution and concentration of cigarette smoke by the "conifuge." J. Colloid Sci. 15:340-356, 1960.

Martonen T.B., and J.E. Lowe. Cigarette smoke pattern in a human respiratory tract model. Proc. Ann. Conf. Eng. Med. Biol. 25:171, 1983 (abstract).

McCusker K., F.C. Hiller, J.D. Wilson, M.K. Mazumder, and R. Bone. Aerodynamic sizing of tobacco smoke particulate from commercial cigarettes. Arch. Environ. Health 38:215-218, 1983.

Muir D.C.F., and C.N. Davies. The deposition of 0.5 μm diameter aerosols in the lungs of man. Ann. Occup. Hyg. 10:161-174, 1967.

Peterson, J.E., and R.D. Stewart. Predicting the carboxyhemoglobin levels resulting from carbon monoxide exposures. J. Appl. Physiol. 39:633-638, 1975.

Sanchis J., M. Dolovich, R. Chalmers, and M.T. Newhouse. Regional distribution and lung clearance mechanisms in smokers and non-smokers, pp. 183-191. In E.H. Walton, Ed. Inhaled Particles, Part III. Surrey, England: Unwin Brothers Ltd., 1971.

Schlesinger R.B., and M. Lippmann. Particle deposition in casts of the human upper tracheobronchial tree. Am. Ind. Hyg. Assoc. J. 33:237-251, 1972.

Schlesinger R.B., and M. Lippmann. Selective particle deposition and bronchogenic carcinoma. Environ. Res. 15:424-431, 1978.

Task Group on Lung Dynamics. Deposition and retention models for internal dosimetry of the human respiratory tract. Health Phys. 12:173-207, 1966.

Weiss S.T., I.B. Tager, M. Schenker, and F.E. Speizer. The health effects of involuntary smoking. Am. Rev. Respir. Dis. 128:933-942, 1983.

8
Assessing Exposures to Environmental Tobacco Smoke Using Biological Markers

Previous chapters have dealt with the formation and composition of tobacco sidestream smoke, its contribution to environmental tobacco smoke (ETS), and the conditions that govern the physicochemistry and toxicity of ETS. Personal monitoring of exposure and analysis of the respiratory environment enable us to estimate the level of toxic agents for individuals exposed to ETS. Studies on the uptake of smoke constituents by individuals and on the metabolic fate of such constituents can provide information relative to epidemiologic observations and the actual exposure levels of different populations.

Exposure to ETS may depend on several factors, including the number of smokers in an enclosed area, the size and nature of the area, and the degree of ventilation. Thus, optimal assessment of exposure should be done by analysis of the physiological fluids of exposed persons rather than by analysis of respiratory environment. The development of new biochemical methods enables us to obtain measurements of exposure to ETS by determining the uptake of specific agents in body fluids and calculating the risk relative to that of the exposure of active smokers. The uptake of individual agents from ETS can be determined by biochemical measures that have been developed for assessment of active smoking behavior, as long as these measures are sensitive and specific enough for quantitating exposure to such agents by nonsmokers.

BIOLOGICAL MARKERS IN PHYSIOLOGICAL FLUIDS

Thiocyanate

The hydrogen cyanide (HCN) absorbed from tobacco smoke is detoxified in the liver, yielding thiocyanate (SCN^-). However, SCN^- in serum and other biological fluids does not exclusively originate from inhaled tobacco smoke. Thiocyanate also can be derived from the diet (Haley et al., 1983; Jarvis, 1985).

Before 1975, primarily two colorimetric methods were used for the manual determination of thiocyanate in biological fluids (Aldridge, 1944; Bowler, 1944). Subsequently, the automatic method by Butts et al. (1974) has found wide application in comparing physiological fluids from smokers and nonsmokers. It entails determination of thiocyanate by its reaction with ferric ions, which yield a color complex with maximal absorbance at 460 nm, the intensity of which can be measured in an autoanalyzer. In sera of nonsmokers, Butts et al. (1974) determined up to 95 μmol/L of SCN^-. The critical value in differentiating between smokers and nonsmokers was 85 μmol/L of SCN^-. In other investigations, 100 μmol/L of SCN^- was found to be the critical level for serum (Junge et al., 1978) and for saliva (Luepker et al., 1981). This fact and the low concentrations of HCN in ETS (Hoffmann et al., 1984) explain why some investigators were unable to distinguish between nonsmokers exposed to ETS and those without any exposure to tobacco smoke (Hoffmann et al., 1984; Jarvis, 1985).

Similarly, the mean serum level of SCN^- in healthy pregnant women at term who were exposed to ETS (35.9 μmol/L) was not distinctly different from that in those without ETS exposure (32.3 μmol/L), nor was there a measureable difference in SCN^- levels in the umbilical cords of the neonates (26 versus 23 μmol/L) (Hauth et al., 1984).

In one study, it appeared that there was a trend toward higher thiocyanate levels in the saliva of nonsmoking children residing with smokers compared to the SCN^- levels in saliva of children without ETS exposure, yet this trend was insignificant (Gillies et al., 1982). In a study of six volunteer nonsmokers exposed to a smoke-filled room for 4 hours, there was a significant increase in salivary SCN^-. However, the SCN^- values of the nonsmokers exposed to ETS were not distinguishable from those nonsmokers free of tobacco smoke exposure (Pekkanen et al., 1976).

In another study, mean serum thiocyanate levels were reported to be significantly higher ($p < 0.002$) for children and adolescents with exposure to cigarette smoke at home ($n = 14$; $SCN^- = 97.3 \pm 45.4$ μmol/L) than for those not exposed ($n = 10$; $SCN^- = 54.2 \pm 11.3$ μmol/L). The authors of the latter study also reported a weak correlation between thiocyanate concentration and number of cigarettes smoked per family (Poulton et al., 1984). This study was criticized because some of the determined thiocyanate levels were within the range reported for heavy cigarette smokers. It is likely that there was deceptive reporting of adolescent smoking status (Jarvis, 1985). Based on the observations to date, the level of thiocyanate in saliva, serum, and/or urine is not useful as an indicator for the uptake of ETS by a nonsmoker.

Carbon Monoxide and Carboxyhemoglobin

Carbon monoxide (CO) in the body originates from endogenous processes as well as environmental sources. The endogenous production of CO is primarily a consequence of the breakdown of hemoglobin and of other heme-containing pigments. Healthy adults produce about 0.4 ml of CO per hour (0.5 mg/h; Coburn et al., 1964). This provides the major portion of CO that is found as carboxyhemoglobin (COHb) in nonsmokers. In nonsmokers without occupational exposure to CO, COHb ranges from 0.5 to 1.5% (National Research Council, 1981; Wald et al., 1981).

The inhalation of CO from the environment is followed by an increase of the CO concentration in the alveolar gas and by diffusion from the gas phase through the pulmonary membrane into the blood. CO is complexed with blood to form COHb and, as such, is transported throughout the body. Complexing it with hemoglobin occurs with a strong coordination bond with the iron of heme, a bond that is about 200 times stronger than that with molecular oxygen. CO is only slowly released from the blood in the process of exhaling. In the case of nonsmokers who have been exposed to elevated levels of CO in the air for a few hours, the half-life of COHb lasts 2-4 hours (National Research Council, 1981).

Monitoring of absorbed CO in the blood is done primarily by the analysis of CO in alveolar gas and by the analysis of COHb in blood. The most widely used technique in the clinical laboratory is the determination of COHb with automated differential spectrophotometry (National Research Council, 1977). The determination of CO in exhaled air by standardized gas analyzers has been used less frequently. However, the portable "Ecolyzer" and other similar instruments have proved to be reliable instruments for the recent validations of the reported smoking habits among populations in field studies (Vogt et al., 1979). The data from both measurements, amount of CO in the alveolar gas and the concentration of COHb in blood, are well correlated. Theoretically, the slope of the graph relating the percent of concentration of COHb to alveolar CO should be about 0.155 at CO concentrations of 0-50 ppm. Most laboratory studies have confirmed this correlation experimentally (National Research Council, 1981). In the case of cigarette smokers who have inhaled puffs of smoke containing 20,000-50,000 ppm of CO, the correlation between exhaled CO and COHb is also in good agreement ($r = 0.97$; Heinemann et al., 1984).

The COHb levels are of value for comparing degrees of smoke inhalation. In a study of men aged 34-64 years, cigarette smokers had on the average 4.7% of COHb; cigar smokers, 2.9%; pipe smokers, 2.2%; and nonsmokers, 0.9% (Wald et al., 1981, 1984). However, measurements of exhaled CO or COHb are not valid indicators of chronic exposure to ETS. A study of 100 self-reported nonsmokers who were divided into four groups—without exposure to ETS, with little, with some, and with a lot—revealed no significant differences in measurements of expired CO (5.0-5.7 ppm; mean, 5.61 ± 2.70 ppm) or COHb (0.80-0.94%; mean, 0.87 ± 0.67%) (Jarvis and Russell, 1984). This observation is also supported by a study of six nonsmoking flight attendants who served in the smokers' section of a trans-Pacific aircraft. Preflight COHb levels were 1.0 ± 0.2% and postflight levels (after serving round-trip) were 0.7 ± 0.2% (Foliart et al., 1983).

Heavily smoke-polluted environments can lead to elevated absorption of CO. This was shown for seven nonsmokers exposed for 2 hours in a pub, whose exhaled air revealed an average of 5.9 ppm of CO, a level that corresponds to the alveolar gas of a smoker after smoking one cigarette (Jarvis et al., 1983). Another study showed that twelve nonsmokers, sharing the nonairconditioned environment of a room with four smokers who smoked four cigarettes each within 30 minutes, had an COHb increase of the same magnitude as that measured in a smoker after consuming one cigarette (Huch et al., 1980).

Even though tobacco smoke is a major source for indoor air pollution, additional sources may contribute to increased CO concentrations in air and, consequently, to higher COHb levels in exposed subjects. Such sources include gas stoves, faulty furnaces, and space heaters (National Research Council, 1981). For example, kerosene heaters can be a major source for indoor pollution. Depending on the model and flame setting, kerosene space heaters generate up to 6.5 mg of CO per minute of operation (Leaderer, 1982).

In summary, CO in alveolar air and as COHb in nonsmokers originates from endogenous processes as well as from environmental sources. ETS is an important pollutant of indoor environments; however, except for highly polluted settings, CO levels in exhaled air and COHb levels in the blood are not statisically significantly elevated following exposure to ETS, although acute short-term exposures from 3-4 hours may be detected if blood or expired air is sampled within 30 minutes of the end of exposure. In sum, however, measurements of exhaled CO and of COHb are not useful indicators of exposure to ambient ETS except in acute exposure studies in the laboratory. CO measures are a marker of gas-phase exposure to ETS.

Nicotine and Cotinine

Disregarding nicotine-containing chewing gum and nicotine aerosol rods as aids for smoking cessation, the presence of nicotine and that of its major metabolite, cotinine, in biological fluids is entirely due to the exposure to tobacco, tobacco smoke, or environmental tobacco smoke. The determination of nicotine and cotinine in saliva, blood, or urine of active and passive smokers is done primarily by gas chromatography (GC) with a nitrogen-sensitive detector and by radioimmunoassay (RIA).

The GC method requires great precaution in order to avoid contamination by traces of nicotine from the environment or from solvents and/or equipment. This is of major importance for samples containing nicotine at levels <20 ng/ml of fluid, as is the case in nonsmokers exposed to ETS (Feyeraband and Russell, 1980). The GC method can be used to measure concentrations of nicotine as low as 1 ng/ml and concentrations of cotinine as low as 5 ng/ml in samples of physiological fluids (Jacob et al., 1981). An experienced chemist can analyze up to 25 samples per day for nicotine and cotinine.

The radioimmunoassays for nicotine and cotinine represent probably the most direct technique available. These assays have only low cross-reactivities with other naturally occurring metabolites of nicotine. The sensitivity of these assays is about 0.5 ng/ml for both nicotine and cotinine and has inter- and intra-assay variations of ±5% (Langone et al., 1973; Hill et al., 1983). An experienced biochemist with automated equipment can analyze up to 80 samples (plus 20 control samples) per day. So far, the RIA method has been used by a limited number of laboratories because it requires the synthesis of specific nicotine and cotinine derivatives for the generation of serum albumin conjugates and the raising of antibodies to these conjugates (Langone et al., 1973). In addition, the RIA method also requires careful drawing and handling of samples to avoid contamination.

Table 8-1 presents results from the major studies on the uptake of nicotine by nonsmokers under acute exposure conditions. These data show that exposure to high levels of ETS in laboratories can lead to a significant uptake of nicotine. This uptake is clearly reflected in the concentrations of nicotine in plasma (up to 0.9 μg/ml for nonsmokers compared with a mean value of 14.8 μg/ml for smokers, an increase of 15-fold) and in urine (84 ng/ml for nonsmokers, compared with 1,750 ng/ml, a increase of 20-fold) (Russell and Feyeraband, 1975; Hoffmann et al., 1984). The significantly higher values for nicotine in the plasma compared to urine may be explained by the short initial half-life in smokers of 9 minutes and relatively short terminal half-life in smokers of 2 hours (Benowitz et al., 1982).

Table 8-2 presents data for nicotine and cotinine uptake as measured in physiological fluids of nonsmokers exposed to ETS under daily life conditions. With the exception of the report by Matsukura et al. (1984), the data demonstrate that the involuntary exposure of the passive smoker amounts to a few percent or less of the amount of nicotine that is inhaled by a cigarette smoker. Table 8-3 compares nicotine and cotinine levels as determined in one laboratory in plasma, saliva, and urine of nonsmokers with and without ETS exposure and of active smokers. This comparison shows that, generally, concentrations of nicotine and cotinine in plasma, saliva, and urine of nonsmokers exposed to ETS amount

TABLE 8-1 Nicotine Uptake by Nonsmokers Exposed to ETS Under Laboratory Conditions

Authors	ETS—Conditions	No. of Nonsmokers	Results	
Harke, 1970	Room—170 m^3	7	Excretion in the urine (6 h after exposure)	
	(1) 11 smokers consumed 100 cigarettes during 2 h; no ventilation (30 ppm CO)		Nicotine: 10 ± 6.8 μg/6 h Cotinine: 35 ± 34.5 μg/6 h	
	(2) as (1)—but with regular ventilation (5 ppm CO)	7	Nicotine: 18 ± 7 μg/6 h Cotinine: 19 ± 9.4 μg/6 h	
Cano et al., 1970	Room—66 m^3 4 smokers and 2 non-smokers		Excretion in the urine	Nicotine, μg/24 h
	(a) lived together for 5 days		Day 1—no smoking	0
			Day 2—98 cigarettes smoked	35-44
			Day 3—121 cigarettes smoked	50-61
			Day 4—98 cigarettes smoked	62.5-70
			Day 5—88 cigarettes smoked	47-50
	(b) lived together for 4 days	2	Day 1—97 cigarettes; 15 μg nic./m^3	23-34
			Day 2—96 cigarettes; 22 μg nic./m^3	22.5-58
			Day 3—94 cigarettes; 35 μg nic./m^3	47.5-69
			Day 4—103 cigarettes; 33 μg nic./m^3	32-65
Russell and Feyerabend, 1975	(1) Room—43 m^3 9 smokers consumed 80 cigarettes and 2 cigars; no ventilation (38 ppm CO)	12	Nicotine Before exposure: 0.73 ± 1.6 μg/ml plasma After 78 min exposure: 0.90 ± 0.29 μg/ml plasma 15 min after ending exposure: 80.0 ± 58.7 ng/ml urine No experimental ETS exposure: 12.4 ng/ml urine 8.9 ng/ml urine	
	(2) Two groups measured after lunch	14 13	No experimental ETS exposure: 12.4 ± 16.9 ng/ml urine 8.9 ± 9.1 ng/ml urine	

TABLE 8-1 *Continued*

Authors	ETS—Conditions	No. of Nonsmokers	Results			
Hoffmann et al., 1984	Room—16 m^3 4 cigarettes concurrently and continuously machine smoked for 80 min; 6 air exchanges/h (200 g nic./m^3 20 ppm CO)	6	Time during exposure		Nicotine	Cotinine
			0	Saliva:	3 ng/ml	1.0 ng/ml
				Plasma:	0.2 ng/ml	0.9 ng/ml
				Urine:	17 ng/mg creat.	14 ng/mg creat.
			80 min	Saliva:	730 ng/ml	1.4 ng/ml
				Plasma:	0.5 ng/ml	1.3 ng/ml
				Urine:	84 ng/mg creat.	28 ng/mg creat.
			Time following exposure			
			30 min	Saliva:	148 ng/ml	1.7 ng/ml
				Plasma:	0.4 ng/ml	1.8 ng/ml
			150 min	Saliva:	17 ng/ml	3.1 ng/ml
				Plasma:	0.7 ng/ml	2.9 ng/ml
				Urine:	100 ng/mg creat.	45 ng/mg creat.
			300 min	Saliva:	7 ng/ml	3.5 ng/ml
				Plasma:	0.6 ng/ml	3.2 ng/ml
				Urine:	48 ng/mg creat.	55 ng/mg creat.

[a]Abbreviations: creat., creatinine; nic., nicotine.

to less than 1% of the mean values observed in physiological fluids of active smokers, even though some nicotine measurements in plasma give a higher reading (Jarvis et al., 1984).

In a large-scale study of 839 nonsmokers (identified by their questionnaire response and also having a cotinine concentration of <20 ng/ml of saliva), cotinine levels increased with the number of smokers in the home for each of three age groups examined independently (<5, 6-17, and >18 years). The cotinine levels in saliva were found to be significantly associated with increasing number of smokers per household within each age group. The median salivary cotinine levels in adult smokers was 287 ng cotinine/ml (Coultas et al., 1986).

Matsukura et al. (1984) report that cotinine in the urine of ETS-exposed nonsmokers reaches an average of 1.56 ± 0.57 μg/mg of creatinine when 40 or more cigarettes per day have been smoked in the home of the exposed subjects. In the case of cigarette smokers, they found cotinine levels of 8.57 ± 0.39 μg/mg of creatinine in urine. This study has been questioned because its findings of cotinine in urine of both active and passive smokers indicate levels substantially higher than those reported in other studies (Adlkofer et al., 1985; Pittenger, 1985) (see Chapter 12).

Nicotine uptake by infants of cigarette-smoking mothers appears to be higher than is generally observed for the adult nonsmoker. The amount of cotinine excreted in the infant's urine has been found to be correlated with the number of cigarettes smoked by the mother in the 24 hours preceding the measurement (Greenberg et al., 1984).

The analysis of nicotine and cotinine in physiologic fluids can be misleading if made on very light smokers or nonsmokers who either sniff tobacco or are tobacco chewers or snuff-dippers. In the case of the very light smoker, nicotine and cotinine values may be similar to those of nonsmokers who had exposure to high levels of ETS (Russell and Feyerabend, 1975; Wald et al., 1984). In the case of individuals who use tobacco nasally, or orally, on a regular basis, the nicotine and cotinine values may approach those of heavy cigarette smokers (Russell et al., 1980; Russell et al., 1981; Palladino et al., in press). In both groups, the analysis of COHb will reveal that these subjects are light smokers or nonsmokers, respectively. However, nicotine and cotinine levels for such persons are clearly not valid for the determination of their exposure to ETS.

TABLE 8-2 Nicotine Uptake by Nonsmokers Exposed to ETS Under Daily Life Conditions[a]

Authors	Group of Nonsmokers	No. of Nonsmokers Examined	Results		
Russell and Feyerabend, 1975	Hospital employees (urine collection 1 h after lunch)			ng/ml	
	(a) Group 1	14	Nicotine in urine:	12.4 ± 16.9	
	(b) Group 2	13	Nicotine in urine:	8.9 ± 9.1	
Feyerabend et al., 1982	Hospital employees and outpatients			ng/ml	
	(a) nonexposed to ETS during the morning (self report)	30	Nicotine in the urine:	7.5 ± 8.5	
			Nicotine in saliva:	5.9 ± 4.4	
	(b) exposed to ETS during the morning (self report)		Nicotine in urine:	21.6 ± 28.9	
			Nicotine in saliva:	10.1 ± 9.7	
Foliart et al., 1983	Flight attendants (San Francisco-Tokyo-San Francisco)	6	Nicotine in serum:	ng/ml	
			(a) before flight	1.6 ± 0.8	
			(b) after flight	3.2 ± 1.0	
Wald et al., 1984	Hospital staff and outpatients			ng/ml	
	(a) nonexposed to ETS	22	Cotinine in urine:	2.0 (0.0–9.3)	
	(b) exposed to ETS (self report)	199	Cotinine in urine:	6.0 (1.4–22.0)	
				ng/ml	
Wald and Ritchie, 1984	(a) husbands of nonsmokers	101	Cotinine in urine:	8.5 ± 1.3	
	(b) husbands of smokers	20	Cotinine in urine:	25.2 ± 14.8	
Jarvis et al., 1983	Employees in an office, sample collection at 11:30 a.m. (I) and 7:45 p.m. (II) (time between collections including 2-h stay in smoking "pub")	7	ng/ml	Before I	After II
			Nicotine in plasma:	0.76	2.49
			Nicotine in saliva:	1.90	43.63
			Nicotine in urine:	10.51	92.63
			Cotinine in plasma:	1.07	7.33
			Cotinine in saliva:	1.50	8.04
			Cotinine in urine:	4.80	12.94

			(Differences between I and II are statistically highly significant; p values range from <0.01 to <0.001) ng/ml	
Jarvis et al., 1985	Nonsmoking school children (11-16-yr-old)			
	I. Neither parent smoked	269	Cotinine in saliva:	0.44 ± 0.68
	II. Only father smoked	96	Cotinine in saliva:	1.31 ± 1.21
	III. Only mother smoked	76	Cotinine in saliva:	1.95 ± 1.71
	IV. Both parents smoked	128	Cotinine in saliva:	3.38 ± 2.45
Matsukura et al., 1984	472 nonsmokers			
	Urine collection in the morning			
	(a) smokers in home	272	μg cot./mg creat.	0.79 ± 0.1
	(b) nonsmokers in home	200		0.51 ± 0.09
	Cigarettes smoked per day in home of nonsmokers			
	1-9	25	μg cot./mg creat.	0.31 ± 0.08
	10-19	57		0.42 ± 0.10
	20-29	99		0.87 ± 0.19
	30-39	38		1.03 ± 0.25
	>40	28		1.56 ± 0.57
	Unspecified	25		0.56 ± 0.16
Greenberg et al., 1984	Infants under 10 months of age (not breastfed)			
	(a) not exposed to ETS	18	Urine ng nic./mg creat.	0 (0-59)
			Urine ng nic./mg creat.	4 (0-145)
			Saliva ng nic./mg creat.	0 (0-3)
	(b) exposed to ETS	28	Urine ng nic./mg creat.	53 (0-370)
			Urine ng cot./mg creat.	351 (41-1,885)
			Saliva ng nic./mg creat.	12.7 (0-166)
			Saliva ng cot./mg creat.	9 (0-25)

[a]Abbreviations: cot., cotinine; creat., creatinine; nic., nicotine.

TABLE 8-3 Approximate Relations of Nicotine as a Parameter Between Nonsmokers, Passive Smokers, and Active Smokers[a]

	Nonsmokers without ETS Exposure No. = 46		Nonsmokers with ETS Exposure No. = 54		Active Smokers No. = 94
Nicotine/Cotinine	Mean Value	% of Active Smokers' Value	Mean Value	% of Active Smokers' Value	Mean Value
Nicotine (ng/ml)					
in plasma	1.0	7	0.8	5.5	14.8
in saliva	3.8	0.6	5.5	0.8	673
in urine	3.9	0.2	12.1*	0.7	1,750
Cotinine (ng/ml)					
in plasma	0.8	0.3	2.0*	0.7	275
in saliva	0.7	0.2	2.5**	0.8	310
in urine	1.6	0.1	7.7**	0.6	1,390

[a]Differences between nonsmokers exposed to ETS compared with nonsmokers without exposure: *$p < 0.01$; **$p < 0.001$.

SOURCE: Jarvis et al., 1984.

Cotinine elimination in the plasma of nonsmokers exposed to ETS was reported to be slower than cotinine elimination in the plasma of active smokers. Cotinine elimination from urine was also significantly slower. In a study of 10 chronic smokers and 4 nonsmokers experimentally exposed to ETS, the half-life of elimination of cotinine from plasma was 49.7 hours in nonsmokers and 18.5 hours in smokers (Sepkovic et al., 1986). Disappearance of cotinine from urine was also significantly slower in nonsmokers than in chronic smokers (32.7 hours versus 21.9 hours). These preliminary data need to be considered when using cotinine to quantify the dose in nonsmokers exposed to ETS.

In summary, the determination of nicotine and, especially, of cotinine in saliva, blood, and/or urine of nonsmokers exposed to ETS represents at present the most appropriate assay for estimating long-term (average daily) exposure. However, venipuncture needed to get serum samples is often impractical, if not impossible. The use of saliva for nicotine and cotinine assays, despite some advantages, also has certain inherent weaknesses, such as uncharacteristically high readings immediately after heavy ETS exposure and the need to wait several hours after exposure for the cotinine concentration to stabilize (Hoffmann et al., 1984). Saliva is a particularly erratic source on which to make nicotine measures. Urinalysis for cotinine is the preferred method for assessment of long-term ETS exposure, because the sampling is noninvasive, the excretion rate of cotinine is only slightly dependent on the pH of urine, and assessment of the average daily exposure on the basis of cotinine levels is independent of the restrictions posed by variations of the half-life of nicotine in smokers and nonsmokers (Beckett et al., 1971; Klein and Gorrod, 1978).

Creatinine—Reference Compound for Urine Analysis

Urine sampling does have some associated problems. Often it is impractical to collect 24-hour urine samples for the analysis of biological markers of direct exposure to tobacco smoke or to ETS unless undertaken under strict medical supervision, such as in a metabolic ward. In this case, the ratio of biological markers to creatinine is often used to allow for variations in fluid intake (and excretion) (see Table 8-1).

Creatinine excretion varies from person to person, but the daily output for each individual is almost constant from day to day. Urinary creatinine bears a direct relation to the muscle mass of the individual. The milligram amount of creatinine excreted during 24 hours per kilogram of body weight is often expressed as the creatinine coefficient. The coefficient varies from 18 to 32 in men (total excretion 1.1-3.2 g/day) and from 10 to 25 in women (total excretion 0.9-2.5 g/day). The coefficient is largely independent of variations in diet, since creatinine in healthy persons is of endogenous origin. In older people, the daily output of creatinine may decrease to 0.5 g/day. In cigarette smokers, urinary output of creatinine in men appears to decrease with greater number of cigarettes smoked per day (Adlkofer et al., 1984). However, this finding needs to be confirmed.

Based on the variations in daily creatinine excretions in the urine, one has to be aware of the limitation of the factor "amount of biological marker per milligram of creatinine." In a study with 15 adult male cigarette smokers, the daily creatinine excretion varied between 1.0 and 2.5 g and the cotinine excretion between 1.3 and 13.1 mg (Hoffmann and Brunnemann, 1983). However, in certain cases, such as with healthy infants, the daily variations in urinary excretion are rather small. Thus, the measured nanograms of cotinine per milligram of creatinine in urine reflect the inhalation of environmental nicotine from ETS rather well (Greenberg et al., 1984).

For the determination in urine, creatinine is complexed with picric acid and the resulting red color is measured spectrophotometrically, a task now predominately done with an autoanalyzer (Faulkner et al., 1976).

Although the determination of cotinine in urine without reference to creatinine has resulted in meaningful data in some studies, the standardized cotinine levels per unit of creatinine may give a more stable measure of ETS exposure—particularly when limited urine samples must be used.

Hydroxyproline

Inhalation of nitrogen dioxide causes degradation of lung collagen and elastin (Kosmidar et al., 1972; Hatton et al., 1977). This degradation results in elevated urinary excretion of hydroxyproline (Lewis, 1980). It is thus possible that the NO_2 in tobacco smoke, and even NO_2 in ETS, has the same lung-damaging effect as pure NO_2.

Kasuga et al. (1981) reported two studies in which healthy cigarette smokers excreted significantly more hydroxyproline than healthy nonsmokers and exsmokers. In the case of 6- to 11-year-old children of smoking parents, Kausga et al. (1981) found elevated hydroxyproline levels in the urine. Because of the relatively low concentration of NO_2 in ETS (see Chapter 2), this finding was unexpected. Adlkofer et al. (1984) were unable to confirm this finding in a study of 23 nonsmokers exposed to ETS.

At present, the question of quantitative aspects of urinary hydroxyproline excretion in nonsmokers exposed to ETS is not settled. It will require additional studies before this compound and its ratio to creatinine can be used as indicators for the degree of ETS exposure.

N-Nitrosoproline

N-nitrosoproline (NPRO) in urine reflects endogenous formation of nitrosamines, many of which are known animal carcinogens (Preussmann and Steward, 1984; Vainio et al., 1985). NPRO appears neither to undergo metabolism in mammals nor to alkylate cellular macromolecules. NPRO is considered to be nonmutagenic and noncarcinogenic and is excreted nearly quantitatively in urine. It has been shown that endogenous formation of NPRO is significantly increased in cigarette smokers (Hoffmann and Brunnemann, 1983; Ladd et al., 1984; Scherer and Adlkofer, in press). The increase is probably due to the high concentrations of nitrogen oxides in tobacco smoke that serve as nitrosating agents and the elevated concentration of thiocyanate in smokers that catalytically enhance the endogenous formation of nitrosamines such as NPRO. These effects are absent in nonsmokers without ETS exposure.

In one 5-day study, four male nonsmokers with controlled diets were exposed to known degrees of ETS for three periods of 80 minutes each on day 3 and day 4. Their 24-hour urine voids were analyzed for NPRO and for cotinine. While the cotinine levels in the urine of these nonsmokers increased from 5-7 ng/ml to 215-360 ng/ml, the NPRO excretion did not significantly change (Brunnemann et al., 1984). In another controlled study with 10 nonsmokers exposed to ETS containing 45 ppb of NO_2, 400 ppb of NO, and 22 ppm of CO, urinary output of NPRO was also not elevated while COHb had increased significantly (Scherer and Adlkofer, in press). Although these two studies require confirmation and should include analytical assessment of nitrosothioproline (NTPRO) (Tsuda et al., 1986), another endogenously formed nitrosamine, at present neither NPRO nor NTPRO measurement in urine can be used to indicate exposure to ETS.

Aromatic Amines

During the burning of cigarettes, 20-30 times more aromatic amines are released into the sidestream smoke than are present in the mainstream smoke (see Chapter 2). Although at this time there is a lack of analytical data, it may be assumed that indoor environments that are strongly polluted with ETS contain measurably higher amounts of aromatic amines than ambient air without tobacco smoke pollution.

Preliminary data indicate that free aniline and *o*-toluidine, serving as surrogates for aromatic amines, are increased, although not significantly, in the 24-hour urine voids of cigarette smokers (3.1 ± 2.6 μg and 6.3 ± 3.7 μg) compared with nonsmokers (2.8 ± 2.5 μg and 4.1 ± 3.2 μg) (El-Bayoumy et al., in press). The next step requires the assay of the metabolites of aniline and *o*-toluidine in the urine of both smokers and nonsmokers. A study of the urinary excretion of aromatic amines in passive smokers would be indicated only if the total amounts of individual amines and their metabolites in smokers' urine are found to be significantly increased.

GENOTOXICITY OF THE URINE

The evaluation of the genotoxicity of urine in nonsmokers with ETS exposure must consider the possibility of confounding effects, because DNA modifiers may be present in urine as a consequence of dietary intake or as a secondary result of the activity of infectious agents in the urine of the host. Nevertheless, urinary constituents may be DNA modifiers, because the inhaled agents are known or suspected mutagens or because the inhaled agents lead to the formation of such biologically active compounds.

Since 1975, the most widely used assay for genotoxicity of human urine is the determination of mutagenicity in bacterial-tested strains with and without activation by enzyme-induced liver homogenate.

In 1977, Yamasaki and Ames reported the presence of mutagens in the urine of cigarette smokers, thus suggesting a correlation between mutagens in smokers' urine and increased risk for bladder cancer. Since publication of these data, other studies have reported an association of urinary mutagens that are active in bacterial tester strains with cigarette smoking (International Agency for Research on Cancer, 1986), but not all results from these studies have been consistent. One reason for the divergent findings could be the influence of dietary factors on the mutagens in the urine of smokers (Sasson et al., 1985) and, perhaps also, nonsmokers exposed to ETS.

Three studies have attempted to explain the possible mutagenic activity of the urine of nonsmokers exposed to ETS. In one study, fractions and subfractions were isolated by high-pressure liquid chromatography (HPLC) from the urine of five passive smokers. Upon metabolic activation by S9 liver homogenates from rats pretreated with 3-methylcholanthrene, these materials were mutagenic in TA-bacterial tester strains (Putzrath et al., 1981). It appeared that these mutagens are a complex mixture of urinary components in the polar lipophilic subfractions. Due to a lack of diet control, these results are ambiguous.

In a second assay of urine for bacterial mutagenicity, 8 male nonsmokers (25 and 35 years of age) were placed in a poorly ventilated room (10 m^3) with 10 smokers for an 8-hour period (Bos et al., 1983). The 12-hour urine samples of the nonsmokers were collected before, during, and after exposure to ETS. Metabolically activated concentrates of the urine samples were analyzed for mutagenic activity in the tester strain, TA 1538. Urine samples collected directly after exposure to ETS were significantly more mutagenic (relative activity: 3.9 ± 1.0) than urine samples of the same nonsmokers prior to (3.1 ± 0.7) or long after ETS exposure (2.5 ± 0.5).

In the third study, six women who were medical students were exposed to ETS in a 10-m^3 exposure chamber on 2 consecutive days for one 3-hour session in the mornings and a 2-hour session in the afternoons. During these sessions, three of the women smoked a total of 30 cigarettes per day of a low-yield filter-tipped brand (5.4 mg tar, 0.4 nicotine, 4.6 mg CO); the other three women did not smoke. After 3 days without exposure and without cigarette smoking by any of the women, the exposure was repeated with reversal of the roles, so that those who had previously been nonsmokers now were smokers, and vice versa. The CO concentration in the chamber averaged 3.0 ± 0.9 ppm. The uptake of smoke was assessed by determination of COHb, cotinine, and thiocyanate in the plasma. Urine samples were collected at the end of the daily smoking periods. Urine was concentrated according to Yamasaki and Ames (1977) and tested for mutagenicity with tested strain TB98 using rat liver homogenate for metabolic activation (Sorsa et al., 1985). As is evident from the data in Table 8-4, COHb values for nonsmokers and passive smokers were indistinguishable, while there was a trend for higher plasma cotinine values in the passive smokers. The authors observed an increase in the mutagenicity of the urine of passive smokers during the period of study. The differences observed were not significant.

On the basis of presently available data, it is likely that the exposure of nonsmokers to heavy ETS increases the potential for metabolically activated genotoxic activity of their urine above and beyond the mutagenic activity that is observed in urine of the same nonsmokers before and long after exposure to ETS. However, before validating the Ames bacterial assay for mutagenicity as an

TABLE 8-4 Pooled Data of Various Biological Parameters Measured in Blood and Urine of Six Subjects After Periods of Nonsmoking, Passive Smoking, and Active Smoking

	COHb		Plasma Cotinine		Plasma Thiocyanate		Mutagenicity in Urine	
Exposure	Number of samples	Mean ± SE, %	Number of samples	Mean ± SE, ng/ml	Number of samples	Mean ± SE, μmol/L	Number of samples	Mean ± SE, number of induced revertants/ml
No smoking	12	0.57 ± 0.04[a]	12	1.4 ± 0.2	12	70.8 ± 9.9	12	4.2 ± 1.2
Passive smoking	12	0.55 ± 0.05[a]	12	2.1 ± 0.4[b]	12	71.8 ± 9.9	24	5.8 ± 1.0
Active smoking	12	3.38 ± 0.54	12	54.4 ± 11.4	12	70.7 ± 10.2	24	6.4 ± 0.8

[a] Values below the detection limit (0.5%) included as 0.4%.

[b] Difference between nonsmoking and passive smoking values not significant but suggestive ($p < 0.10$; t-test).

SOURCE: Sorsa et al., 1985.

appropriate method for estimating the genotoxic effect of the urine of ETS-exposed nonsmokers, the method itself and the diet of test subjects have to be standardized. Research in this area is needed, as are studies on the isolation and identification of the active agents in the urine of ETS-exposed nonsmokers.

Adducts Formed in Passive Smokers upon Exposure to ETS

Since about 1975, highly sensitive methods have been developed for the determination of protein- or DNA-adducts of environmental carcinogens and toxic agents in circulating blood. Methods probing these reactions for the toxic agents known to occur in tobacco smoke and ETS include determination of hemoglobin adducts of nitrosodimethylamine, methyl chloride, vinyl chloride, and benzene (National Institute of Environmental Health Sciences, 1984), as well as 4-aminobiphenyl (Green et al., 1984). DNA adducts with the smoke carcinogen, benzo[*a*]pyrene (B*a*P), have been described (Santella et al., 1985), and the tobacco-specific 4-(*N*-methyl-*N*-nitrosamino)-1-(3-pyridyl)-1-butanone (NNK) leads to O^6-methylguanine in DNA (Hoffmann and Hecht, 1985). RIA's have been developed for quantitative determination of both the B*a*P-DNA adduct and O^6-methylguanine (Perera et al., 1982; Foiles et al., 1985). So far, the method for the determination of the DNA adducts has been applied to the analysis of benzo[*a*]pyrene in smokers (Shamsuddin et al., 1985). In addition, the hemoglobin-4-aminobiphenyl assay has been used for the analysis of the blood of smokers (Tannenbaum et al., in press). In both cases, only a limited number of samples have been analyzed for these adducts. Nevertheless, the data appear encouraging. Another sensitive method for quantifying DNA adducts is the P^{32}-postlabelling technique, which has been applied to human tissues (Gupta et al., 1982; Everson et al., 1986).

Validation and quantitative determination of the uptake of tobacco smoke carcinogens is urgently needed. Assays of adducts of B*a*P, aromatic amines, and tobacco-specific nitrosamines with protein or DNA in the circulating blood are the most promising tests of exposure to tobacco smoke. Once such assays have been advanced to yield reproducible, informative methods in smokers, they may be subsequently refined to such sensitivities that they will also furnish reliable data on such adducts in the blood of passive smokers.

FUTURE NEEDS

At present, the best method for quantifying human exposure to ETS is the assay of nicotine and cotinine in urine and possibly saliva. Nicotine and cotinine can also be determined in serum samples, but these samples require invasive techniques. In smoke-polluted environments, nicotine is present in the vapor phase as a free base, thus its uptake by the passive smoker may not be representative of the uptake of acidic and neutral smoke components from the vapor phase nor of any component in the particulate phase. Thus, future studies should be concerned with developing techniques to measure the uptake by the nonsmoker of various other types of tobacco-specific ETS components. This may include assays for the vapor-phase 3-vinylpyridine or flavor components that are indigenous to tobacco. Particulate-phase agents to be traced could include solanesol, tobacco-specific nitrosamines, and polyphenols such as chlorogenic acid or rutin. These components are likely to be found only in trace amounts in ETS, and, thus, only minute quantities would be found in the circulating blood of passive smokers, making the development of assays difficult. The development of new trace methods for quantifying the levels of some tobacco-specific materials in nonsmokers may require the identification of adducts formed between the ETS components and the proteins in blood. This approach would require the development of highly sensitive methods such as immunoassays (e.g., RIA, ELISA) or postlabelling with radioisotopes or other markers.

The epidemiological studies on the effects of exposure to ETS by nonsmokers have to consider a number of non-ETS-related factors. This fact underlines the urgent need for the development of highly sensitive dosimetric methods for ETS-specific carcinogens that can be applied in field studies.

SUMMARY AND RECOMMENDATIONS

Passive smokers are exposed to trace amounts of toxic agents including tumor initiators, tumor promoters, carcinogens, and organ-specific carcinogens when inhaling ETS. The determination of thiocyanate, nicotine, and cotinine in body fluids such as saliva, serum, and urine, as well as quantitication of CO in alveolar air and COHb in blood, has been useful for the assessment of the habits of individuals and groups of smokers of cigarettes, cigars, and pipes. Currently, for measuring the exposure to ETS by nonsmokers, nicotine and cotinine appear useful. In acute exposure studies, COHb can be a useful marker.

Nicotine and cotinine, however, may not be directly related to the carcinogenic potential of the smoke. Indicators that are related to the carcinogenic risk are needed. To assess the risks involved in the exposure to carcinogenic agents from ETS, sensitive dosimetry methods for tobacco-specific compounds are urgently needed. During the last decade, immunoassays and postlabelling methods have been developed for tracing toxic and carcinogenic agents in circulating blood. These methodologies should be used for the development of dosimetry studies in nonsmokers exposed to ETS. Protein and DNA adducts may provide exposure measures that could be effectively used in epidemiologic studies.

What Is Known

1. Determinations of thiocyanate, nicotine, and cotinine in saliva, serum, and urine, as well as quantification of CO in alveolar air and carboxyhemoglobin in blood, have been shown to be useful parameters for the assessment of the habits of individuals and groups of active smokers of cigarettes, cigars, and pipes. However, in general, only nicotine and its metabolite cotinine have proven useful for measuring the exposure to ETS of nonsmokers.

2. Assessment of average daily exposure on the basis of cotinine levels in saliva and urine is independent of the restrictions posed by variations of the half-life of nicotine in smokers and nonsmokers.

3. The determination in urine of the amount of cotinine per milligram of creatinine should provide a more stable measure of recent environmental exposure to nicotine from ETS than cotinine without reference to creatinine, particularly when limited volumes of urine are available.

4. It is likely that the exposure of nonsmokers to ETS increases the mutagenic activity of their urine over the activity observed in urine of the same nonsmokers when not exposed to ETS.

What Scientific Information Is Missing

1. The question of urinary hydroxyproline excretion in nonsmokers exposed to ETS is not settled.

2. A study on the urinary excretion of aromatic amines in nonsmokers exposed to ETS is needed in order to correlate the total amounts of individual amines and their metabolites in the urine of nonsmokers exposed to ETS.

3. Where exposure histories can be specified clearly, validation of the use of adduct assays to determine and quantify uptake of tobacco smoke carcinogens is needed.

4. Information is needed on certain tobacco-specific constituents and their fate in the ETS-exposed nonsmoker, including solanesol, tobacco-specific nitrosamines, and polyphenols such as chlorogenic acid or rutin.

5. Knowledge of the levels of nitrosothioproline following exposure to ETS as well as nitrosoproline is needed.

6. Knowledge of the effects of diet is needed when interpreting results of the Ames bacterial assay for mutagenicity of the urine of ETS-exposed nonsmokers.

7. Identification of the mutagenic agents in the urine of ETS-exposed nonsmokers needs to be made.

8. Future studies should be concerned with methodologies that enable us to assay the uptake by the nonsmoker of various other types of ETS components that are tobacco-specific.

9. New trace methods will have to be developed for dosimetry studies of carcinogens involving adducts (DNA and protein) and the development of highly sensitive methods such as immunoassays or postlabelling for other products.

10. The epidemiological studies on the effects of ETS exposure in nonsmokers should consider a number of non-ETS-related factors. This fact underlines the urgent need for the development of highly sensitive dosimetric methods for ETS-specific carcinogens that can be applied in field studies.

REFERENCES

Adlkofer, F., G. Scherer, and W.D. Heller. Hydroxyproline excretion in urine of smokers and passive smokers. Prev. Med. 13:670-679, 1984.

Adlkofer, F., G. Scherer, and U. von Hees. Passive smoking. N. Engl. J. Med. 312:719-720, 1985.

Aldrige, W.N. A new method for the estimation of micro quantities of cyanide and thiocyanate. Analyst 69:262-265, 1944.

Beckett, A.H., J.W. Gorrod, and P. Jenner. The analysis of nicotine—1′-N-oxide in urine, in the presence of nicotine and cotinine, and its application to the study of *in vivo* nicotine metabolism in man. J. Pharm. Pharmacol. 23:55S-61S, 1971.

Benowitz, N.L., F. Kuyt, and P. Jacob III. Circadian blood nicotine concentrations during cigarette smoking. Clin. Pharmacol. Ther. 32:758-764, 1982.

Bos, R.P., J.L.G. Theuws, and P.Th. Henderson. Excretion of mutagens in human urine after passive smoking. Cancer Lett. 19:85-90, 1983.

Bowler, R.G. The determination of thiocyanate in blood serum. Biochem. J. 38:385-388, 1944.

Brunnemann, K.D., J.C. Scott, N.J. Haley, and D. Hoffmann. Endogenous formation of N-nitrosoproline upon cigarette smoke inhalation. IARC Sci. Publ. 57:819-828, 1984.

Butts, W.C., M. Kuehneman, and G.M. Widdowson. Automated method for determining serum thiocyanate to distinguish smokers from nonsmokers. Clin. Chem. 20:1344-1348, 1974.

Cano, J.-P., J. Catalin, R. Badre, C. Dumas, A. Viala, and R. Guillerme. Determination de la nicotine par chromatographie en phase gazeuse. II. Applications. Ann. Pharm. Fr. 28:633-640, 1970.

Coburn, R.F., W.J. Williams, and R.E. Forster. Effects of erythrocyte destruction on carbon monoxide production in man. J. Clin. Invest. 43: 1098-1103, 1964.

Coultas, D.B., J.M. Samet, C.A. Howard, G.T. Peake, and B.J. Skipper. Salivary cotinine levels and passive tobacco smoke exposure in the home. Am. Rev. Respir. Dis. 133:A157, 1986.

El-Bayoumy, K., J.M. Donahue, S.S. Hecht, and D. Hoffmann. Identification and quantitative determination of aniline and toluidines in human urine. Cancer Res., in press.

Everson, R.B., E. Randerath, R.M. Santella, R.C. Cefalo, T.A. Avitts, and K. Randerath. Detection of smoking-related covalent DNA adducts in human placenta. Science 231:54-57, 1986.

Faulkner, W.R., and J. W. King. Renal function, pp. 981, 997-999. In N.W. Tietz, S. Berger, and W.T. Caraway, Eds. Fundamentals of Clinical Chemistry. Philadelphia: Saunders, 1976.

Feyerabend, C., T. Higgenbottam, and M.A.H. Russell. Nicotine concentrations in urine and saliva of smokers and nonsmokers. Br. Med. J. 284:1002-1004, 1982.

Feyerabend, C., and M.A.H. Russell. Assay of nicotine in biological materials: Sources of contamination and their elimination. J. Pharm. Pharmacol. 32:178-181, 1980.

Foiles, P.G., N. Trushin, and A. Castonguay. Measurement of 0^6-methyldeoxyguanosine in DNA methylated by the tobacco-specific carcinogen 4-(methylnitrosamino)-1-(3-pyridyl)-1-butanone using a biotin-avidin enzyme-linked immunosorbent assay. Carcinogenesis 6:989-993, 1985.

Foliart, D., N.L. Benowitz, and C.E. Becker. Passive absorption of nicotine in airline flight attendants. N. Engl. J. Med. 308:1105, 1983.

Gillies, P.A., B. Wilcox, C. Coates, F. Kristmundsdöttir, and D.J. Reid. Use of objective measurement in the validation of self-reported smoking in children aged 10 and 11 years: Saliva thiocyanate. J. Epidemiol. Comm. Health 36:205-208, 1982.

Green, L.C., P.L. Skipper, R.J. Turesky, M.S. Bryant, and S.R. Tannenbaum. *In vivo* dosimetry of 4-aminobiphenyl in rats via a cysteine adduct in hemoglobin. Cancer Res. 44:4254-4259, 1984.

Greenberg, R.A., N.J. Haley, R.A. Etzel, and F.A. Loda. Measuring the exposure of infants to tobacco smoke: Nicotine and cotinine in urine and saliva. N. Engl. J. Med. 310:1075-1078, 1984.

Gupta, R.C., M.V. Reddy, and K. Randerath. ^{32}P-postlabeling analysis of non-radioactive aromatic carcinogen-DNA adducts. Carcinogenesis 9:1081-1092, 1982.

Haley, N.J., C.M. Axelrad, and K.A. Tilton. Validation of self-reported smoking behavior: Biochemical analyses of cotinine and thiocyanate. Am. J. Public Health 93:1204-1207, 1983.

Hatton, D.V., C.S. Leach, A.E. Nicogossian, and N.N. Ferrante. Collagen breakdown and nitrogen dioxide inhalation. Arch. Environ. Health 32:33-36, 1977.

Harke, H.-P. Zum Problem des Passiv-Rauchens. Münch. Med. Wochenschr. 112:2328:2334, 1970.

Hauth, J.C., J. Hauth, R.B. Drawbaugh, L.C. Gilstrap III, and W.P. Pierson. Passive smoking and thiocyanate concentrations in pregnant women and newborns. Obstet. Gynecol. 63:519-522, 1984.

Heinemann, G., H. Schievelbein, and F. Richter. Die analytische und diagnostische Validität der Bestimmung von Carboxyhämoglobin im Blut und Kohlenmonoxid in der Atemluft von Rauchern und Nichtrauchern. J. Clin. Chem. Clin. Biochem. 22:229-235, 1984.

Hill, P., N.J Haley, and E.L. Wynder. Cigarette smoking: Carboxyhemoglobin, plasma nicotine, cotinine and thiocyanate levels vs. self-reported data and cardiovascular disease. J. Chron. Dis. 36:439-449, 1983.

Hoffmann, D., and K.D. Brunnemann. Endogenous formation of N-nitrosoproline in cigarette smokers. Cancer Res. 43:5570-5574, 1983.

Hoffmann, D., N.J. Haley, J.D. Adams, and K.D. Brunnemann. Tobacco sidestream smoke: Uptake by nonsmokers. Prev. Med. 13:608-617, 1984.

Hoffmann, D., and S.S. Hecht. Nicotine-derived N-nitrosamines and tobacco-related cancer: Current status and future directions. Cancer Res. 45:935-944, 1985.

Huch, R., J. Danko, L. Spatling, and R. Huch. Risks the passive smoker runs. Lancet 2:1376, 1980.

International Agency for Research on Cancer (IARC) Monograph. Evaluation of the Carcinogenic Risk of Chemicals to Humans, Vol. 38, pp. 163-314. Tobacco Smoking. Lyons: IARC, 1986. 421 pp.

Jacob, P., III, M. Wilson, and N.L. Benowitz. Improved gas chromatographic method for the determination of nicotine and cotinine in biologic fluids. J. Chromatogr. 222:61-70, 1981.

Jarvis, M.J. Serum thiocyanate in passive smoking. Lancet 1:169, 1985.

Jarvis, M.J., and M.A.H. Russell. Measurement and estimation of smoke dosage to non-smokers from environmental tobacco smoke. Eur. J. Respir. Dis. 65(Suppl. 133):68-75, 1984.

Jarvis, M.J., M.A.H. Russell, and C. Feyerabend. Absorption of nicotine and carbon monoxide from passive smoking under natural conditions of exposure. Thorax 38:829-833, 1983.

Jarvis, M., H. Tunstall-Pedoe, C. Feyerabend, C. Vesey, and Y. Saloojee. Biochemical markers of smoke absorption and self reported exposure to passive smoking. J. Epidemiol. Comm. Health 38:335-339, 1984.

Jarvis, M.J., M.A.H. Russell, C. Feyerabend, J.R. Eiser, M. Morgan, P. Gammage, and E.M. Gray. Passive exposure to tobacco smoke: Saliva cotinine concentrations in a representative population sample of non-smoking schoolchildren. Br. Med. J. 291:927-929, 1985.

Junge, B., D. Borges, M.-B. Berkholz, W. Thefeld, and H. Hoffmeister. Thiocyanat im Serum als Indikator für die Schadstoffbelastung durch Tabakrauch. Arbeitsmed. Sozialmed. Praeventivmed. 13:13-18, 1978.

Kasuga, H., H. Matsuki, and F. Osaka. Smoking effects and urinary hydroxyproline. Presented at the 9th International Scientific Meeting of International Epidemiological Association, Edinburgh, Scotland, 1981. 14 pp.

Klein, A.E., and J.W. Gorrod. Metabolism of nicotine in cigarette smokers during pregnancy. Eur. J. Drug Metab. Pharmocokinet. 3:87-93, 1978.

Kosmidar, S., K. Ludyga, A. Misiewica, M. Drozda, and J. Sagan. Experimental and clinical investigations on the emphysema forming action of nitrogen oxides. Zentralbl. Arbeitsmed. Arbeitsschutz 22:326-368, 1972.

Ladd, K.F., H.L. Newmark, and M.C. Archer. N-Nitrosation of proline in smokers and nonsmokers. J. Natl. Cancer Inst. 73:83-87, 1984.

Langone, J.J., H. Gjika, and H. VanVunakis. Nicotine and its metabolites. Radioimmunoassays for nicotine and cotinine. Biochemistry 12:5025-5030. 1973.

Leaderer, B.P. Air pollutant emissions from kerosene space heaters. Science 218:1113-1115, 1982.

Lewis, T.R. Criteria relevant to an occupational health standard for nitrogen dioxide, pp. 361-375. In S.D. Lee, Ed. Nitrogen Oxides and Their Effects on Health. Ann Arbor: Ann Arbor Science Publications, 1980.

Luepker, R.V., T.F. Pechacek, D.M. Murray, C.A. Johnson, F. Hund, and D.R. Jacobs. Saliva thiocyanate: A chemical indicator of cigarette smoking in adolescents. Am. J. Public Health 71:1320-1324, 1981.

Matsukura, S., T. Taminato, N. Kitano, Y. Seino, H. Hamada, M. Uchihashi, H. Nakajima, and Y. Hirata. Effects of environmental tobacco smoke on urinary cotinine excretion in nonsmokers. N. Engl. J. Med. 311:828-832, 1984.

National Research Council, Committee Medical and Biologic Effects of Environmental Pollutant. Carbon Monoxide. Washington, D.C.: National Academy Press, 1981. 239 pp.

National Institute of Environmental Health Sciences (NIEHS). Biochemical and cellular markers of chemical exposure and preclinical indicators of disease, pp. 197-257. In Human Health in the Environment. Some Research Needs: Report of the Third Task Force for Research Planning in Environmental Health Science. Bethesda, Maryland: National Institutes of Health, 1984. 407 pp. (Available from the U.S. Government Printing Office as NIH Publ. No. 86-1277.)

Palladino, G., J.D. Adams, K.D. Brunnemann, N.J. Haley, and D. Hoffmann. Snuff-dipping in college students: A clinical profile. Military Med., in press.

Pekkanen, T.J., O. Elo, and M.L. Hanninen. Changes in non-smokers' saliva thiocyanate levels after being in a tobacco smoke-filled room. World Smoking Health 1:37-39, 1976.

Perera, F.P., M.C. Poirier, S.H. Yuspa, J. Nakayama, A. Jaretzki, M.M. Curnen, D.M. Knowles, and I.B. Weinstein. A pilot project in molecular cancer epidemiology: Determination of benzo(a)pyrene-DNA adducts in animal and human tissues by immunoassays. Carcinogenesis 3:1405-1410, 1982.

Pittenger, D.J. Passive smoking. N. Engl. J. Med. 312:720, 1985.

Poulton, J., G.W. Rylance, A.W.J. Taylor, and C. Edwards. Serum thiocyanate levels as indicator of passive smoking in children. Lancet 2:1405-1406, 1984.

Preussmann, R., and B.W. Stewart. N-nitroso carcinogens, pp. 643-828. In C. Stearle, Ed. Carcinogens. American Chemical Society Monograph 182. Washington, D.C.: American Chemical Society, 1984.

Putzrath, R.M., D. Langley, and E. Eisenstadt. Analysis of mutagenic activity in cigarette smokers' urine by high performance liquid chromatography. Mutat. Res. 85:97-108, 1981.

Russell, M.A.H., and C. Feyerabend. Blood and urinary nicotine in non-smokers. Lancet 1:179-181, 1975.

Russell, M.A.H., M. Raw, and M.J. Jarvis. Clinical use of nicotine chewing-gum. Br. Med. J. 280:1599-1602, 1980.

Russell, M.A.H., M.J. Jarvis, G. Devitt, and C. Feyerabend. Nicotine intake by snuff users. Br. Med. J. 283:814-817, 1981.

Santella, R.M., L.-L. Hsieh, C.-D. Lin, S. Viet, and I.B. Weinstein. Quantitation of exposure to benzo(a)pyrene with monoclonal antibodies. Environ. Health Perspect. 62:95-99, 1985.

Sasson, I.M., D.T. Coleman, E.J. LaVoie, D. Hoffmann, and E.L. Wynder. Mutagens in human urine: Effects of cigarette smoking and diet. Mutat. Res. 158:149-157, 1985.

Scherer, G., and F. Adlkofer. Endogenous formation of N-nitrosoproline in smokers and nonsmokers. In D. Hoffmann and C. Harris, Eds. Mechanisms in Tobacco Carcinogenesis (Banbury Report 23). Cold Spring Harbor, New York: Cold Spring Harbor Laboratories, in press.

Sepkovic, D.W., N.J. Haley, and D. Hoffmann. Elimination from the body of tobacco products by smokers and passive smokers. J. Am. Med. Assoc. 256:863, 1986 (letter).

Shamsuddin, A.K.M., N.T. Sinopoli, K. Hemminki, R.R. Boesch, and C.C. Harris. Detection of benzo(a)pyrene: DNA adducts in human white blood cells. Cancer Res. 45:66-68, 1985.

Sorsa, M., P. Einistö, K. Husgafvel-Pursianinen, H. Järventaus, H. Kivistö, Y. Peltonen, T. Tuomi, and S. Valkonen. Passive and active exposure to cigarette smoke in a smoking experiment. J. Toxicol. Environ. Health 16:523-534, 1985.

Tannenbaum, S.R., M.S. Bryant, P.L. Skipper, and M. Maclure. Hemoglobin adducts of tobacco-related aromatic amines: Application to molecular epidemiology. In D. Hoffmann and C. Harris, Eds. Mechanisms in Tobacco Carcinogenesis (Banbury Report 23). Cold Spring Harbor, New York: Cold Spring Harbor Laboratories, in press.

Tsuda, M., J. Niitusuma, S. Sato, T. Hirayama, T. Kakizoe, and T. Sugimura. Increase in the levels of N-nitrosoproline, N-nitrothioproline, and N-nitro-2-methylthioproline in human urine by cigarette smoking. Cancer Lett. 30:177-124, 1986.

Vainio, H., K. Hemminki, and J. Wilbourn. Data on the carcinogenicity of chemicals in the IARC monographs programme. Carcinogenesis 6:1653-1665, 1985.

Vogt, T.M., S. Selvin, and J.H. Billings. Smoking cessation program: Baseline carbon monoxide and serum thiocyanate levels as predictors of outcome. Am. J. Public Health 69:1156-1159, 1979.

Wald, N.J., and C. Ritchie. Validation of studies on lung cancer in non-smokers married to smokers. Lancet 1:1607, 1984.

Wald, N.J., M. Idle, J. Boreham, A. Bailey, and H. Van Vunakis. Serum cotinine levels in pipe smokers: Evidence against nicotine as cause of coronary heart disease. Lancet 2:775-777, 1981.

Wald, N.J., J.Boreham, A. Bailey, C. Ritchie, J.E. Haddow, and G. Knight. Urinary cotinine as marker for breathing other people's tobacco smoke. Lancet 1:230-231, 1984.

Yamasaki, E., and B.N. Ames. Concentration of mutagens from urine by adsorption with the nonpolar resin XAD-2: Cigarette smokers have mutagenic urine. Proc. Natl. Acad. Sci. USA 74:3555-3559, 1977.

III
HEALTH EFFECTS POSSIBLY ASSOCIATED WITH EXPOSURE TO ENVIRONMENTAL TOBACCO SMOKE BY NONSMOKERS

9
Introduction

Epidemiologic and experimental studies seek to determine if a relationship exists between a particular exposure and particular health effects. When the exposure is via the air, as is the case with environmental tobacco smoke (ETS) exposure to nonsmokers, the organs that are directly exposed include the eyes, nose, throat, and lungs. Clinical, epidemiologic, and animal studies have shown, generally speaking, that air pollutants can have major health effects on the respiratory system (National Research Council, 1985). Experimental research using animals (Chapter 3) and research with biological markers in humans (Chapter 8) indicate that various constituents of the smoke are absorbed into the blood and, therefore, are transported to organs and tissues of the body. Consequently, the range of possible health effects of exposure to ETS may be very broad and vary enormously in their effect on the individual. Effects may be reversible or irreversible, discomforting, or life-threatening.

In the following chapters, several possible health effects that have received substantial attention are reviewed. Many of the health effects associated with active smoking have been evaluated in studies of nonsmokers exposed to ETS. These include: acute, noxious sensory irritation; nonmalignant respiratory symptoms and disease; decrease in pulmonary function; lung and other cancers; cardiovascular disease; relative growth, ear infections in children; and low birthweight of children of nonsmoking women.

Nonsmokers commonly complain of the perception of tobacco smoke and its irritating, noxious, or annoying qualities. However, in most such spontaneous instances, these complaints are voiced because the subjects can *see* another person actively smoking in their vicinity. Chapter 10 reviews experimental studies that evaluate these acute comfort aspects under controlled conditions.

Chapters 11 and 12 assess and evaluate possible nonneoplastic and neoplastic pulmonary effects of exposure to ETS by nonsmokers. Over the past 15 years, a number of studies in children and in adults have assessed various possible acute and chronic pulmonary effects subsequent to long-term exposure to ETS. Individuals who have chronic lung diseases, such as patients with asthma, alpha-l-antitrypsin deficiency, or cystic fibrosis, are potentially hypersensitive to the effects of ETS exposures.

Chapter 13 reviews and evaluates reports of cancers other than lung that may be associated with exposure to ETS in nonsmokers.

Chapter 14 discusses the possible association of exposure to ETS with chronic and acute cardiovascular responses and cardiovascular diseases in nonsmokers. Individuals with chronic disease that compromise the cardiovascular system, such as patients with a history of angina pectoris, are at a high risk for developing abnormal cardiovascular responses following exposure.

Chapter 15 considers evidence that a number of other health effects are linked to ETS exposure in children of smokers, including lower relative growth, frequency of ear infections, and low birthweight (with nonsmoking pregnant mothers).

The studies reviewed here are epidemiologic and experimental. Epidemiologic studies include case-control studies, in which subjects are selected according to whether or not they have the health outcome being studied, and cohort (or prospective) studies, in which subjects are classified according to whether or not they have been exposed to ETS. Cross-sectional studies are those in which an assessment is made of a population at one point in time. Longitudinal studies follow a group of persons over time. In experimental studies, subjects are exposed to ETS under controlled conditions often using chamber studies. Most studies of ETS have been cross-sectional rather than longitudinal. To be informative, a study must evaluate a sufficient number of people to provide a precise estimate of the effect; obtain valid information regarding the history of exposure and health status of the individuals; and, of course, the statistical analyses must be appropriate to the study design. The appropriate design and use of these epidemiologic methods for the study of air pollution and possible health effects are discussed in general terms in the monograph "Epidemiology and Air Pollution" (National Research Council, 1985).

REFERENCE

National Research Council, Committee on the Epidemiology of Air Pollutants. Epidemiology and Air Pollution. Washington, D.C.: National Academy Press, 1985. 224 pp.

10
Sensory Reactions to and Irritation Effects of Environmental Tobacco Smoke

In this chapter, the acute sensory reactions from exposure to ETS are discussed. These reactions include perception of odor and irritation of eyes and upper airways. Methods for evaluating these psychosensory phenomena include controlled chamber studies, where ventilation and smoking rates are manipulated and evaluated in terms of reported perception by a small number of subjects.

ODOR

The perception of odor is often the earliest indicator of exposure to many airborne contaminants, but not for all. For some individuals, odor may merely be a nuisance. For others, odor is an early indicator of a complex reaction to exposure to ETS involving allergic and other physiologic responses.

Considerations of sensory reactions have a central role in the development of guidelines for ventilation requirements for occupied spaces. The amount of ventilation, or number of air exchanges, needed to eliminate unacceptable odors and irritation commonly exceeds that required to meet any other needs, such as control of carbon dioxide. For a number of years, quite apart from concerns about possible adverse health from exposure to ETS, ventilation engineers have viewed ETS as the most problematic common indoor contaminant (Leonardos and Kendall, 1971).

Efforts to derive functional relationships between the amount of a contaminant generated in a space and the amount of outdoor air, i.e., ventilation, necessary to control its odor began in the

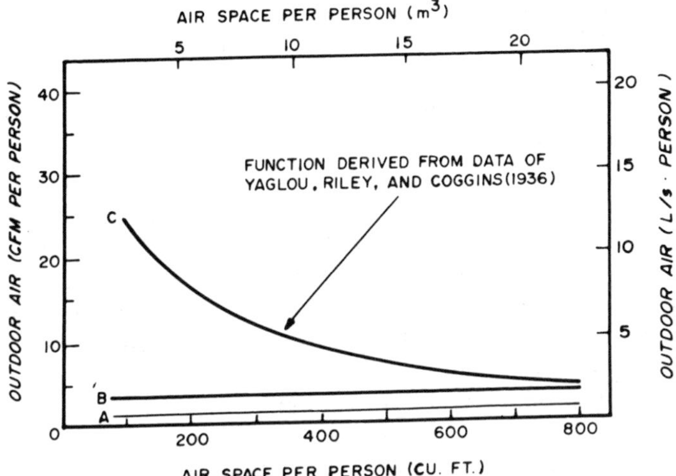

FIGURE 10-1 Relationships between ventilation rate and air space per person in an environmental chamber according to three criteria: (A) maintenance of oxygen concentration; (B) control of carbon dioxide to a level of 0.6% (2.5 cubic feet per minute); and (C) control of body odor at a moderate level under sedentary conditions of occupancy, no smoking.

1930s (Yaglou et al., 1936). Function C in Figure 10-1 is derived from experiments of Yaglou et al. (1936), where judges assessed the odor generated by occupants sitting quietly in an environmental chamber. The function depicts the combination of air space per person and ventilation rate of the air space (outdoor air) per person necessary to maintain odor at a moderate, acceptable level under steady-state conditions. Theoretical functions A and B, which fall below C, implying less need for ventilation, represent the outdoor air needed to maintain oxygen at a minimum of 20% and the air necessary to hold carbon dioxide at a maximum 0.6%, respectively.

The decrease in curve C at low occupancy density (large air space per person) resulted most likely from the instability of occupancy body odor in Yaglou's chamber. That is, occupancy odor decays relatively rapidly on its own (Yaglou and Witheridge, 1937; Clausen et al., 1984). Tobacco smoke odor, on the other hand, exhibits relative stability. When smoking has ceased in an unventilated room, the odor will remain at the about same level over many hours (Yaglou and Witheridge, 1937; Clausen et al., 1985). In a diagram such as Figure 10-1, a function for tobacco smoke odor, like functions A and B, would be independent of the size of the space or of air space per occupant. In this respect, tobacco smoke odor behaves as a simple contaminant and ventilation requirements for reducing tobacco smoke odor should depend strictly on rate of smoking.

Twenty years after his study on occupancy odor, Yaglou (1955) reported a small experiment on tobacco smoke odor. Studying the very high smoking rate of 24 cigarettes per hour generated by six of nine occupants in his 1,410-cubic-foot chamber, he reported the need for 40 cfm (cubic feet per minute) per smoker, or 600 cubic feet per cigarette, in order to achieve moderate, acceptable odor. At about the same time, Kerka and Humphreys (1956), using similar psychophysical techniques, estimated the requirement at 2,250 cubic feet per cigarette, or 300 cfm per smoker smoking 8 cigarettes per hour. At a smoking rate of 2 cigarettes per hour, this would be 75 cfm per smoker.

Recent results have estimated ventilation needs closer to those of Kerka and Humphreys (1956) than those of Yaglou (1955), but have also uncovered limitations on ventilation as a solution to the odor problems produced by ETS. Figure 10-2 shows how tobacco smoke odor varied over time for three smoking rates and various ventilation rates (Cain et al., 1983). The line connecting the open squares in the left panel depicts the level of odor generated by nonsmoking occupancy with low ventilation. It shows that even in the presence of higher ventilation rates, smoking generated more odor than simple occupancy.

The psychophysical judges in the experiment, a mixed group of smokers and nonsmokers, assessed acceptability in addition to perceived intensity. Figure 10-3 shows the percent of dissatisfaction as a function of ventilation rate per cigarette. The ventilation rate that would lead to 20% of judges dissatisfied is 4,240 cubic feet per cigarette (shown by the vertical dashed line). Twenty percent dissatisfied is the maximum level allowed by recommendation of the American Society of Heating, Refrigeration and Air-Conditioning Engineers (ASHRAE, 1981). On the realistic assumption that the percentage of people actually smoking in a space at any given time will equal about 10%, ventilation rate per person (smokers and nonsmokers) would need to be 53 cfm (see Figure 10-3) to reduce odors to a level that would satisfy 80% of the judges.

Despite ASHRAE's goal of satisfying at least 80% of visitors to a space, none of its recommendations for ventilation are as high

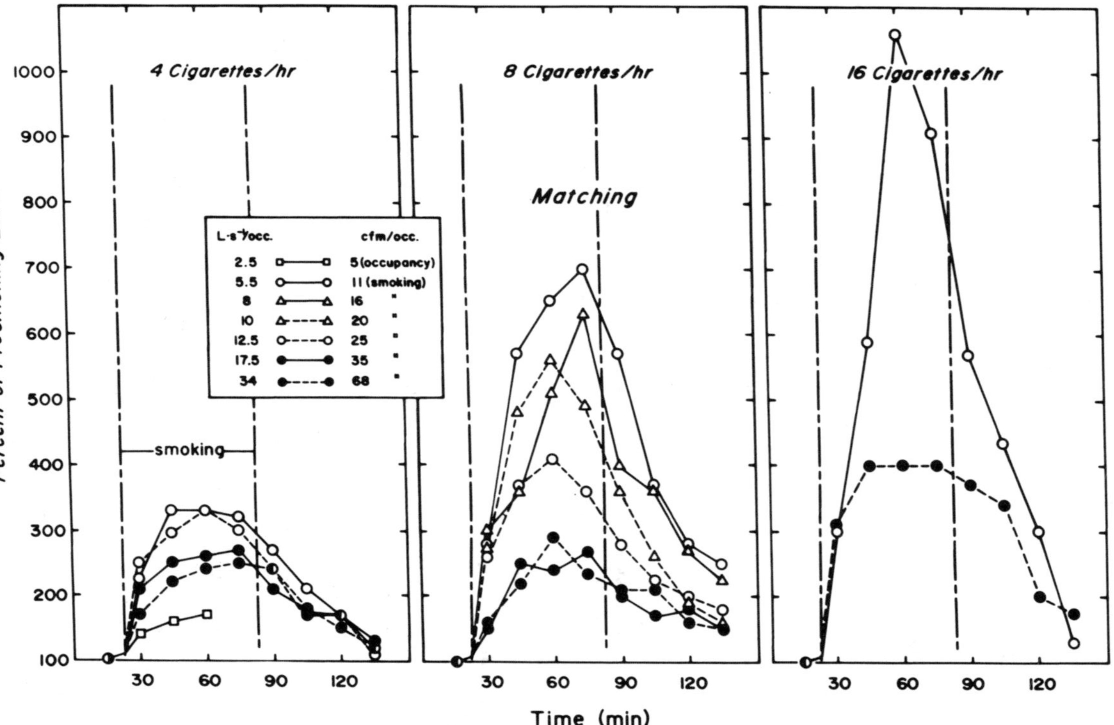

FIGURE 10-2 Intensity of odor during and after smoking in an environmental chamber for three different rates of cigarettes smoked per hour. Measurement of odor intensity was parts per million butanol matched to the test odor according to ASTM standard E544-75. Each point represents judgments taken over a 15-minute period. From Cain et al. (1983).

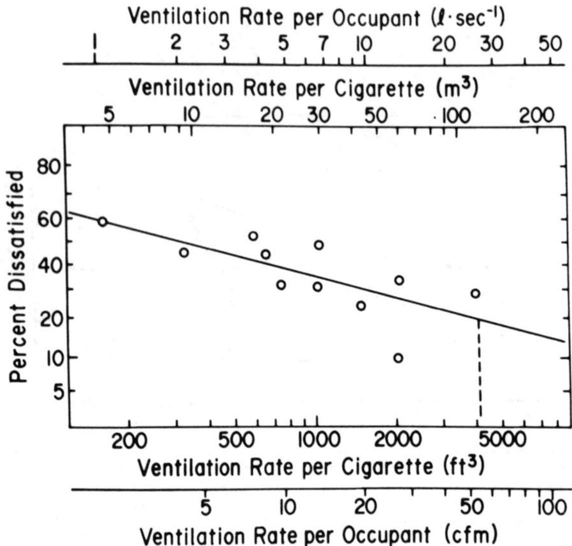

FIGURE 10-3 Percent of judgments of *unacceptable* odor quality of air versus ventilation per cigarette and ventilation per occupant, assuming that 10% of occupants in a space will be smoking at any time. Data from Cain et al. (1983).

as 53 cfm per occupant. For offices where smoking is allowed, the ASHRAE recommendation is 20 cfm per occupant. For many other smoking areas, however, the ASHRAE recommendation is 35 cfm per occupant. Such recommendations did not result from experiment, but rather from a consensus procedure of expert heating and refrigerating engineers that weighed available information. The bulk of the data on the acceptability of odor and irritation from ETS was not available at the time ASHRAE prepared its standard in 1981. The standard was, however, the first to specify the need for 4 to 5 times greater ventilation rates during smoking occupancy as compared with nonsmoking occupancy. The most common rate specified for smoking occupancy is 35 cfm per occupant, whereas 7 cfm per occupant is the most common rate specified for nonsmoking occupancy. This means that in a space where smoking is allowed, the pollution generated by smoking creates the greatest need for ventilation.

According to the data of Cain et al. (1983) (Figure 10-3), ASHRAE's proposed ventilation rate of 35 cfm per occupant during smoking will lead to 25% of visitors being dissatisfied (75%

satisfied) with the odor. Data suggest that the difference in satisfaction between smoking and nonsmoking occupancy, and hence the difference in recommended ventilation rates, arises largely because of the intensity of the odors (Figure 10-4), rather than the quality of the odors. At equal odor intensity, the occupancy odor and tobacco smoke odor are disliked about equally.

An additional factor affecting annoyance with odor is that nonsmokers are much more likely than smokers to object to tobacco smoke odor. Figure 10-5 depicts relative dissatisfaction with tobacco smoke odor at various intensities, expressed in terms of equivalent levels of butanol. At 32 ppm (butanol level 2), 1% of smokers found the odor unacceptable, while 20% of nonsmokers found it so. The odor had to rise to 256 ppm (level 5) before as

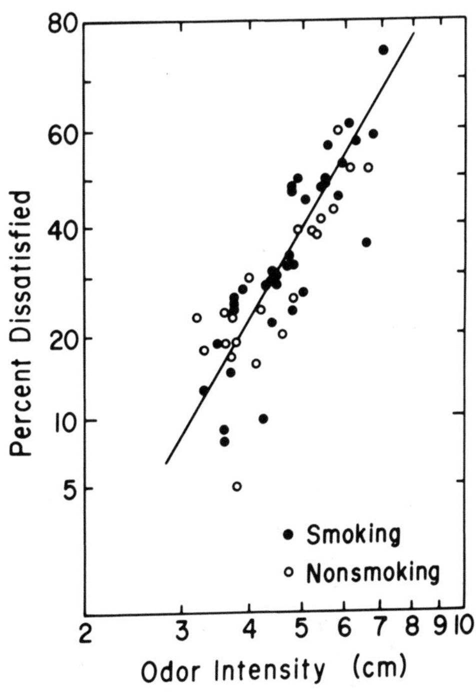

FIGURE 10-4 Percent of judgments of *unacceptable* odor quality of air versus odor intensity assessed by means of a graphic rating procedure during various conditions of smoking and nonsmoking occupancy. Each point represents the outcome from a particular combination of contaminant generation (number of occupants or rate of smoking) and ventilation rate. Data from Cain et al. (1983).

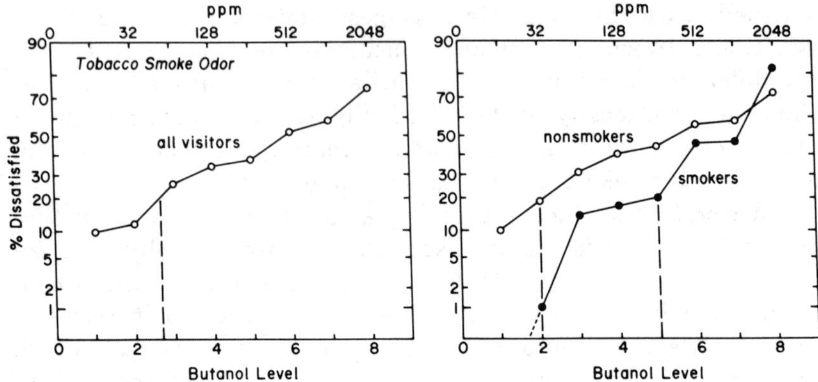

FIGURE 10-5 Percent of judgments of *unacceptable* odor quality of air derived from tobacco smoke odor related to equivalent level of butanol (parts per million at top; $\log_2$ at bottom). Judgments accumulated across all conditions of smoking (2,357 judgments). Left: Data from all visitors. Right: Data from smokers and nonsmokers plotted separately. Data from Cain et al. (1983).

many as 20% of smokers found the odor unacceptable. In terms of practical solutions to the odor problem caused by tobacco smoke, the difference between smokers and nonsmokers may prove insurmountable. Under usual levels of smoking, no realistic level of ventilation will drive tobacco smoke odor as low as the equivalent of 32 ppm butanol (butanol level 2).

IRRITATION

Ventilating and air-conditioning engineers have typically concerned themselves with the reactions of visitors to enclosed spaces on the assumption that visitors will exhibit more sensitivity than occupants. As society has become more concerned with the health risks of smoking in the recent past, research on consequences of ETS exposure has focused on the occupant. Included within this concern have been the sensory reactions of occupants.

Figure 10-6 illustrates changes in tobacco smoke odor and irritation over time for occupants. Whereas perceived odor magnitude may fade due to olfactory adaptation, irritation may increase. Also apparent in this figure is a relationship between relative humidity and odor or irritation perception. In the low relative humidity conditions, both odor and irritation were exacerbated.

Receptors for irritation exist throughout the nasal, pharyngeal, and laryngeal areas and on the surface of the eyes. The receptors comprise free nerve endings of the fifth, ninth, and tenth cranial nerves and form the mediating elements of what is known as the *common chemical sense*. Although particularly sensitive to corrosive stimuli, the common chemical sense responds to almost any airborne organic material at high concentration (Cain, 1981).

The common chemical sense (or irritation perception) is characterized by a tendency to respond more vigorously over time (Cometto-Muniz and Cain, 1984). A person in an environment with a low-level irritant may even fail to notice any irritation at first. Once irritation has begun, however, it may persist even after removal of the stimulus.

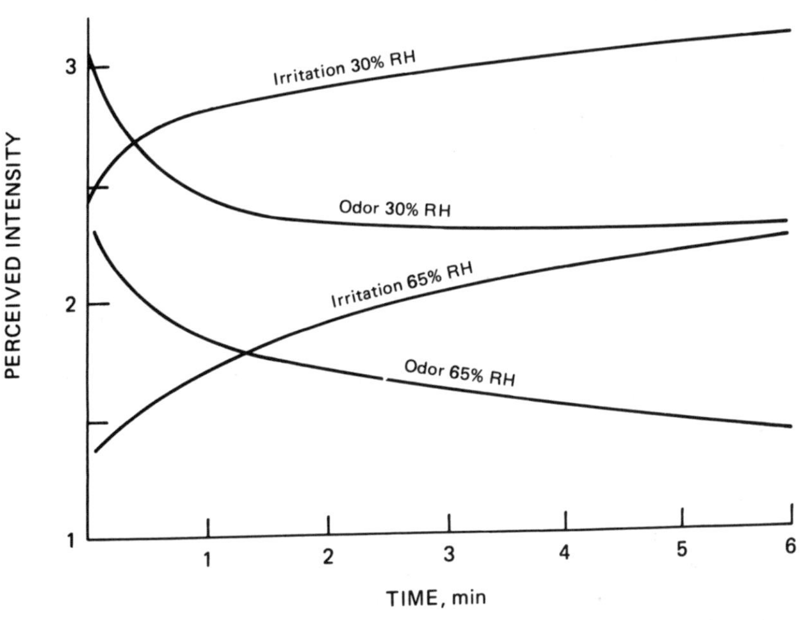

FIGURE 10-6 Changes in odor and irritation during continuous, short-term exposure to cigarette smoke generated in a chamber. Ventilation equalled 14 cfm per cigarette and ambient temperature equalled 25°C. Relative humidity (RH) was 30% in one condition and 65% in the other. Adapted from Kerka and Humphreys (1956).

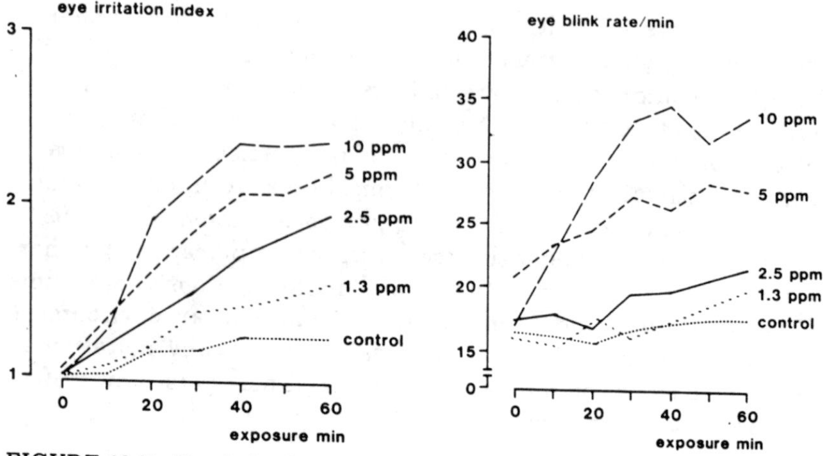

FIGURE 10-7 Eye irritation related to duration of exposure and concentration (parts per million carbon monoxide) of ETS. Left: Eye irritation index. Right: Eye blink rate. From Weber (1984).

Chamber Studies

A number of chamber studies have examined irritation and odor from tobacco smoke (Weber et al., 1976a,b; Weber et al., 1979a,b; Weber and Fischer, 1980; Muramatsu et al., 1983; Weber, 1984). The major findings include:

- Irritation from ETS varies with both concentration (measured as an increment in carbon monoxide as a surrogate for ETS) and time over long durations, as shown in Figure 10-7.
- The eyes are the most readily affected site for irritation, with the nose second.
- Rate of eye blinking correlates well with estimates of eye and nose irritation when the level of ETS is high (i.e., level of ETS such that the carbon monoxide concentration is at least 5 ppm), though eye blinking seems a less sensitive index than psychophysical judgments (Figure 10-7).
- Degree of annoyance (a composite index of impressions as defined by Weber) reaches a steady state much more rapidly than irritation, presumably because odor contributes to annoyance.
- Degree of annoyance depend almost entirely on the gas phase of ETS. Filtration of the particles is followed by only a small, though relatively constant, reduction in annoyance.

• Eye irritation and increased eye blink rate depend almost entirely on the particulate phase of ETS. Particle filtration diminishes the sense of irritation greatly.

• Weber (1984) suggested that ETS corresponding to CO concentrations of 1.5 to 2.0 ppm should form the maximum permissible level of exposure in environmentally realistic circumstances. At about 2 ppm of CO, almost 20% of occupants report "strong" or "very strong" eye irritation. Cain et al. (1983) and Clausen et al. (1985) found that incremental CO concentrations of 1 to 2 ppm led to 20% of visitors becoming dissatisfied with the air.

One of the more important issues with respect to control of ETS is whether filtration of the particles will reduce discomfort. As indicated above, Weber and colleagues found only a small reduction of annoyance when they filtered the particles with Cambridge pads. Since their criteria for annoyance largely assessed odor, their data largely agree with those of Clausen et al. (1985), who found that electrostatic precipitation of the particles caused no significant reduction in odor perceived by visitors to a chamber. Nevertheless, Weber and associates did find that filtration reduced reported eye irritation considerably. This led them to draw the conclusion that eye irritation derived largely from the particulate phase of ETS. Cain et al. (in press), on the other hand, found only a slight reduction of irritation following electrostatic precipitation of the particles. This disparity suggests the need for a more direct comparison of the sensory effects of the two filtration methods and for chemical analysis in order to determine whether Cambridge pads remove a vapor-phase constitutent of ETS that is left airborne by electrostatic precipitation.

Field Studies

Winnecke et al. (1984) argued that when people engage in social activities (e.g., playing cards or games) they become somewhat less critical of the environment and will tolerate a level corresponding to more than a 5-ppm increment in CO. It is suggested that when undistracted, occupants of chambers in experimental studies might complain about circumstances that would go unnoticed in life situations. On the other hand, irritation may prove relatively resistant to distraction. Restaurants would seem to offer a realistic proving ground for the interpretation of the chamber studies.

Weber et al. (1979a) found that more than 20% of occupants in restaurants included in a Zurich study reported eye irritation when CO, used as a surrogate for tobacco smoke levels, increased by 2 ppm above background. There was a direct relationship between reported irritation and CO concentration in four restaurants surveyed. In a study of more than 40 workrooms, Weber and Fischer (1980) also found a similar association between the concentration of CO and reported eye irritation.

Judgments of dissatisfaction, whether taken inside a chamber or in the field, may well vary as the social acceptance of certain odors, including ETS, changes with time. For this reason, judgments of some attribute, such as eye irritation, or judgments of odor intensity, particularly those that entail a reference such as butanol, should form the information of interest for long-term considerations. Dissatisfaction measures may be more variable.

HYPERSENSITIVE INDIVIDUALS

Individuals with chronic lung diseases, such as asthma and vasomotor rhinitis, may be more sensitive to the acute irritating effects of exposure to ETS (see Chapter 11). In addition, many people without active diseases report allergic or allergic-like symptoms as a result of exposure to ETS (e.g., Speer, 1968; Zussman, 1974). Reported symptoms include eye irritation, nasal symptoms, headache, cough, wheezing, sore throat, and nausea. The percent of people who report these responses varies with the nature of the exposure. These reports have led to the belief that a tobacco smoke allergy may exist.

Several investigators have studied immediate cutaneous hypersensitivity to extracts of tobacco leaves. Zussman (1974) found that 16% of 200 atopic patients reported that they were clinically sensitive to ETS exposure. All of them did develop erythema during the intradermal tests. Becker et al. (1976) found that one-third (11 out of 31) of human volunteers, including smokers, exhibit hypersensitivity to a glycoprotein purified from cured tobacco leaves (TGP-L) and from cigarette smoke condensate (TGP-CSC). Reports of immediate skin reactivity suggest an immunological basis for clinical sensitivity to tobacco smoke.

Tobacco smoke has been shown to contain immunogens that can stimulate immune responses to tobacco leaf extract in experimental animals (Lehrer et al., 1978; Becker et al., 1979; Gleich and

Welsh, 1979). However, the extracts differ and there is controversy concerning the purity of tobacco glycoprotein isolates (Becker et al., 1981; Bick et al., 1981).

In a recent study of Lehrer et al. (1984), skin prick tests of 93 subjects were done, including 60 of whom claimed clinical sensitivity to tobacco smoke. The group included atopic and nonatopic individuals. Approximately 50% of the atopic subjects had positive skin tests to leaf extracts or cigarette smoke condensate (CSC). Fewer than 5% of nonatopic individuals had a positive reaction, independent of whether they claimed to be sensitive to ETS exposure. Radioallergosorbent tests (RAST) were also conducted. Forty-five percent of atopic individuals and 6% of nonatopic individuals were positive for leaf extracts. There were no significant differences in specific serum IgE antibodies among smokers, exsmokers, or nonsmokers. Fewer than 6% of either group responded to CSC. Because there was no relationship between subjective tobacco smoke sensitivity and reaction to the various tests, the authors concluded that the reported subjective sensitivity is probably not related to hypersensitivity to tobacco leaf or smoke antigens.

In summary, experimental and clinical studies have indicated that there are immunogens in ETS and that a portion of the population is sensitive as shown by dermatological tests. However, the specific agent responsible for this reactivity has not been conclusively identified. Furthermore, there is some question as to whether reactions to skin tests are correlated with subjective complaints. It is clear, however, that a substantial number of atopic individuals will have positive skin tests to tobacco smoke or tobacco leaf extracts. More research needs to be done to characterize the immunogens and explain the relationship between subjective symptoms and skin tests.

SUMMARY AND RECOMMENDATIONS

There are a number of acute, noxious effects of exposure to ETS by nonsmokers that may occur. These include annoyance with odor, eye irritation, throat irritation, and immunological responses. The specific constituents that elicit these responses are not known.

What Is Known

Odor

1. ETS arouses odor responses. The objectionable odor generated by ETS greatly exceeds that generated by simple occupancy under comparable conditions of occupancy, density, temperature, and relative humidity, and is more persistent.

2. Tobacco smoke odor is stable over time. Ventilation requirements for tobacco smoke odor will therefore vary in strict proportion to the number of cigarettes smoked.

3. Rooms (and other spaces) where there is smoking require much more ventilation than spaces with nonsmoking occupancy. During smoking, ventilation requirements that satisfy at least 80% of visitors to a room exceed 50 cfm per occupant.

4. Nonsmokers and visitors to rooms appear to set a more stringent criterion than smokers for acceptability of tobacco smoke odor. Current ventilation guidelines for smoking occupancy will apparently fail to satisfy a criterion level of 80% of visitors (mixed group). It is not clear that any practical ventilation rate could satisfy 80% or more nonsmokers under typical conditions of smoking occupancy.

Irritation

5. Low humidity may exacerbate odor and irritation responses to ETS.

6. Whereas odor will govern the reactions of visitors to a smoking space, irritation will largely govern the reactions of occupants. Over time, eye irritation grows to become the most important negative response of the occupant. Dissatisfaction observed in chamber studies is commensurate with that found in field studies.

7. Eye blink offers a reasonable correlate of sensory irritation at high levels of smoke (i.e., levels of ETS such that the concentration of CO is at least 5 ppm), but not at low levels.

8. Filtration of particles from ETS via an electrostatic precipitator causes no decline in odor to visitors and no meaningful decline in odor or irritation to occupants. This suggests that irritation and odor derive primarily from gas- or vapor-phase constituents.

9. Filtration of particles via a Cambridge pad reduced irritation, but not odor, to occupants. Perhaps the Cambridge pad

removes some critical vapors from the smoke along with the particles.

10. A substantial portion of atopic individuals are sensitive to tobacco leaf or tobacco smoke extracts as shown by skin tests. However, cutaneous sensitivity appears not to correlate with subjective symptoms.

What Scientific Information Is Missing

1. The outcomes obtained in chambers regarding dissatisfaction created by the odor and irritation of ETS should be further verified in field situations. The chamber studies imply that there must be considerably more than 20% dissatisfaction in places where smoking occurs even when current ventilation standards are met.
2. Prospects for abatement of discomfort through filtration of the vapor or particulate phases of ETS should receive attention.
3. Objective physiological or biochemical indices should be sought to validate reports of chronic irritation of the eyes, nose, and throat.
4. Research is needed to determine specific constituents that are the irritants in ETS.
5. Information is needed on the prevalence and severity of allergic and hypersensitive responses to tobacco smoke in the general population and in atopic individuals.
6. Further research needs to be done to determine the specific elements that are immunogenic in extracts of tobacco smoke and to relate immune response on skin tests to subjective complaints of sensitivity to tobacco smoke.
7. Research is needed to evaluate the medical importance of positive reactions to RAST tests of tobacco leaf products for atopics.

REFERENCES

ASHRAE Standard 62-81. Ventilation for Acceptable Indoor Air Quality. Atlanta: ASHRAE, 1981. 19 pp.

Becker, C.G., T. Dubin, and H.P. Wiedemann. Hypersensitivity to tobacco antigen. Proc. Natl. Acad. Sci. USA 73:1712-1716, 1976.

Becker, C.G., R. Levi, and J. Zavecz. Induction of IgE antibodies to antigen isolated from tobacco leaves and from cigarette smoke condensate. Am. J. Pathol 96:249-254, 1979.

Becker, C.G., N. Van Hamont, and M. Wagner. Tobacco, cocoa, coffee, and ragweed: Cross-reacting allergens that activate factor-XXI-dependent pathways. Blood 58:861-867, 1981.

Bick, R.L., R.L. Stedman, P.L. Kronick, E. Hillman, and J. Fareed. Studies related to tobacco glycoprotein: A claimed activator of coagulation fibrolysis, complement, kinin and a claimed allergen. Thromb. Haemostasis 46:231, 1981.

Cain, W.S. Olfaction and the common chemical sense: Similarities, differences, and interactions, pp. 109-121. In H.R. Moskowitz and B. Warren, Eds. Order Quality and Intensity as a Function of Chemical Structure. American Chemical Society Symposium 148. Washington, D.C.: American Chemical Society, 1981.

Cain, W.S., B.P. Leaderer, R. Isseroff, L.G. Berglund, R.J. Huey, E.D. Lipsitt, and D. Perlman. Ventilation requirements in buildings. I. Control of occupancy odor and tobacco smoke odor. Atmos. Environ. 17:1183-1197, 1983.

Cain, W.S., T. Tosun, L.C. See, and B.P. Leaderer. Environmental tobacco smoke: Sensory reactions of occupants. Atmos. Environ., in press.

Clausen, G. P.O. Fanger, W.S. Cain, and B.P. Leaderer. Stability of tobacco smoke odor in enclosed spaces, pp. 437-441. In B. Berglund, T. Lindvall, and J. Sundell, Eds. Indoor Air, Vol. 3. Sensory and Hyperreactivity Reactions to Sick Buildings. Stockholm, Sweden: Swedish Council for Building Research, 1984.

Clausen, G., P.O. Fanger, W.S. Cain, and B.P. Leaderer. The influence of aging, particle filtration and humidity on tobacco smoke odor, pp. 345-350. In P.O. Fanger, Ed. Clima 2000, Vol. 4. Indoor Climate. Copenhagen, Denmark: VVS Kongress-VVS Messe, 1985.

Cometto-Muniz, J.E., and W.S. Cain. Temporal integration of pungency. Chem. Senses 8:315-327, 1984.

Gleich, G.J., and P.W. Welsh. Immunochemical and physicochemical properties of tobacco extract. Am. Rev. Respir. Dis. 120:995-1001, 1979.

Kerka, W.F., and C.M. Humphreys. Temperature and humidity effect on odor perception. ASHRAE Trans. 61:531-552, 1956.

Lawther, P.J., and B.T. Commins. Cigarette smoking and exposure to carbon monoxide. Ann. N.Y. Acad. Sci. 174:135-147, 1970.

Leonardos, G., and D.A. Kendall. Questionnaire study on odor problems of enclosed space. ASHRAE Trans. 77, 101-112, 1971.

Lehrer, S.B., M.R. Wilson, and J.E. Salvaggio. Immunogenic properties of tobacco smoke. J. Allergy Clin. Immunol. 62:368-370, 1978.

Lehrer, S.B., F. Barbandi, J.P. Taylor, and J.E. Salvaggio. Tobacco smoke "sensitivity"—Is there an immunological basis? J. Allergy Clin. Immunol. 73:240-245, 1984.

Muramatsu, T., A. Weber, S. Muramatsu, and F. Akermann. An experimental study on irritation and annoyance due to passive smoking. Int. Arch. Occup. Environ. Health 51:305-317, 1983.

Speer, F. Tobacco and the nonsmoker. Arch. Environ. Health 16:443-446, 1968.

Viessman, W. Ventilation control of odor. Ann. N.Y. Acad. Sci. 116:630-637, 1964.

Weber, A. Acute effects of environmental tobacco smoke. Eur. J. Respir. Dis. 68(Suppl. 133):98-108, 1984.

Weber, A., and T. Fischer. Passive smoking at work. Int. Arch. Occup. Environ. Health 47:209-221, 1980.

Weber, A., T. Fischer, and E. Grandjean. Passive smoking in experimental and field conditions. Environ. Res. 20:205-216, 1979a.

Weber, A., T. Fischer, and E. Grandjean. Passive smoking: Irritating effects of the total smoke and the gas phase. Int. Arch. Occup. Environ. Health 43:183-193, 1979b.

Weber, A., C. Jermini, and E. Grandjean. Irritating effects on man of air pollution due to cigarette smoke. Am. J. Public Health 66:672-676, 1976a.

Weber, A., T. Fischer, and E. Grandjean. Objektive und subjektive physiologische Wirkungen des Passivrauchens. Int. Arch. Occup. Environ. Health 37:277-288, 1976b.

Winnecke, G., K. Plischke, A. Roscovanu, and H.W. Schlipkoeter. Patterns and determinants of reaction to tobacco smoke in an experimental exposure setting, pp. 351-356. In B. Berglund, T. Lindvall, and J. Sundell, Eds. Indoor Air, Vol. 2. Radon, Passive Smoking, Particulates, and Housing Epidemiology. Stockholm, Sweden: Swedish Council for Building Research, 1984.

Yaglou, C.P. Ventilation requirements for cigarette smoke. ASHRAE Trans. 61:25-32, 1955.

Yaglou, C.P., and W.N. Witheridge. Ventilation requirements, Part 2. ASHRAE Trans. 43:423-436, 1937.

Yaglou, C.P., E.C. Riley, and D.I. Coggins. Ventilation requirements. ASHRAE Trans. 42:133-162, 1936.

Zussman, B.M. Tobacco sensitivity in the allergic population. J. Asthma Res. 11:159-167, 1974.

11
Effects of Exposure to Environmental Tobacco Smoke on Lung Function and Respiratory Symptoms

This chapter discusses epidemiologic studies of nonsmokers exposed to tobacco product smoke that have evaluated lung function or respiratory symptoms, most of which have evaluated children. The effects of active cigarette smoking are briefly reviewed to recount the reasons why certain aspects of lung function have been studied in nonsmokers. The plausibility of finding similar effects in nonsmokers exposed to ETS is discussed and the studies found in the literature are assessed.

LUNG FUNCTION AND SYMPTOMS IN ACTIVE SMOKERS

Cross-sectional studies of smokers have demonstrated that smokers, compared with nonsmokers, have (1) an increased prevalence of chronic cough, chronic sputum production, and wheezing and (2) decreased lung function (see U.S. Public Health Service, 1984, for an extensive review). The effects of smoking on both respiratory symptoms and lung function may be seen within a few years of the onset of regular smoking (U.S. Public Health Service, 1979, 1984; Woolcock et al., 1984). Longitudinal studies have demonstrated that the mean rate of decline with age of the 1-second forced expiratory volume (FEV_1) is greater in smokers than in nonsmokers. In some smokers, the rate of decline of FEV_1 is rapid, leading to clinically important chronic airflow obstruction.

The structural changes associated with active cigarette smoking are seen in both the conducting airways and the pulmonary parenchyma (for a more detailed description, see U.S. Public

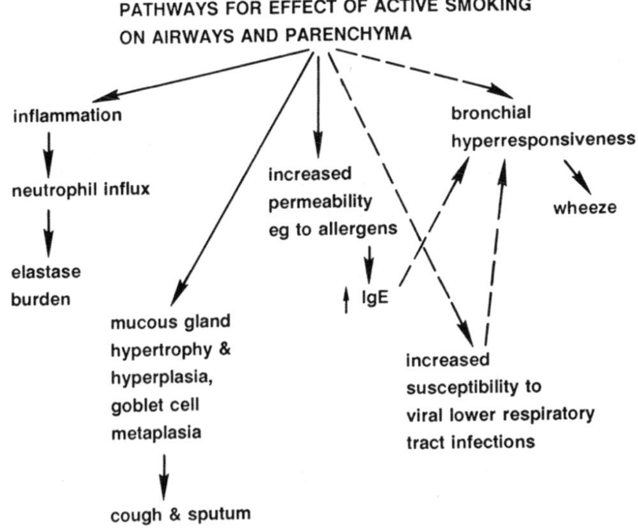

FIGURE 11-1 Known and suspected mechanisms for effects of tobacco smoke on airways. Solid lines = known mechanisms; dashed lines = suspected mechanisms.

Health Service, 1984). In the large airways there is hypertrophy and hyperplasia of the mucous glands. These changes are followed by an increase in mucus production that leads to increased cough and sputum production. Structural changes in smaller airways range from relatively mild inflammation to narrowing and closure of airways due to inflammation, goblet cell hyperplasia, and intraluminal mucus. Changes in the parenchyma include increased numbers of inflammatory cells and ultimately destruction of the alveolar walls, most commonly in the central part of the lobule, i.e., the development of centrilobular emphysema (see Figure 11-1).

The link between airway disease and parenchymal disease is poorly understood. Smokers with severe functional impairment usually have an appreciable amount of emphysema (U.S. Public Health Service, 1984).

Cessation of smoking leads to a rapid decrease in respiratory symptoms, an improvement in lung function, and a shift towards the nonsmoker's rate of decline of FEV_1 (U.S. Public Health Service, 1979, 1984). These improvements are usually seen regardless of the functional level at which cessation occurs.

Population-based studies of adults have generally shown a strong dose-response relationship between FEV_1 with dose measured either in terms of years smoked, the number of cigarettes per day, or the integrated dose, i.e., pack-years (U.S. Public Health Service, 1984). It is worthwhile noting, however, that in two major studies (Burrows et al., 1977a; Beck et al., 1981) the active smoking dose accounted for only about 15% of the variation of FEV_1 even after age and height adjustment. Most of the variance could be attributed to the naturally occurring large variability in pulmonary function. Another reason the active smoking dose did not explain much of the variance is that the number of cigarettes an individual smokes cannot readily be translated into the dose of smoke that is delivered into the airways and parenchyma. Many factors, such as puff volume and lung volume at which inhalation starts, clearance rates, and airway geometry of the lungs of exposed individuals, will influence the dose and the distribution of the smoke within the lungs. Variability in individual susceptibility to the effects of chemicals deposited in the lung has been demonstrated in studies of animals (Evans et al. 1971, 1975, 1978).

PLAUSIBILITY FOR AN EFFECT DUE TO PASSIVE SMOKING

The dose of cigarette smoke delivered to the lungs of nonsmokers exposed to ETS is both qualitatively and quantitatively different from mainstream smoke, being a small fraction of that delivered to the lungs of an active smoker (see discussions in Chapter 7). Exposure to constituents of tobacco smoke may begin in utero and continue throughout childhood through ETS exposure. During these periods, the lung is undergoing both growth and remodeling. Therefore, the lung of the fetus and young child may be particularly susceptible to environmental insults.

Despite qualitative differences between mainstream smoke, sidestream smoke, and ETS, it has been customary to assume that exposure to ETS approximates a low-dose exposure to tobacco smoke. The ability to measure responses to low doses depends on the shape of the dose-response curves, the sensitivity and specificity of the measurement tools available, and whether there is a threshold of exposure below which there is no response in any individual.

The assumed shape of the dose-response curve determines what kinds of effects would be expected and the estimates of the probability of detecting them. If the dose-response curve were linear with a shallow slope, or a slope concave to the dose axis, the response at low doses might be so small that it would be difficult to detect. In such a situation, only the very susceptible portion of the population might have detectable effects. It is likely that there is a distribution of susceptibility to the effects of ETS within the population, such that there will be some persons who will respond at low doses and some persons for whom many years of heavy exposure may be needed to cause the same symptoms or change in lung function (Cockcroft et al., 1983).

If individuals who are most susceptible to the irritating effects of cigarette smoke on the lower respiratory tract do not start to smoke or, having started, soon quit as smokers, then a population of nonsmokers would be more likely to include the most susceptible individuals than a population of smokers. The existence of different subpopulations introduces an additional complication to the extrapolation from high-dose exposure in active smokers to the low-dose exposures of nonsmokers.

In addition, it is likely that the development of respiratory disease or symptoms, lung function level, and rate of decline reflect the cumulative burden of many environmental exposures and other insults, such as respiratory infections (Purvis and Ehrlich, 1963) to the lung. Furthermore, it might be hypothesized that the cumulative burden may interact with the individual's genetically determined susceptibility.

METHODOLOGIC CONSIDERATIONS FOR EPIDEMIOLOGIC STUDIES

A recent report of the National Research Council (1985) is devoted to methodologic issues of epidemiology and air pollution. In this section, many of the problems are reviewed briefly.

Study Design and Analysis

Chronic pulmonary effects of ETS have been the subject of several recent reviews (Lee, 1982; Weiss et al., 1983; Surgeon General, 1984; Guyatt and Newhouse, 1985; Taylor et al., 1985) and symposium or workshop reports (U.S. Public Health Service,

1983; Gammage and Kaye, 1984; Rylander, 1984). Many of the studies reported in these reviews had not been originally designed to study chronic pulmonary effects of ETS exposure. Instead, these data sets were reanalyzed to address the question of the pulmonary effects of ETS. This use of these studies suggests the need for caution when interpreting their results.

Several analytic approaches were used in the reported studies. Independent risk factors, such as age and sex, usually need to be taken into account, but this was not always done. Several statistical approaches, such as stratification or regression analysis, are used to take into account the effects of potentially confounding variables. For most of the potentially confounding variables, researchers do not agree on the nature of the roles of the variables as confounders and, hence, on the appropriate ways to introduce these variables into the data analyses.

Assessing Exposure

Interpretation of epidemiological studies is hampered by the existence of factors that interact with and modify the response to exposure and by confounding factors that are associated with the same symptom complex as exposure to ETS, such as coughing, production of sputum, and wheezing (see Table 11-1). These variables must be assessed and accounted for in the statistical analyses where possible.

Unreported active smoking could lead to a large bias. Underreporting of smoking is likely in studies of older children, particularly when parents answer questionnaires for their children. Children who have parents who smoke are themselves more likely to smoke. Therefore, because active smoking is likely to have a considerably greater impact on respiratory symptoms and lung function than exposure to ETS, misclassification of the children who smoke will tend to overestimate the effect of exposure to ETS.

For blue collar males, occupational exposure can also be important and may interact with both direct cigarette smoke and ETS. Many pulmonary toxicants can exist in the workplace. Furthermore, ETS exposure can occur in the workplace. Similarly, comparison of inner-city-dwelling persons with less urban, or suburban, controls can lead to biases.

TABLE 11-1 Potentially Confounding and Effect Modifying Factors in Epidemiologic Studies of Exposure to Environmental Tobacco Smoke

- Unreported active smoking
  - Tobacco products
  - Marijuana
  - Clove cigarettes
- Developmental factors
  - Maternal smoking during pregnancy
- Factors related to outdoor environment
  - Outdoor temperature, humidity
  - Respirable and nonrespirable particulates, e.g., fugitive dust
  - Pollens and other allergens
- Factors related to indoor environment
  - Crowding
  - Number and age of siblings
  - Total number of people/animals in dwelling unit
  - Total number of smokers in dwelling unit
  - Household conditions
  - Frequency of air exchanges
  - Temperature and humidity
  - Use and condition of air conditioning units
  - Conditions of child care facilities
  - Unvented combustion products from heating/cooking stoves
  - Respirable and nonrespirable particulates, e.g., wood smokes
  - Pollens, molds, mites
  - Allergens and infectious organisms
  - Formaldehyde
- Factors related to work/hobbies
  - Work/hobby-related exposure to gases, fumes, particulates
- Miscellaneous factors
  - Annoyance response to tobacco smoking
  - Reporting biases

Assessing Respiratory Variables

Methods commonly used to assess the effect of passive smoking on the respiratory system, such as respiratory symptom questionnaires and measurement of lung function, may lead to some error.

The problems associated with the respiratory symptom questionnaires include:

- Different questionnaires are used in studies. Differences in how the questions are asked can sometimes lead to large differences in answers. For instance, asking "Are you a smoker?" may elicit a "No" response from an exsmoker whereas the question "Have you ever smoked?" would be answered "Yes".

- Some studies use a self-administered questionnaire, whereas other studies use a trained interviewer. Trained interviewers can determine whether the subject understands the questionnaire and can follow a prescribed set of probing questions that may help to resolve the specific nature of not-well-described symptoms.
- Some studies have parents complete the questionnaires for the children, whereas other studies have the child answer the questionnaire. For older children, parents may not be aware of active smoking by the child and exposures to ETS in environments outside the home.
- Questionnaires necessarily involve some subjective elements that are prone to recall bias. For example, a smoker who is symptomatic may be more likely to report the same symptom in his/her child (Schenker et al., 1983; Ferris et al., 1985).

Many tests are prone to measurement error, which tends to obscure differences between groups of subjects. For example, it may be necessary to repeat lung function measurements for a given individual and to average results to get a reliable estimate. Lung function tests are often not sensitive to the structural and functional changes associated with lung disease (Drill and Thomas, 1980).

CROSS-SECTIONAL STUDIES

In the following sections, selected cross-sectional studies of respiratory symptoms, lung function, and respiratory infections and longitudinal studies of lung functions are reviewed. The studies reviewed here are larger studies in which attempts have been made to standardize assessments and many of the data-gathering techniques, including interviews.

Studies of Respiratory Symptoms in Children

Almost all of the cross-sectional studies that have compared children of parents who smoke with the children of parents who do not smoke have reported increased prevalences of respiratory symptoms, usually cough, sputum, or wheezing, in the children of smoking parents. Some studies, including some that have not found a statistically significant increase in the prevalence of respiratory symptoms in ETS exposed children, have demonstrated an increase in respiratory symptom prevalence with an increasing *number* of parents or other adults who smoke in the home (see below).

Three problems are especially important for studies of respiratory symptoms in children, i.e., underreported active smoking on the part of children, recall bias leading to overreporting of symptoms by parents, and the confounding variables of infections in parents. All three may lead to overestimation of symptom prevalences among children of smokers. Recall bias would occur if parents who have respiratory symptoms are more likely to report those symptoms in the children. (The possiblity also exists that parents with these symptoms would look upon them as so commonplace as not to be worthy of mention). Parents who are smokers are also more likely to have more respiratory symptoms and respiratory infections. Respiratory infections (and, as a consequence, symptoms) among children of smokers may be the result of direct transmission of infectious agents from the parent or may be caused by inflammation and irritation of lung tissues due to ETS exposure and consequent increase in susceptibility to infection. It has been observed that parents, especially mothers, who have a history of severe respiratory illness report higher rates of respiratory symptoms in their children (Schenker et al., 1983; Ferris et al., 1985).

Various ways of dealing with these potential sources of bias have been proposed. Restricting the study or analysis to children below age 8 is likely to eliminate bias due to underreporting of children who currently smoke. It is more difficult to handle the overreporting of symptoms in children when the parents have respiratory symptoms.

An additional problem for interpretation of parental reports of respiratory symptoms was noted by Schenker et al. (1983). In their study, children whose questionnaires were completed by fathers had significantly fewer symptoms reported than children with mother-completed questionnaires. There was no comparison of questionnaires completed separately by both mother and father for the same child. Because the rates for symptoms as reported by the mother were similar to what was found in other studies and because the fathers reported significantly fewer symptoms, the investigators suggested that fathers underreported symptoms in their children.

Table 11-2 reviews several selected cross-sectional studies of respiratory symptoms in children and adults. Lebowitz and Burrows (1976), reporting on children in the Tucson Epidemiologic Study of Obstructive Lung Disease, emphasized the need for controlling for parental symptoms. They reported that children had a higher prevalence of respiratory symptoms if they lived in households with adults with the same symptom, regardless of the family smoking habits. When the presence of symptoms in the adults was taken into account by partitioning households based on presence or absence of adult symptoms(s), the odds ratio that remained was greater than unity but was no longer statistically significant [Mantel-Haenszel odds ratio for all respiratory symptoms calculated from data presented is 1.35 (95% confidence limits of 0.91 to 1.98)]. Most symptoms were reported more frequently for children in currently smoking families.

Ferris et al. (1985) have argued that correcting for parental symptoms represents an overcorrection for respiratory symptoms in children since it also corrects for the parents' smoking habits. In the Harvard Air Pollution Respiratory Health Studies (Six-Cities Study) of 10,106 white children aged 6-9 years, the variable indicating whether the parent had a history of bronchitis, emphysema, or asthma was found to be a highly significant independent risk factor for cough and wheeze and a history of respiratory illness among children (Figure 11-2). Children whose parents had a positive history had 72-155% higher symptom and illness rates than children whose parents had no history of these illnesses. Adjustment for parental respiratory history reduced the size of the estimated effects of maternal smoking on respiratory symptoms and illnesses by 20 to 30%, but the associations remained statistically significant for most of the outcome symptom and respiratory illness variables (odds ratios of 1.23 and 1.28, respectively).

In both the Lebowitz and Ferris studies, adjustment for parental symptoms or respiratory illness decreased the strength of the apparent association between exposure to ETS and respiratory symptoms, but did not eliminate it. This finding leads to the reasonable conclusion that the exposures typical of ETS are sufficient to cause respiratory symptoms in some children. The increases in frequency of cough were 20 to 50%, and as high as 90%, when there were smoking parents. The increases in frequency of wheezing were more variable, which may indicate the difficulty in

TABLE 11-2 Effects of Passive Smoking on Respiratory Symptoms: Selected Cross-sectional Studies Involving Children/Adolescents

Study	Source of Subjects	Subjects	Exposure Assessment	Findings	Comments
Colley, 1974	Aylesbury, UK; seven public schools; 1971	1,328 boys, 270 girls; ages 6–14	Self-administered questionnaire from parents	1. Close association of child cough and parent winter morning phlegm 2. Prevalence of cough, 15.6% no smokers, 22.2% both parents smoke (ns)	Suggested cross-infection may be important cause; used different question from U.S. studies
Lebowitz and Burrows, 1976	Tucson, Ariz.; stratified cluster random sample of households; 1972–1973	1,655 households; Anglo-white; 1,252 children <16, 2,516 children >15	Self-administered NHLBI questionnaire from children >15; otherwise from parents	1. Prevalence of cough in young children, 7.8% no smokers, 10.4% smokers ($p < 0.05$) 2. Significance gone when parental symptoms considered	Less than 15 years old assumed to be nonsmokers; concluded familial aggregation important, potential confounder
Schilling et al., 1977	Survey of towns in Connecticut and South Carolina	816 children in 376 families; 607 children < 16, 109 children > 15	Respiratory Symptom Questionnaire, administered by interviewer	1. No effect of parental smoking on children's cough or wheeze 2. Prevalence of wheeze in young children related to parental wheeze ($p < 0.01$)	Tried to account for active smoking in children
Bland et al., 1958	Derbyshire, UK; 48 secondary schools; 1974	2,847 boys, 2,988 girls; 12 years old	Self-administered questionnaire by child	Prevalence of cough, 16% no smokers, 19% one smoker, 23.5% two smokers ($p < 0.01$)	Effects of child's and parent's smoking independently analyzed.

TABLE 11-2 *Continued*

Study	Source of Subjects	Subjects	Exposure Assessment	Findings	Comments
Tager et al., 1979	East Boston, Mass.; random sample in schools; 1975–1977	444 children; ages 5–9 years	NHLBI questionnaire administered by interviewer; if age <10, parent answered	No increase in respiratory illness with parental smoking	Controlled for family size
Weiss et al., 1980	See Tager et al., 1979	650 children; ages 5–9 years	See Tager et al., 1979	Persistent wheeze, 1% no smokers, 6.8% one smoker, 11.8% two smokers ($p < 0.02$)	See Tager et al., 1979
Dodge, 1982	Three towns in Arizona; survey of schools; 1978–1979	558 children; ages 8–10 years	Self-administered by parents	Child's wheeze ($p < 0.05$), sputum ($p < 0.05$), and cough ($p < 0.01$) related to parental smoking	
Schenker et al., 1983	Pennsylvania; survey of schools	4,071 children; ages 5–14	Self-administered by parents	Trend with number of smoking parents not significant for any symptoms	Not adjusted for parental symptoms although found to influence no. symptoms reported
Ware et al., 1984	Six U.S. cities; different regions survey of schools; 1974–1979	10,106 children; ages 6–13	Self-administered by parents	20–35% increased risk of all respiratory illness and symptoms with maternal smoking	Multiple logistic regression with gas cooking as other predictor

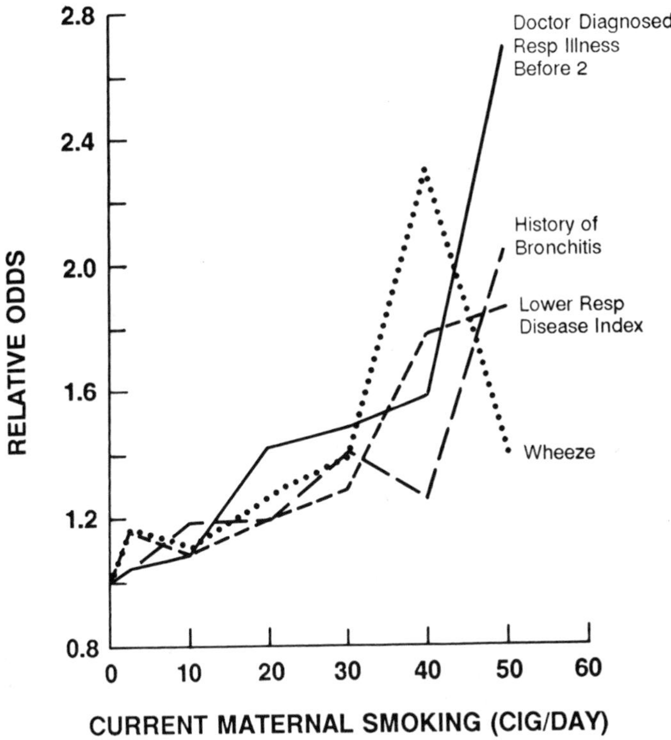

FIGURE 11-2 Relative odds of respiratory illness or symptoms versus average daily cigarette smoking by the child's mother. Reference value is zero cigarettes per day. From Ferris et al. (1985).

assessing this symptom. Furthermore, there appears to be a dose-response relationship between exposure and the likelihood of the child's developing respiratory symptoms or a respiratory illness. In the Harvard Study, a significant dose-response relationship was reported; the more mothers who smoked, the greater the risk of respiratory symptoms and illnesses among their children.

Studies of Lung Function in Children

A more quantitative measure of the impact of ETS on the lung is obtained by measures of lung function. Many of the studies that have examined the relationship between passive smoking and lung function have been cross-sectional.

Most studies have examined the effect of exposure to parental smoking rather than ETS exposure outside the immediate family. It is assumed that children are less likely than adults to be exposed to occupational irritants. The cumulative burden of respiratory insults is, therefore, likely to be smaller in children than in adults. It is often difficult (but not impossible) to measure lung function in young children and also hard to dissect out the relative contribution of ETS and that of natural variation and the effect of respiratory infections to pulmonary damage.

A majority of the studies (reviewed in Table 11-3) has shown a small decrease (up to 0.5% FEV_1 per year) in rate of increase in lung function associated with normal growth in children living with one or more parents who smoke compared with those living with nonsmoking parents (Table 11-3 and Figure 11-3). These differences have usually been statistically significant. Although the mean effect is small, there are individuals in each study who have large decrements in growth of lung function. Some studies have found a dose-response relationship with the number of smokers in the home or the amount smoked (Hasselblad et al., 1981). Ware (1984) shows (see Figure 11-4) a highly significant negative association between maternal smoking level and FEV_1 at both the baseline and follow-up examinations. For a child of a mother who smoked one pack of cigarettes per day compared with a child of a nonsmoking mother, the FEV_1 was $0.7 \pm 0.2\%$ lower at the baseline examination and $0.8 \pm 0.2\%$ lower at the follow-up examination 1 year later. This amounts to a 10- to 20-ml difference for a child with an FEV_1 between 1.5 and 2.5 L. In most studies, only the maternal effect was statistically significant. This may be because mothers usually spend more time with their young children than fathers.

A study carried out in Shanghai in the People's Republic of China reported a clear paternal effect. Chen and Li (1986), in a cross-sectional study of 303 boys and 268 girls aged 8-16, found that the number of cigarettes smoked by fathers was linearly related to a decrease in FEV_1 and $FEF_{25-75\%}$, the average forced expiratory flow during the middle half of the period of expiration. None of the mothers in this study were smokers; therefore, there was no maternal effect in that population. Differences in father's smoking status accounted for 0.5% of the variation among individuals in FEV_1 and 1.2% of the variation in $FEF_{25-75\%}$.

TABLE 11-3 Effects of Passive Smoking on Pulmonary Function: Selected Cross-sectional Studies Involving Children/Adolescents

Study	Source of Subjects	Subjects	Exposure Assessment	Findings	Comments
Lebowitz et al., 1982	Tucson, Ariz.; stratified cluster random sample of households; 1972–1973	1,655 households; Anglo-white; 1,252 children <16, 2,516 children >15	Self-administered NHLBI questionnaire from children >15; otherwise from parents	No relationship of FEV_1 with parental smoking when household aggregation of body mass taken into account	Less than 15-year-olds assumed to be nonsmokers; concluded familial aggregation important, potential confounder
Schilling et al., 1977	Survey of towns in Connecticut and South Carolina	816 children in 376 families; 607 children < 16, 209 children > 15	Respiratory Symptom Questionnaire, administered by interviewer	MEF 50% lower in younger children with maternal smoking ($p < 0.05$); FEV_1, PEF not significant	Tried to account for active smoking in children
Tager et al., 1979	East Boston, Mass.; random sample in schools; 1975–1977	444 children; ages 5–9 years	NHLBI questionnaire administered by interviewer; if age <10, parent answered	Lower z-scores for $FEF_{25-75\%}$ in children with smoking parents	Controlled for family size
Weiss et al., 1980	See Tager et al., 1979	650 children; ages 5–9 years	See Tager et al., 1979	Lower z-scores for $FEF_{25-75\%}$ with maternal smoking ($p < 0.005$); FVC, FEV_1 not significant	See Tager et al., 1979; also controlled for wheeze in child
Hasselblad et al., 1981	CHESS study, seven cities; survey of schools; 1970–1973	16,689 children; ages 5–13 years	Self-administered by parent (usually mother)	$FEV_{0.75}$ dose-response relationship with mother's smoking	No information on child's smoking; small effect of maternal smoking (0.1% of variance)

TABLE 11-3 *Continued*

Study	Source of Subjects	Subjects	Exposure Assessment	Findings	Comments
Dodge, 1982	Three towns in Arizona; survey of schools; 1978–1979	558 children; ages 8–10 years	Self-administered by parents	No effect of parental smoking on any parameters, cough ($p < 0.01$) related to parental smoking	Lung function tests not standardized
Ware et al., 1984	Six U.S. cities; different regions; survey of schools; 1974–1979	10,106 children; ages 6–13	Self-administered by parents	FEV_1 significantly negative; FVC positive relation to maternal smoking	Multiple logistic regression with gas cooking as other predictor
Chen and Li, 1986	Shanghai, PRC; survey of two schools; 1984	571 children; ages 8–16 years	Self-administered questionnaire by parents	Paternal lifetime smoking related to z-scores of FEV_1, MMEF, and $FEF_{62.6-87.5\%}$	No effect of maternal smoking, probably due to low prevalence of female smokers in PRC
Tashkin et al., 1984	Los Angeles County survey of four areas in city; 1973	971 nonsmoking, nonasthmatic children, ages 7–17	Modified NHLBI questionnaire administered by interviewer	Inconsistent effect of maternal smoking in younger boys and older girls	Effect in older girls probably due to unreported smoking by child
Ferris et al., 1985	See Ware et al., 1984	See Ware et al., 1984	See Ware et al., 1984	Significant effect of parental smoking on FEV_1	See Ware et al., 1984

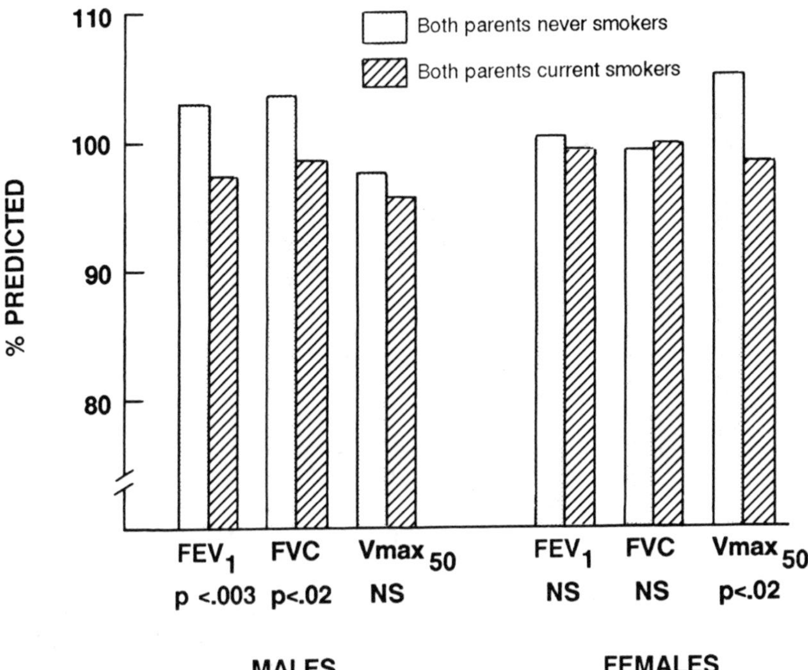

FIGURE 11-3 Mean percent lung function, by parental smoking, of nonsmoking males and females, ages 10-19, 1962-1965, from Tecumseh, Michigan. Burchfiel et al. (1986).

The most important contributors to variation in lung function among children are size-related factors such as sex, age, and height. These account for about 50-60% of the variation (Comroe et al., 1962).

It is not possible to determine whether ETS is directly causing the decreased lung function observed in children of smoking parents or if an increased infection rate in these children (see below) is responsible for the decrease. The annual small decrease in FEV_1, which is related to exposure to ETS, is unlikely to be clinically significant. However, the effect may be important in two respects. First, the existence of statistically significant differences related to parental smoking leads to the conclusion that there are pathophysiologic effects of exposure to ETS in the lungs of the growing child. It may be an in utero effect, an effect on the growing and remodeling lung, or both. Second, it raises the question of whether the child who is adversely affected by parental smoking

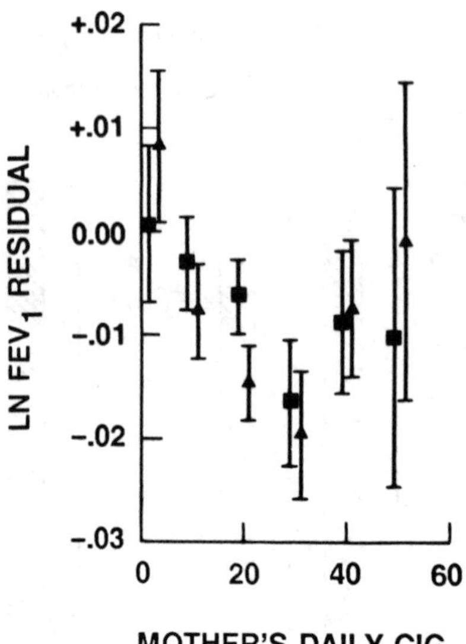

FIGURE 11-4 Mean of pulmonary function residual (± 1 SD) by mothers' reported daily cigarette smoking, compared with children whose mothers have never smoked. Squares represent the first examination ($n = 7{,}112$) and triangles represent the second examination ($n = 6{,}278$). From Ware et al. (1984).

may be at an increased risk for the development of chronic airflow obstruction in adult life. An accelerated decline in lung function could increase the risk of chronic pulmonary disease (Samet et al., 1983).

Studies of Lung Function in Adults

White and Froeb (1980) studied 800 nonsmoking, middle-aged subjects, out of a total population size of 2,100, and found a small statistically significant decrease (8%) in $FEF_{25-75\%}$ in both men and women who were nonsmokers exposed to ETS. The reported reduction in $FEF_{25-75\%}$ for ETS exposed nonsmokers was almost identical to that of the smokers of 1-10 cigarettes per day. This raises questions about their findings. This study may suffer from problems of selection bias in the allocation of subjects to categories and the absence of any exsmokers (Adlkofer, et al., 1980; Aviado, 1980; Huber, 1980; Lee, 1982).

A cross-sectional study from France (Kauffmann et al., 1985) supports the conclusions that exposure to ETS may have an effect on lung function in nonsmoking adults. The French Cooperative Study surveyed more than 7,800 adult residents of seven cities in France in 1975 and found 1,675 were true nonsmokers. In men and women over 40, nonsmokers of either sex who had a spouse who smoked had a significantly lower $FEF_{25-75\%}$ than those living with a nonsmoker. These differences were not explained by social class, educational level, air pollution, or family size. Among the women, there was also a significant difference in FEV_1 and a dose effect was seen with the amount smoked by their husbands. These differences, only apparent in persons over 40, were small and were uncovered only following detailed examination of the data after the population had been stratified by age.

Two other cross-sectional studies involving adult women have found an effect of exposure to ETS on lung function. In a study of 220 married women aged 25 to 69 years from five U.S. cities, Kauffmann and coworkers (1986) reported that standardized residuals for FEV_1 and FEV_1/FVC* for the group identified as passive smokers were intermediate between the results of nonsmokers and current smokers. In a study of 163 nonsmoking women living in a rural area of the Netherlands, Brunekreef and coworkers (1985) found that those exposed to ETS tended to have slightly lower mean values for all of the lung function variables measured. These differences reached statistical significance for peak flow and $FEF_{25-75\%}$ in the 40- to 60-year-olds. The numbers in each of their groups were small. No information was given on possible childhood exposures to cigarette smoke of the women studied.

Kentner and coworkers (1984), in a study of 1,351 white collar workers (941 men and 410 women) in northern Bavaria, and Comstock et al. (1981), a study that included 1,724 adults residents of Washington County, Maryland, examined the potential effects of ETS. In these studies, information was collected from subjects using questionnaires and the subjects were then classified as never smoked, exsmokers, and current smokers. The Kentner et al. study evaluated home and workplace exposures, whereas the Comstock et al. study evaluated only home exposures. In the Kentner et al. (1984) study, an additional classification was made for other smokers, representing those who were cigar and pipe smokers. These

* FVC is the forced vital capacity.

investigators found no significant reductions in lung function with ETS exposure.

In view of the large number of factors that affect lung function, it is not surprising that it is difficult to document the extent to which a single type of exposure affects lung function. The lungs of adults have been subjected to many environmental exposures and potential insults over a lifetime, making it unlikely that a specific effect could be isolated. The variability in lung function due to differences of the other factors tends to obscure effects of a single variable. In addition, results in adults should be evaluated for possible misclassification of exsmokers or occasional smokers as nonsmokers, as well as possible confounding by occupational exposures to other pollutants or to ETS.

LONGITUDINAL STUDIES OF LUNG FUNCTION IN CHILDREN AND ADULTS

An important unanswered question is whether exposure to ETS affects the way the lungs grow and develop during childhood. Respiratory symptoms, by themselves, may have little clinical significance but would be important if associated with a change in the rate of lung growth and development or the development of pulmonary pathology at older ages.

There is evidence from two cohort studies (Table 11-4) that parental smoking may affect the rate of lung growth during childhood. Tager and coworkers (1983), who have followed 1,156 elementary school children in East Boston, Massachusetts, over a 7-year period, reported that maternal smoking was associated with a reduced rate of annual increase in FEV_1 and $FEF_{25-75\%}$. There was a reported 3-5% decrease in expected lung growth over the 7-year period.

Burchfiel and coworkers (1986) examined pulmonary function in 3,482 children in Tecumseh, Michigan. Children 0 to 19 years old were followed for 15 years, during which time questionnaire information was collected from both parents. FEV_1 and FVC values were significantly lower by 5% in male nonsmokers 10 to 19 years of age whose parents were current smokers.

The Harvard Air Pollution Respiratory Health Studies (Ferris et al., 1985; Berkey et al., 1986) (Figure 11-5) show a relatively smaller effect than that reported by Tager and coworkers (1983). The Harvard study included 7,834 children between the ages of

TABLE 11-4 Effects of Passive Smoking on Pulmonary Function: Selected Longitudinal Studies Involving Children/Adolescents

Study	Source of Subjects	Subjects	Exposure Assessment	Findings	Comments
Tager et al., 1983	East Boston, Mass.; random sample in schools; 1975–1981	1,156 children from 404 families; ages 5–9 years	NHLBI questionnaire completed by parents	1-year change in FEV_1 reduced in smoking families ($p < 0.02$); 9% decrease over 2 years, 7% decrease over 5 years	Tried to account for child's smoking; change scores corrected for age, sex, height, first FEV_1
Ferris et al., 1985	Six U.S. cities; different regions; survey of schools; 1974–1981	8,380 white children; ages 5–19 years; 6 annual visits	Self-administered by parents	Growth rate in FEV_1 reduced with maternal smoking ($p < 0.02$), dose related	Assumed children did not smoke; controlled for city and SES
Berkey et al., 1986	Same as Ferris et al., 1985	7,867 white children ages 6–10 years	Same as Ferris et al., 1985	Maternal and paternal smoking not significantly related to FEV_1 growth rate; however, number of cigarettes smoked by mother significant effect ($p < 0.05$)	Corrected for parental education

6 and 10 years who were followed over a 5-year period. Children whose mothers smoked one pack of cigarettes per day had FEV_1 levels, at age 8, that were 0.81% lower than children with nonsmoking mothers. Growth rates for FEV_1 were approximately 0.17% per year lower. For a child aged 8 years with an FEV_1 of 1.62 L, this corresponds to a deficit in rate of growth of FEV_1 of approximately 3 ml per annum and a deficit of 13 ml by age 8. In contrast to the lower FEV_1 seen in children whose mothers smoked, higher levels for FVC were observed in children with smoking mothers compared with children whose mothers did not smoke. For example, average FVC at age 8 for a child whose mother smoked one pack per day, was 0.33% higher than a child with a nonsmoking mother. On the other hand, the growth rate for FVC was 0.17% lower for a child with a smoking mother. This would be equivalent to a 2.8 percent decrease in pulmonary development throughout childhood and implies a decrease in the development of pulmonary function in children of smoking parents.

In view of the effects that climatic conditions can have on housing characteristics, and subsequent ventilation rates, it would be advantageous to conduct longitudinal studies in regions of the United States other than the Northeast. In any future studies, great care should be taken, as it was in the two cohort studies, to account for potential confounding variables in the analyses, such as socioeconomic status and gas cooking. Another aspect that deserves more attention in future studies is the effect on children's pulmonary function when parents stop smoking.

THE EFFECT OF PASSIVE SMOKING ON RESPIRATORY INFECTIONS

There is now strong evidence that bronchitis, pneumonia, and other lower-respiratory-tract illnesses occur more frequently (at least during the first year of life) in children who have one or more parents who smoke (see Table 11-5). Evidence that this increased frequency of acute respiratory infections continues into later childhood is less convincing, although the evidence from both cross-sectional studies and cohort studies shows such a trend.

Harlap and Davies (1974) followed a cohort of 10,672 infants born in Israel between 1965 and 1968. Admissions to the hospital during the first year of life were recorded. Information about maternal smoking was obtained during the pregnancy only. Infants

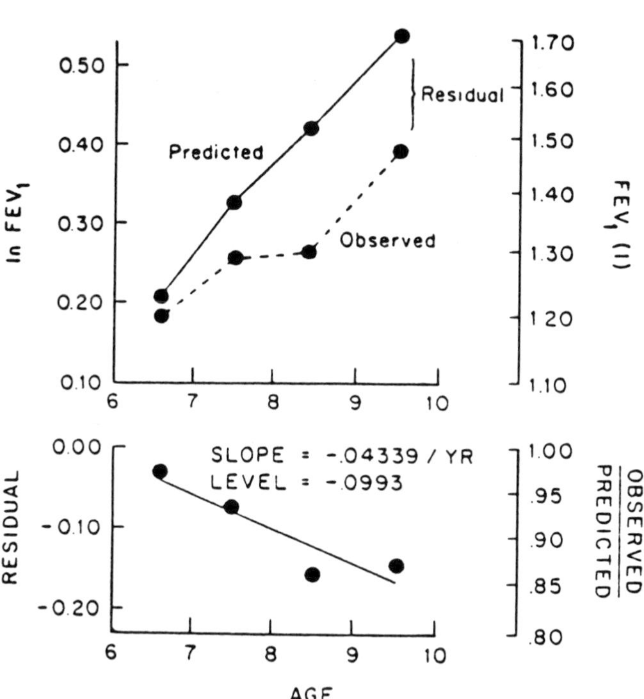

FIGURE 11-5 Calculation of growth rate and level of $\ln(\text{FEV}_1)$ for an individual child. The residuals in the upper panel, i.e., the difference between observed and predicted $\ln(\text{FEV}_1)$, were regressed on age in the lower panel. From Berkey et al. (1986).

with major congenital malformations and those dying before their first birthday were excluded from the study. For the total population studied, there were 25.4 admissions per 100 babies under 1 year of age. The infants of mothers who smoked had a 27.5% greater hospital admission rate for pneumonia and bronchitis than children of nonsmoking mothers. A dose-response relationship was also found between the amount of maternal smoking and admissions to hospital for pneumonia and bronchitis.

Colley (1974; Leeder et al., 1976) carried out a similar study in London. The study involved a birth cohort of 2,205 infants born between 1963 and 1965. In this group of children, the incidence of pneumonia and bronchitis in the first year of life was associated with the parents' smoking habits. This was true whether or not the parent has respiratory symptoms. The incidence was lowest for children of nonsmoking parents, highest in families where both

TABLE 11-5 Childhood Respiratory Tract Illness and Passive Smoking

Study	Source of Subjects	Subjects	Exposure Assessment and Health Information	Findings	Comments
Harlap and Davies, 1974	Birth cohort; West Jerusalem; 1965–1969	All infants in cohort of 10,672 admitted to hospital in Jerusalem	Antenatal interview of mothers	1. Significantly more admissions for bronchitis or pneumonia, especially in winter, in infants whose mothers smoke 2. Dose-response for number of cigarettes by mother and excess of bronchitis and pneumonia	Information about mother's smoking obtained prenatally, not concurrent with child's admission; no information about father's smoking obtained
Colley, 1974; Leeder et al., 1976	Birth cohort; Harrow, UK; 1963–1965	2,205 infants	Annual follow-up by health visitors for 5 yr; questionnaire administered by trained health visitor	1. Incidence of pneumonia and bronchitis in first year associated with parental smoking: incidence lowest with both nonsmokers, highest with both smokers, intermediate with one smoker 2. Associations inconsistent after 1 yr 3. In first year of life, ETS exposure doubled risk for pneumonia/bronchitis	Most important determinant of respiratory illness was bronchitis or pneumonia in sibling; analysis not controlled for number of siblings

Rantakallio, 1978	Birth cohort; Northern Finland; 1966	1,821 exposed, 1,821 unexposed; ages 0–5	Smoking determined in interview during pregnancy	Significant increase in hospitalization for respiratory illness	Only maternal smoking evaluated; categories based on smoking during pregnancy
Said et al., 1978	Cohort; France; 1975–1976	3,920 children; ages 10–20	Self-administered by children	Increase in tonsillectomy and/or adenoidectomy	Smoking by parents may not have coincided or preceded operations
Fergusson et al., 1981	Birth cohort; Christchurch, New Zealand; 1977	1,265 infants	Follow-up by structured interviews with mother at birth, 4 mo, 1, 2, and 3 yr; diaries kept by mothers on child's history of medical care; check with hospital records	1. Lower respiratory illness significantly related to mother's smoking in first year of life, equivocal in second and absent in third 2. No effect of paternal smoking 3. Linear dose-response between maternal smoking and incidence of lower respiratory infections	Analysis controlled for maternal age, education, family size, family living conditions
Pedreira, 1985	Birth cohort from practice of four pediatricians in suburb of Washington, D.C.; 1976–1981	1,144 infants followed for 1 yr after birth	Interview with mother at first well baby exam carried out by doctor; all subsequent office visits in first year of life for lower respiratory tract infection	1. Tracheitis and bronchitis significantly related to maternal smoking 2. No dose-response relationship 3. Bronchiolitis not related to parental smoking	No adjustment made for potentially confounding variables; relatively affluent area and low maternal smoking rate (19%)

TABLE 11-5 *Continued*

Study	Source of Subjects	Subjects	Exposure Assessment and Health Information	Findings	Comments
Speizer et al., 1980	Six U.S. cities; 1974–1979	8,120 children; ages 6–10	Questionnaire completed by parents	Parental smoking and sex of child related to respiratory disease before age 2	Recall bias a potential problem because children aged 6–10 at time of survey
Dutau et al., 1981	Survey in south of France; 1979–1980	892 children; ages 0–6 seen by pediatrician or admitted to hospital	Questionnaire administered to parents	Significant relationship between annual incidence of lower respiratory infections and total number of cigarettes smoked inside home	Pointed out importance of day care centers and nursery schools in increasing rates of lower respiratory infections and difficulty of adjustment for this

parents smoked, and intermediate where one parent smoked. This effect was not seen consistently over age 1.

A third birth-cohort study, involving 1,265 children in New Zealand, was reported by Fergusson et al. (1981). They studied the children from birth to age 3 years and found an increase in both bronchitis/pneumonia and lower respiratory illness during the first year in children whose mothers smoked. During the second year, the relationship between maternal smoking and lower respiratory illness was equivocal. The relationship disappeared by the third year. There was no effect observed of paternal smoking on the incidence of lower respiratory illness. Using logistic regression, they found that the rates of lower respiratory illness were related to maternal smoking. For each five cigarettes smoked per day by the mother, there was an increase of 2.5-3.5 lower respiratory "events" per 100 children at risk. Adjustment for maternal age, education, family size, and family living conditions did not change the relationship.

Rantakallio (1978) studied the effect of maternal smoking during pregnancy on morbidity and mortality of children to age 5 based on 12,068 births. Smoking status on the mother was only available from antenatal interview. Perinatal mortality was not higher among children of smokers, however, postneonatal mortality (between 28 days and 5 years) was significantly increased. Children of smokers were hospitalized for respiratory illness significantly more often than children of nonsmokers and the average duration of hospitalization was longer among children of smokers.

Two case-control studies evaluated smaller groups of children hospitalized for respiratory infection and nonhospitalized controls. Pullan and Hay (1982) studied 130 children who were hospitalized with a documented respiratory syncytial virus (RSV) infection in infancy and 111 controls. They found that children hospitalized with documented RSV infections were more likely to have mothers who smoked and that the children had an excess of wheeze and asthma and lower levels of pulmonary function, which persisted to age 10. Sims et al. (1978) also suggested that cigarette smoking by parents during a baby's first year of life is associated with an increased risk of RSV infections.

Speizer et al. (1980) studied approximately 8,000 children, aged 6-10 years, from six communities in the United States as part of a prospective study of the health effects of air pollution (Harvard Air Pollution Respiratory Health Studies). Parental smoking and sex of the child was associated with respiratory disease before age 2, after other variables had been taken into account. Children from households with gas cooking also gave a history of more frequent respiratory illness before age 2 than children from households with electric cooking.

Dutau et al. (1981) studied 892 children under age 6 in the south of France who were seen by a pediatrician or hospitalized for various reasons. They found a significant correlation between the annual incidence of pulmonary infections and the total number of cigarettes smoked inside the house.

Pedreira et al. (1985) followed all newborns (1,144 infants) seen by a group of pediatricians for a first well-baby examination between 1976 and 1981. They found that tracheitis and bronchitis occurred significantly more frequently (89% and 44%, respectively) in infants whose parents smoked and that maternal smoking imposed greater risks upon the infants than paternal smoking.

One study looked at the frequency of tonsillectomies and/or adenoidectomies in children (Said et al., 1978). They found the frequency was significantly increased among children with smoking parents. However, the smoking status reported for the parent may have been current smoking status, even though the operations had occurred 5 to 15 years previously.

All the studies that have examined the incidence of respiratory illnesses in children under the age of 1 year have shown a positive association between such illnesses and exposure to ETS. The association is very unlikely to have arisen by chance. It may represent a direct association between ETS exposure and disease (a causal explanation) and/or an indirect one (noncausal) arising because children living in homes of smokers are at risk of such diseases for other reasons. Some of the studies have examined the possibility that the association is indirect by allowing for confounding factors—such as social class, parental respiratory illnesses and birthweight—and have concluded that such factors do not explain the results. This argues, therefore, in favor of the causal explanation. Such an explanation is supported by the evidence of a dose-response relationship specific for respiratory disease (Tables 11-6 and 11-7). Also, the mother's smoking is more likely to affect the infant than the father's smoking, since the proximity of mother and child is closer during the child's first year when the effect is more marked and consistent than later in childhood (see Fergusson et al., 1981). This also supports a causal, rather than an indirect, explanation. Therefore, the evidence indicates that smoking in the home does increase the incidence of respiratory illness in infants.

The mechanism for this increase is less certain. It could represent a direct effect of ETS on the respiratory tract of the infant or it could be due to such infants' being exposed to more parental respiratory infections as a result of their parents' smoking. Either way, smoking in the home appears to increase the rate of respiratory illness in young children.

WHEN DO PULMONARY EFFECTS OF PASSIVE SMOKING OCCUR?

The weight of evidence is that there are clearly observable effects of ETS on the respiratory system. These effects include an increase in the incidence of acute respiratory infections in early infancy; increased prevalance of cough, sputum production, and wheezing; and a decrease both in lung function measured at an instant in time and in the growth of lung function. The finding of differences in symptom prevalence, respiratory infection rates, and lung function among children exposed and not exposed to ETS is often interpreted as evidence of a chronic effect of ETS on the airways. This is probably true, and it is unlikely that ETS is not an upper- and lower-respiratory-tract irritant in children.

The possibility that there is an effect of maternal smoking in utero as well must be considered. Evidence of an in utero effect in pregnant rats exposed to whole tobacco smoke has been reported by Collins et al. (1985). These investigators reported that pregnant rats exposed to smoke daily from day 5 to day 20 of gestation, when compared with control rats, showed reduced lung volume at term and saccules that were reduced in number and increased in size. The internal surface area of the lung was decreased. The relevance of this study to maternal smoking during pregnancy in humans is not yet clear and deserves further investigation.

Other factors that may alter the time when ETS effects during childhood include the relative immaturity of the immunologic system and the growth and remodeling that are occurring in the immature lung. The infant lung differs in a number of important ways from the adult lung: (1) T-lymphocyte and macrophage function are not fully developed at birth, (2) there is increased susceptibility to infection as a result of comparatively immature

TABLE 11-6 Experimental Studies of Acute ETS Exposures for Asthmatic Patients

Study	Population	Exposure	Findings	Comments
Shephard et al., 1979a	Fourteen patients from the Gage Research Institute (nine male, five female); mean age 37 years	Room: 14.6 m^3 Time: 2 h Cig.: 7 CO: 24 ppm	Changes in pulmonary function slight; slight decrease in total lung capacity (helium mixing, $p < 0.02$)	Patients on medication; associated chronic bronchitis or pulmonary emphysema in some patients; four patients claimed smoke sensitivity
Dahms et al., 1981	Ten patients from St. Louis Univ. Hospital Allergy Clinic; ages 16–39; 10 controls, ages 24–53	Room: 30 m^3 Time: 1 h Cig.: n.g. CO: 15–20 ppm	Linear decrease in pulmonary function over time in patients; FEV_1 decreased 21.4%; $FEF_{25-75\%}$, 19.2%; FVC, 20%; no change in controls	Patients on medication with restricted use of bronchodilators 4 h prior to test; five patients and five controls complained of irritation to ETS
Knight and Breslin, 1985	Six patients (4M, 2F); mean age 25.5 yr	Details not given	Significant decrease in 3/6 subjects; $PC_{20}FEV_1$ significantly decreased with histamine	No correlation of decreased function with chest symptoms
Wiedemann et al., 1986	Nine patients with near normal lung function; ages 19–30	Room: 4.25 m^3 Time: 1 h Cig.: n.g. CO: 40–50 ppm	No change in expiratory flow rates; small decrease in bronchial reactivity; $PD_{20}FEV_1$ increased from 0.25 to 0.79 with methylcholine	Patients off medication; six patients with history of reaction to ETS

Abbreviations: n.g. = not given.

TABLE 11-7 Admission Rates in the First Year of Life for Bronchitis and Pneumonia per 100 Infants by Maternal Smoking and Number of Cigarettes Smoked Daily (Number of Infants in Parentheses)

Nonsmokers					
Never Smoked	Former Smokers	Smokers (Cigarettes per day)			Total
(8,900)	(786)	1-10 (747)	11-20 (179)	21+ (60)	(10,672)
9.6	7.8	10.8	16.2	31.7	9.8

NOTE: Differences among three categories of smoker $p < 0.001$.

SOURCE: Harlap and Davies (1974).

lung defenses, (3) the internal diameter of the small airways is extremely small and vulnerable to obstruction, and (4) the newborn child has its full complement of airways at birth but only a small proportion of the alveoli. During childhood the airways grow in internal diameter, and the alveoli both multiply and increase in size.

The question of the timing of the effect of ETS on the growing and developing lung remains to be elucidated. If the effect is in utero, the question of how this carries over into infancy and childhood must be addressed. Likewise, the carryover effects of increased incidence of respiratory infections in infancy must be determined. In this regard, there is already some information relating early childhood respiratory illness to subsequent respiratory symptoms and impaired lung function later in childhood (Woolcock et al., 1984; McConnochie, 1985). Evidence is also accumulating that respiratory infections in early childhood are related to an accelerated decline of FEV_1 in adult life (Burrows et al., 1977b; Lebowitz and Burrow, 1976). If this is so, and if exposure to ETS increases susceptibility to acute respiratory infections in infancy, ETS may have a carryover effect into adult life.

From the evidence to date, it appears that the effects of exposure to ETS may start in utero by altering the growth pattern of the fetal lung. In infancy, exposure to ETS may increase susceptibility to viral respiratory infections that in turn may have a carryover effect into later childhood and adult life. Direct effects of ETS as an airway irritant are also likely, although the dose by itself may be insufficient except for the most susceptible individuals to cause symptoms and/or functional impairment. It is unlikely that exposure to ETS can cause much emphysema. As one of the many pulmonary insults, however, ETS may add to the total burden of environmental factors that become sufficient to cause chronic airway or parenchymal disease.

STUDIES OF ACUTE PULMONARY EFFECTS

Several studies have examined acute responses to ETS. Because asthmatics may be hypersensitive to exposures to noxious agents, a number of studies have also searched for acute effects of exposure to ETS among asthmatic populations. Other studies have been conducted on normal healthy adults.

Normal Subjects

Pimm et al. (1978) compared various physiologic responses of nonsmokers to either room air or room air plus machine-generated cigarette smoke. Each smoke exposure consisted of combustion of four cigarettes to produce an extremely polluted room with high levels of carbon monoxide (24 ppm) and particles (greater than 4 mg/m^3). Pulmonary function tests, nitrogen washout curves, blood carboxyhemoglobin levels, and heart rates were measured before, during, and after a 2-hour exposure. A few statistically significant differences between smoke and ambient air exposure days were found. The differences were small and were considered by the investigators to be of questionable importance. Subjective complaints were common in this and other acute cigarette smoke exposure studies, particularly eye irritation and cough. CO and suspended particles are thought to be less important than the phenols, aldehydes, and organic acids in producing this symptomatology (Hinds and First, 1975).

Shephard et al., (1979b) utilized a protocol similar to Pimm et al. (1978) but under conditions of intermittent moderate exercise (increasing the respiratory volume per minute 2.5 times). Moderate and heavy ETS exposures were considered, associated with CO concentrations of 20 and 31 ppm, respectively. Neither exercise

TABLE 11-8 Pneumonia and Bronchitis by Parents Smoking in First Year of Follow-up, Annual Incidence per 100 Children (Number of Infants in Parentheses)

Both Nonsmokers	Both or One Exsmokers or Smoking Habits Changed	One Smoker	Both Smokers	All
7.8	9.2	11.4	17.6	11.5
(372)	(675)	(552)	(478)	(2,077)

SOURCE: Colley et al. (1974).

nor exposure level significantly influenced symptomatology. Small decrements (3-4%) in FVC, FEV_1, $V_{max50\%}$, and $V_{max25\%}$ (the volumes of air expired during the first half of the period of forced expiration or first quarter of the period, respectively) were noted in response to smoke exposures; however, static lung volumes were unaffected. Eye irritation and odor complaints were very common. One subject complained of wheezing and chest tightness, although his pulmonary function was not significantly impaired. Subjective symptom scores were higher overall for the higher smoke exposure (13.8 versus 10.3 points/subject at the lower exposure). A few subjects reported cough, nasal discharge, or stuffiness and throat irritation.

Asthmatic Subjects

A number of studies have examined acute pulmonary responses of asthmatic patients to exposure to ETS (Table 11-8). However, the mechanisms for bronchoconstriction among asthmatics differ. Therefore, the comparison between study populations and between individuals within studies is difficult.

Shephard et al. (1979a) examined asthmatic persons to determine whether their response to ETS exceeded that of normal subjects in a previous study. The subjects (9 men and 5 women; average age, 37 years) were exposed for 2 hours to machine-generated smoke (CO, 24 ppm). None of the patients had current respiratory infections, but some may have had associated chronic bronchitis or pulmonary emphysema. No significant alterations in dynamic lung volumes (FEV_1, $V_{max50\%}$, and $V_{max25\%}$) were detected when the asthmatics' responses to ambient air and cigarette smoke were compared. A small, but significant, decrease in total lung capacity (TLC) was noted, although preexposure TLC was slightly higher than that on the same exposure day (96.5% and 103.5% relative to ambient air TLC, respectively). The lack of measurable change was interesting in light of a reported history of exacerbation with exposure to ETS by four subjects. Acute symptomatic responses during the experimental study were similar to those seen in the investigators' previous study of normal individuals; however, more complaints of tightness in the chest (43% of subjects) and wheezing (36%) were made by asthmatic subjects. It was concluded that asthmatics did not have unusual measurable responsiveness to ETS exposure in this study.

The findings of Dahms et al. (1981) contrast with those of Shephard et al. (1979a). The exposure in this study was less intense, i.e., 1 hour at CO levels of 15-20 ppm. The patients were 16 to 39 years old, had mild impairment, and were on medication, except for the restriction that no bronchodilators might be used within 4 hours previous to the test. Five of the patients reported specific complaints when exposed to ETS. When compared with control subjects, asthmatics showed significant pulmonary function changes following 1 hour of smoke exposure. FVC decreased 20% and FEV_1 declined 21.4% in the asthmatic subjects. These decreases are very large compared with the other studies. Based on a 0.40% increase in blood carboxyhemoglobin, the environmental CO concentration was calculated to be between 15 and 20 ppm—compared with approximately 24 ppm in the Shephard et al. (1979a) studies. Reasons for the discrepancy between the Dahms and Shephard studies results are not clear, nor do Dahms et al. (1981) cite or discuss the earlier Shephard et al. (1979a) findings.

Knight and Breslin (1985) evaluated six nonsmoking patients. The details of the subject population and exposure conditions were not specified. They measured a mean fall in FEV_1 of 11% following exposure to ETS. Using a histamine inhalation test, they found that the provocative concentration (or dose) that produced a 20% fall in FEV_1 ($PC_{20}FEV_1$ or $PD_{20}FEV_1$) decreased following exposure to ETS. This indicates an increased bronchial reactivity to histamine. The authors hypothesized that the airways may be primed to react more vigorously to other triggers.

Wiedemann et al. (1986) evaluated nine asthmatic individuals (aged 19 to 30 years) with normal or nearly normal lung function for both lung function and airway reactivity following exposure to ETS. Six patients reported a history of reaction to ETS. These subjects, all of whom were off medication, were exposed for 1 hour (CO between 40 and 50 ppm). Their carboxyhemoglobin levels increased an average of 0.86% ($p < 0.001$), FVC decreased 2% ($p < 0.01$), and FEV_1 declined 1% (not statistically significant). Airway reactivity was assessed using a methylcholine challenge test. The $PD_{20}FEV_1$ increased from 0.25 ± 0.22 on the day before exposure to 0.79 ± 1.13 postexposure ($p < 0.05$), indicating a decrease in airway reactivity following exposure. The magnitude of this decrease was small, and the clinical meaning of the change is uncertain.

There are a number of possible reasons for the apparent inconsistency among these studies, not the least of which is small sample sizes. The subjects have not been characterized fully. As noted by the authors, the stability of patients and mechanisms of bronchoconstriction differ among subjects. For instance, patients were included in several of these studies, regardless of whether they were hypersensitive on the methylcholine challenge test. Further, some studies were performed on medicated patients. None of the studies could be performed blind to the presence of ETS. Therefore, the authors could not exclude the possibility that pulmonary function changes could be emotionally related to cigarette smoke exposure, especially in those patients who reported previous histories of adverse response to ETS exposure.

There are several issues that are unresolved by these studies. For instance, what proportion of a clearly defined population of asthmatics do react to ETS? If the patients are selected according to methylcholine or histamine responsiveness, criteria should be given for the extent of responsiveness, since it is a continuum. To address the issue of degrees of sensitivity, the appropriate case-control or cross-over studies, with carefully selected populations, need to be done.

Mechanisms of Response

The mechanisms responsible for eye irritation and rhinitis, as well as possible changes in airway size, are almost entirely unknown. They could represent irritant effects from gases such as oxides of nitrogen, acrolein, ammonia, and other reactive constituents. Lundberg et al. (1983) reported that throat irritation and local edema may be due to vapor-phase components that stimulate substance P release from local capsaicin-sensitive afferent neurons in the airway mucosa. It is also possible that an allergic mechanism could be involved. Several authors have described allergic reactions to cigarette smoke (see, for example, Zussmann, 1970). Cutaneous hypersensitivity to tobacco antigens has been described in clinical settings (Becker et al., 1976). Constituents of tobacco smoke have also been shown to be immunogenic in laboratory animals (Becker et al., 1979; Gleich and Welsh, 1979).

During the last 10 years, Becker and colleagues (1979, 1981; Becker and Dubin, 1977) have isolated a tobacco glycoprotein both from cured tobacco leaves as well as from cigarette smoke condensate. Animals that were previously sensitized to this antigen had both pulmonary and cardiovascular changes when challenged (Levi et al., 1982). However, the role, if any, of this antigen, as well as other antigens that may be present in tobacco smoke, in the pathogenesis of cardiopulmonary disease in active smokers, let alone nonsmokers exposed to ETS, remains controversial.

SUMMARY AND RECOMMENDATIONS

There have been many studies of respiratory effects of exposure to ETS to children. In view of the weight of the scientific evidence that ETS exposure in children increases the frequency of pulmonary symptoms and respiratory infection, it is prudent to eliminate smoking and resultant ETS from the environments of small children.

What Is Known

1. Children of parents who smoke compared with the children of parents who do not smoke show increased prevalences of respiratory symptoms, usually cough, sputum, and wheezing. The odds ratios from the larger studies, adjusted for the presence of parental symptoms, were 1.2 to 1.8, depending on the symptoms. These findings imply that ETS exposures cause respiratory symptoms in some children.

2. Estimates of the magnitude of the effect of parental smoking on FEV_1 function of children range from zero to approximately 0.5% decrease per year. This small effect is unlikely by itself to be clinically significant. However, it may reflect pathophysiologic

effects of exposure to ETS in the lungs of the growing child and, as such, may be a factor in the development of chronic airflow obstruction in later life.

3. Bronchitis, pneumonia, and other lower-respiratory-tract illnesses occur up to twice as often during the first year of life in children who have one or more parents who smoke than in children of nonsmokers.

What Scientific Information Is Missing

1. ETS exposure during childhood may influence the development of airway hyperresponsiveness in adult life. Research is needed to address this issue. To evaluate the timing of physiologic changes during development may require animal studies.

2. Future cross-sectional studies of ETS exposure and lung function in adults need to be designed to control for other factors that may affect lung function.

3. Little information is available from long-term longitudinal studies of the effect of exposure to ETS by nonsmokers on lung function in either children or adults. Studies need to be carried out in areas with different climates and characteristics of housing over long enough periods of time to assess the effects of changing smoking patterns. Animal studies may also be required to address these longitudinal questions. Intervention studies, in which parents stop smoking in the presence of children, should be done to assess the reversibility of these effects.

4. The pathophysiologic mechanism of increased susceptibility to viral infections in very young children exposed to ETS has not been clarified.

5. The extent to which normal and asthmatic adults are affected by short-term exposures to ETS needs to be studied further.

6. The few studies of the effect of short-term ETS exposure of asthmatic patients and of nonasthmatics are not consistent. This may be because they have not been conducted under adequate control and have examined persons with considerable variability in the severity of asthmatic disease and airway responsiveness. Future studies should carefully define the populations when addressing issues of frequency of reaction to ETS and should be done separately on hyperresponsive and nonhyperresponsive patients when addressing issues of severity of reaction to ETS.

7. Studies of other patients with obstructive lung disorders, such as cystic fibrotic and alpha-1-antitrypsin patients, need to be done. Future studies need to identify susceptible subpopulations, if they exist, who are unusually vulnerable to the acute effects of ETS exposure.

8. There is no consensus on how to deal with data on parental respiratory symptoms. Investigations should report on rates of childhood illness/symptoms using analyses that are both adjusted and unadjusted for parental symptoms.

9. There is need for information on changes in pulmonary function between the end of the peak growth period and adult life to assess the possible reversibility of effects.

REFERENCES

Adlkofer, F., G. Scherer, and H. Weimann. Small-airways dysfunction in passive smokers. N. Engl. J. Med. 303:392, 1980.

Aviado, D.M. Small-airway dysfunction in passive smokers. N. Engl. J. Med. 303:393, 1980.

Beck, G.J., C.A. Doyle, and E.N. Schachter. Smoking and lung function. Am. Rev. Respir. Dis. 123:149-155, 1981.

Becker, C.G., T. Dubin, and H.P. Wiedemann. Hypersensitivity to tobacco antigen. Proc. Natl. Acad. Sci. USA 73:1712-1716, 1976.

Becker, C.G,. and T. Dubin. Activation of factor XII by tobacco glycoprotein. J. Exp. Med. 146:457-467, 1977.

Becker, C.G., R. Levy, and J. Zavecz. Induction of IgE antibodies to antigen isolated from tobacco leaves and from cigarette smoke condensate. Am. J. Pathol. 96:249-254, 1979.

Becker, C.G., N. Van Hamont, and M. Wagner. Tobacco, cocoa, coffee, and ragweed: Cross-reacting allergens that activate factor-XII-dependent pathways. Blood 58:861-867, 1981.

Berkey, C.S., J.H. Ware, D.W. Dockery, B.G. Ferris, Jr., F.E. Speiger. Indoor air pollution and pulmonary function growth in preadolescent children. Am. J. Epidemiol. 123:250-260, 1986.

Bland, M., B.R. Bewley, V. Pollard, and M.H. Banks. Effect of children's and parents' smoking on respiratory symptoms. Arch. Dis. Child. 53:100-105, 1978.

Brunekreef, B., P. Fischer, B. Remijn, R. Van der Lende, J. Schouten and P. Quanjer. Indoor air pollution and its effect on pulmonary function of adult non-smoking women. III. Passive smoking and pulmonary function. Int. J. Epidemiol. 14:227-230, 1985.

Burchfiel, C.M., M.W. Higgins, J.B. Keller, W.J. Butler, W.F. Howatt, and I.T.T. Higgins. Passive smoking, respiratory symptoms and pulmonary function: A longitudinal study in children. Am. Rev. Respir. Dis. 133:A157, 1986.

Burrows, B., R.J. Knudson, M.G. Cline, and M.D. Lebowitz. Quantitiative relations between cigarette smoking and ventilatory function. Am. Rev. Respir. Dis. 115:195-205, 1977a.

Burrows, B., R.J. Knudson, and M.D. Lebowitz. The relationship of childhood respiratory illness to adult obstructive airway disease. Am. Rev. Respir. Dis. 115:751-760, 1977b.

Chen, Y., and W.X. Li. The effect of passive smoking on children's pulmonary function in Shanghai. Am. J. Public Health 76:515-518, 1986.

Chen, Y., W. Li, and S. Yu. Influence of passive smoking on admissions for respiratory illness in early childhood. Br. Med. J. 293:303-306, 1986.

Cockcroft, D.W., B.A. Berscheid, and K.Y. Murdock. Unimodal distribution of bronchial responsiveness to inhaled histamine in a random human population. Chest 83:751-754, 1983.

Colley, J.R.T. Respiratory symptoms in children and parental smoking and phlegm production. Br. Med. J. 2:201-204, 1974.

Colley, J.R.T., W.W. Holland, and R.T. Corkhill. Influence of passive smoking an parental phlegm on pneumonia and bronchitis in early childhood. Lancet 2:1031-1034, 1974.

Collins, M.H., A.C. Moessinger, J. Kleinerman, J. Bassi, P. Rosso, A.M. Collins, L.S. James, and W.A. Blanc. Fetal lung hypoplasia associated with material smoking: Morphometric analysis. Pediatr. Res. 19:408-412, 1985.

Comroe, J.H., R.E. Forster II, A.B. Dubois, W.A. Briscoe, and E. Carlsen. The Lung: Clinical Physiology and Pulmonary Function Tests. Chicago: Year Book Medical Publ., Inc., 1962. pp. 323-364.

Comstock, G.W., M.B. Meyer, K.J. Helsing, and M.S. Tockman. Respiratory effects on household exposures to tobacco smoke and gas cooking. Am. Rev. Respir. Dis. 124:143-148, 1981.

Dahms, T.E., J.F. Bolin, and R.G. Slavin. Passive smoking: Effects on bronchial asthma. Chest 80:530-534, 1981.

Dodge, R. The effects of indoor pollution on Arizona children. Arch. Environ. Health 37:151-155, 1982.

Drill, S., and R. Thomas. Evaluation of Short-Term Bioassays to Predict Functional Impairment. Virginia: The MITRE Corp., 1980.

Dutau, G., C. Enjaume, M. Petrus, P. Darcos, P Demeurisse, and P. Rochiccioli. Enquete epidemiologue sur la tabagisme passif des enfants de 0 a 6 ans. Arch. Fr. Pediatr. 38:721-725, 1981.

Evans, M.J., W. Mayr, R.F. Bils, and C.G. Loosli. Effects of ozone on cell renewal in pulmonary alveoli of aging mice. Arch. Environ. Med. 22:450-453, 1971.

Evans, M.J., L.J. Cabral, R.J. Stephens, and G. Freeman, 1975. Transformation of alveolar type 2 cells to type 1 cells following exposure to NO_2. Exp. Mol. Pathol. 22:142-150, 1975.

Evans, M.J., N.P. Dekker, L.J. Cabral-Anderson, and G. Freeman. Quantitation of damage to the alveolar epithelium by means of type 2 cell proliferation. Am. Rev. Respir. Dis. 118:787-790, 1978.

Fergusson, D.M., L.J. Horwood, F.T. Shannon, and B. Taylor. Parental smoking and lower respiratory illness in the first three years of life. J. Epidemiol. Comm. Health 35:180-184, 1981.

Ferris, B.G., Jr., J.H. Ware, C.S. Berkey, D.W. Dockery, A. Spiro III, and F.E. Speizer. Effects of passive smoking on health of children. Environ. Health Perspect. 62:289-295, 1985.

Gammage, R.B. and S.V. Kaye. Indoor air and human health, pp. 195-200. Proceedings of the Seventh Life Sciences Symposium, Knoxville, Tennessee, Oct. 29-31, 1984. 430 pp.

Gleich, G.J., and P.W. Welsh. Immunochemical and physicochemical properties of tobacco extracts. Am. Rev. Respir. Dis. 120:995-1001, 1979.

Guyatt, G.H., and M.T. Newhouse. Are active and passive smoking harmful? Determining causation. Chest 88:445-451, 1985.

Harlap, S., and A.M. Davies. Infant admissions to hospital and maternal smoking. Lancet 1:529-532, 1974.

Hasselblad, V., C.G. Humble, M.G. Graham, and H.S. Anderson. Indoor environmental determinants of lung function in children. Am. Rev. Respir. Dis. 123:479-485, 1981.

Hinds, W.C., and M.W. First. Concentrations of nicotine and tobacco smoke in public places. N. Engl. J. Med. 292:844-845, 1975.

Huber, G.L. Small-airways dysfunction in passive smokers. N. Engl. J. Med. 303:392, 1980.

Kauffmann, F. Selection bias of PiMZ subjects. Am. Rev. Respir. Dis. 131:800-801, 1985.

Kauffmann, F., D.W. Dockery, F.E. Speizer and B.G. Ferris, Jr. Respiratory symptoms and lung function in women with passive and active smoking. Am. Rev. Respir. Dis. 133:A157, 1986.

Kentner, M., G. Triebig, and D. Weltle. The influence of passive smoking on pulmonary function—A study of 1,351 office workers. Prev. Med. 13:656-659, 1984.

Knight, A., and A. B. Breslin. Passive cigarette smoking and patients with asthma. Med. J. Aust. 4:194-195, 1985.

Lebowitz, M.D., and B. Burrows. Respiratory symptoms related to smoking habits of family adults. Chest 69:48-50, 1976.

Lebowitz, M.D., D.B. Armet, and R. Knudson. The effect of passive smoking on pulmonary function in children. Environ. Int. 8:371-373, 1982.

Lee, P.N. Passive smoking. Food Chem. Toxicol. 20:223-229, 1982.

Leeder, S.R., R. Corkhill, L.M. Irwig, W.W. Holland and J.R.T. Colley. Influence of family factors on the incidence of lower respiratory illness during the first year of life. Br. J. Prev. Soc. Med. 30:203-212, 1976.

Levi, R., J.H. Zavecz, J.A. Burke, and C.G. Becker. Cardiac and pulmonary anaphylaxis in guinea pigs and rabbits induced by glycoprotein isolated from tobacco leaves and cigarette smoke condensate. Am. J. Pathol. 106:318-325, 1982.

Lundberg, J.M., C.R. Martling, A. Saria, K. Folkers, and S. Rosell. Cigarette smoke-induced airway oedema due to activation of capsaicin-sensitive vagal afferents and substance P release. Neuroscience 10:1361-1368, 1983.

McConnochie, K.M., and K.J. Roghmann. Predicting clinically significant lower respiratory tract illness in childhood following mild bronchiolitis. Am. J. Dis. Child. 139:625-631, 1985.

McConnochie, K.M., and K.J. Roghmann. Parental smoking, presence of older sibling, and family history of asthma increase risk of bronchiolitis. Am. J. Dis. Child. 140:806-812, 1986.

National Research Council, Committee on the Epidemiology of Air Pollutants. Epidemiology and Air Pollution. Washington, D.C.: National Academy Press, 1985. 224 pp.

Pedreira, F.A., V.L. Guandolo, E.J. Feroli, G.W. Mella, and I.P. Weiss. Involuntary smoking and incidence of respiratory illness during the first year of life. Pediatrics 75:594-597, 1985.

Pimm P.E., F. Silverman, and R.J. Shephard. Physiological effects of acute passive exposure to cigarette smoke. Arch. Environ. Health 33:201-213, 1978.

Purvis, M.R., and R. Ehrlich. Effects of atmospheric pollutants on susceptibility to respiratory infection. II. Effect of nitrogen dioxide. J. Infect. Dis. 113:72-76, 1963.

Pullan, C.R., and E.N. Hey. Wheezing, asthma, and pulmonary dysfunction 10 years after infection with respiratory syncytial virus in infancy. Br. Med. J. 284:1665-1669, 1982.

Rantakallio, P. Relationship of maternal smoking to morbidity and mortality of the child up to the age of five. Acta Paediatr. Scand. 67:621-631, 1978.

Rylander, R. Environmental tobacco smoke and lung cancer. Eur. J. Respir. Dis. 133(Suppl.):127-133, 1984.

Said, G., J. Zalokar, J. Lellouch, and E. Patois. Parental smoking related to ademoidectomy and tonsillectomy in children. J. Epidemiol. Comm. Health 32:97-101, 1978.

Schenker, M.B., J.M. Samet, and F.E. Speizer. Risk factors for childhood respiratory disease. The effect of host factors and home environmental exposures. Am. Respir. Dis. 128:1038-1043, 1983.

Schilling, R.S.F., A.D. Letai, S.L. Hui, G.J. Beck, J.B. Schoenberg, and A. Bouhuys. Lung function, respiratory disease, and smoking in families. Am. J. Epidemiol. 106:274-283, 1977.

Shephard, R.F., R. Collins, and F. Silverman. "Passive" exposure of asthmatic subjects to cigarette smoke. Environ. Res. 20:392-402, 1979a.

Shephard, R.J., R. Collins, and F. Silverman. Responses of exercising subjects to acute "passive" cigarette smoke exposure. Environ. Res. 19:279-291, 1979b.

Sims, D.G., M.A. Downham, P.S. Gardner, J.K. Webb, and D. Weightman. Study of 8-year old children with a history of respiratory syncytial virus bronchiolitis in infancy. Br. J. Med. 1:11-14, 1978.

Speizer, F.E., B. Ferris, Y.M. Bishop, and J. Spengler. Respiratory disease rates and pulmonary function in children associated with NO_2 exposure. Am. Rev. Respir. Dis. 121:3-10, 1980.

Tager, I.B., S.T. Weiss, A. Munoz, B. Rosner, and F.E. Speizer. Longitudinal study of the effects of maternal smoking on pulmonary function in children. N. Engl. J. Med. 309:699-703, 1983.

Tager, I.B., S.T. Weiss, B. Rosner, and F.E. Speizer. Effect of parental cigarette smoking on the pulmonary function of children. Am. J. Epidemiol. 110:15-26, 1979.

Tashkin, D.P., V.A. Clark, M. Simmons, C. Reems, A.H. Coulson, L.B. Bourque, J.W. Sayre, R. Detels, and S. Rokaw. The UCLA population studies of chronic obstructive respiratory disease. Am. Rev. Respir. Dis. 129:891-897, 1984.

Taylor, L.D., S.D. Greenberg, and P.A. Buffler. Health effects of indoor passive smoking. Tex. Med. 81:35-41, 1985.

U.S. Public Health Service. Smoking and Health. A Report of the Surgeon General. DHEW (PHS) Publ. No. 79-50066. Rockville, Maryland: U.S. Department of Health and Human Services, Public Health Service, Office on Smoking and Health, 1979.

U.S. Public Health Service. The Health Consequences of Smoking: Cardiovascular Disease. A Report of the Surgeon General. DHHS(PHS) Publ. No. 84-50204. Rockville, Maryland: U.S. Department of Health and Human Services, Public Health Service, Office on Smoking and Health, 1983. 384 pp.

U.S. Public Health Service. The Health Consequences of Smoking: Chronic Obstructive Lung Disease. A Report of the Surgeon General. DHHS (PHS) Publ. No. 84-50205. Rockville, Maryland: U.S. Department of Health and Human Services, Public Health Service, Office on Smoking and Health, 1984. 545 pp.

Ware, J.H., D.W. Dockery, A. Spiro III, F.E. Speizer, and B.G. Ferris, Jr. Passive smoking, gas cooking, and respiratory health of children living in six cities. Am. Rev. Respir. Dis. 129:366-374, 1984.

Weiss, S.T., I.B. Tager, F.E. Speizer, and B. Rosner. Persistent wheeze: Its relation to respiratory illness, cigarette smoking, and level of pulmonary function in a population sample of children. Am. Rev. Respir. Dis. 122:697-707, 1980.

Weiss, S.T., I.B. Tager, M. Schenker, and F.E. Speizer. The health effects of involuntary smoking. Am. Rev. Respir. Dis. 128:933-942, 1983.

White, J.R., and H.F. Froeb Small-airways dysfunction in nonsmokers chronically exposed to tobacco smoke. N. Engl. J. Med. 302:720-723, 1980.

Wiedemann, H.P., D.A. Mahler, J. Loke, J.A. Virgulto, P. Snyder, and R.A. Matthay. Acute effects of passive smoking on lung function and airway reactivity in asthma subjects. Chest 89:180-185, 1986.

Woolcock, A.J., J.K. Peat, S.R. Leeder, and C.R.B. Blackburn. The development of lung function in Sydney children: Effects of respiratory illness and smoking. A ten-year study. Eur. J. Respir. Dis. 65(Suppl.132):1-137, 1984.

Zussman, B.M. Tobacco sensitivity in the allergic patient. Ann. Allergy 28:371-377, 1970.

12
Exposure to Environmental Tobacco Smoke and Lung Cancer

The risk of lung cancer in cigarette smokers is directly related to the number of cigarettes smoked. At low-to-average levels of smoking, this relationship is approximately linear and with no apparent threshold, although there are good theoretical reasons to believe that the true dose-response curve should be curvilinear and probably quadratic (Doll and Peto, 1978; Gart and Schneiderman, 1979). Among smokers, an increase in exposure leads to an increase in risk, as long as the additional tobacco smoke, whether through active or passive smoking, reaches the bronchial epithelium. Passive smoking would, therefore, be expected to cause some increase in risk of lung cancer in active smokers, as well as in any other persons in whom the appropriate tissues are exposed.

The studies reviewed in this chapter have attempted to address the questions of whether an increase in risk of lung cancer does occur in nonsmokers exposed to ETS and whether the dose-response relationship is similar to that in smokers. In part, this depends on whether there is a threshold dose of cigarette smoke exposure below which there is no increase in risk. Biological theory and current evidence on low-dose exposure to carcinogens do not provide evidence for such a threshold, and it is generally thought that one is unlikely (Office of Science and Technology Policy, 1985). If there is no threshold, it follows that exposure to tobacco smoke at low concentrations, such as that experienced by nonsmokers exposed to ETS, will cause an increased risk of lung cancer. The risk, of course, will be expected to be very much smaller than that associated with active smoking because of the much lower exposure of the bronchial epithelium to tobacco smoke.

TABLE 12-1 Urinary Cotinine (ng/ml) in Nonsmokers According to Number of Reported Hours of Exposure to Other People's Tobacco Smoke Within the Past 7 Days (Including Day Urine Sample Was Collected)

Duration of Exposure			
Quintile	Limits (h)	No.	Urinary Cotinine, mean ± SD[a]
1st	0.0–1.5	43	2.8 ± 3.0
2nd	1.5–4.5	47	3.4 ± 2.7
3rd	4.5–8.6	43	5.3 ± 4.3
4th	8.6–20.0	43	14.7 ± 19.5
5th	20.0–80.0	45	29.6 ± 73.7
All	0.0–80.0	221	11.2 ± 35.6

[a]Trend with increasing exposure was significant ($p < 0.001$).

SOURCE: Wald et al. (1984).

USING BIOLOGICAL MARKERS TO ESTIMATE RISK

Cotinine, a metabolite of nicotine, while of itself not considered a carcinogen, is a useful marker of exposure to tobacco smoke, whether through active or passive smoking. Table 12-1 shows that the mean urinary cotinine concentration increases with the estimated exposure to other people's tobacco smoke over the past 7 days. Much of these data, collected in the United Kingdom (Wald et al., 1984), showed that nonsmokers had, on average, about 0.4% of the concentration of urinary cotinine found in active smokers. Similar work done in Japan suggested that nonsmokers had relatively high cotinine levels, about one-seventh the levels in average Japanese smokers (Matsukara et al., 1984). The reason for this difference is not known and it needs to be investigated. However, in both countries studies showed increasing urinary cotinine levels in proportion to the estimated increasing ETS exposure.

In most of the epidemiologic studies that assessed the relationship of lung cancer to ETS-exposed nonsmokers, the measure of exposure used was "living with a smoking spouse." The observed risks of lung cancer for nonsmokers were compared for those living with a smoking spouse and those living with nonsmokers. While it is reasonable to believe that people living with smokers would be more heavily exposed to ETS than people living with nonsmokers, this would seem to be a relatively insensitive measure of exposure. Many people who are exposed to other peoples' smoke may not always be married to smokers. Even if they are married to smokers, they are likely to be exposed to their spouses' smoke for only a relatively small proportion of the day. The possibility exists that they may be exposed to other people's smoke, for instance, at work, or while in other public places.

A study using urinary cotinine levels as a measure of exposure, however, showed that "marriage to a smoker" may identify individuals who are more exposed to tobacco smoke in general, not simply from their spouses (Wald and Ritchie, 1984). Table 12-2 shows that the exposure to other people's smoke was greater for men married to smokers than for men married to nonsmokers (median hours of reported exposure of 21.1 and 6.5 hours per week, respectively). Of particular relevance for epidemiologic studies is the fact that exposure is greater outside the home as well as within the home. A reasonable interpretation of this fact is that men married to smokers might be more tolerant of other people's smoke than men married to nonsmokers and are less likely to seek out smoke-free environments outside the home. Similar results, based on questionnaire information, have been reported by others (Friedman et al., 1983).

These results corroborate the use of a spouse's smoking history as a method of classifying nonsmokers into groups that have different exposure levels to tobacco smoke. Using data from the

TABLE 12-2 Urinary Cotinine Concentration and Number of Reported Hours of Exposure to Other People's Tobacco Smoke Within the Past 7 Days in Nonsmoking Married Men According to Smoking Habits of Their Wives

Smoking Category of Wife	No. of Men	Urinary Cotinine Concentration, ng/ml		Exposure to Other People's Smoke in Preceding Week, h			
				Total		Outside Home	
		Mean (SE)	Median	Mean (SE)	Median	Mean (SE)	Median
Nonsmoker	101	8.5(1.3)[a]	5.0	11.0(1.2)[b]	6.5	10.0(1.2)[c]	6.0
Smoker	20	25.2(14.8)	9.0	23.2(4.1)	21.1	16.4(3.3)	10.7

NOTE: Differences (nonsmoking wife versus smoking wife): [a]$p < 0.05$; [b]$p < 0.001$; [c]$p < 0.06$ (Wilcoxin rank sum test).

SOURCE: Wald and Ritchie (1984).

British study (Table 12-2), the relative urinary cotinine levels in three groups—nonsmoking men married to nonsmoking women, nonsmoking men married to smoking women, and men who were themselves active smokers—were in the ratio of 1:3:215 (actual mean values were 8.5, 25.2, and 1,826 ng/ml, respectively; Wald and Ritchie, 1984, and personal communication). Assuming a similar half-life of cotinine in smokers and nonsmokers, this suggests that exposure to ETS among nonsmokers who are exposed is about 1% (i.e., 25.2/1826) of that of active smokers. Similar results were reported by another United Kingdom study (Jarvis et al., 1984) and one from the United States (Haley et al., 1986). However, the half-life of cotinine in nonsmokers may be roughly 50% longer than in active smokers (Kyerematen et al., 1982; Sepkovic et al., 1986), thereby changing the estimate of relative exposure by up to 50%. Assuming a usage of 20 cigarettes (one pack) per day by active (male) smokers and assuming a linear relationship between number of cigarettes smoked per day and urinary cotinine level, this represents exposure to smoke equivalents of roughly 0.1 to 0.2 cigarettes per day. Others have estimated cigarette equivalent exposures of 0.2 to 1 cigarettes per day (Klosterkötter and Gono, 1976; Hugod et al., 1978; Vutuc, 1984).

Urinary cotinine is at present the best marker of tobacco smoke intake for passive smoking dosimetry because it is highly sensitive and specific for tobacco smoke. Because it can be measured directly in nonsmokers as well as active smokers, it makes it possible to estimate the relative exposures of the two groups (see Chapter 8). With other markers or with other substances in tobacco smoke, this is not currently possible. Estimates must be made of the extent to which these substances are inhaled in mainstream smoke, on the one hand, and released into room air, diluted, and then inhaled by nonsmokers, on the other (Chapter 7). Both of these estimates involve more assumptions in estimating the actual intake.

Whether a urinary cotinine measurement can provide a reasonable basis for computing a first estimate of the risk of lung cancer arising from ETS exposure depends in part on whether the intake of the relevant carcinogens in active and passive smokers is directly proportional to the relevant intake of nicotine, from which cotinine is derived. Our lack of knowledge of which specific smoke components are responsible for causing lung cancer and our present inability to measure their intake directly creates uncertainty. But, as a first approximation, it is reasonable to assume proportionality.

Based on the above dosimetric considerations, the risk of lung cancer from ETS exposure among nonsmokers in the United Kingdom and United States would be small. Assuming linearity in the dose-response relationships, the risk would be about 1% of the excess risk in active smokers. This is equivalent to a relative risk of 1.14 in males, given that the relative risk in average male active smokers is 10 to 15 times greater than in nonsmokers (Hammond, 1966; Doll and Peto, 1978). For ETS-exposed women, the average relative risk may be less. If the cotinine data suggesting greater ETS exposures in Japan are correct, the excess risk in Japan would be greater.

ASSESSING THE RISK FROM EPIDEMIOLOGIC STUDIES OF LUNG CANCER AND EXPOSURE TO ETS

Some of the epidemiologic studies on the possible relationship between ETS exposure of nonsmokers and lung cancer have been discussed elsewhere (Rylander, 1984; Samet, 1985; IARC, 1986). The majority of studies of lung cancer in nonsmokers and ETS exposure classify subjects on the basis of whether the nonsmoker lives with a smoker. Eighteen such studies were identified, and the analysis presented below is based on 13 studies listed in Tables 12-3 and 12-4. The other 5 studies were excluded for the following reasons:

- Knoth et al. (1983), no reference population was given;
- Miller (1984), study reported all cancers but did not report on lung cancers separately;
- Sandler et al. (1985), included very few lung cancer cases;
- Koo et al. (1984), a more recent analysis of the population was presented in Koo et al. (1986); and
- Wu et al. (1985), raw data were not presented.

Otherwise our analysis used data from all the studies, thereby reducing the possibility of bias arising out of selecting only some of the studies that met minimal standards.

Table 12-3 gives the characteristics of the 13 studies included in the analysis. The relative risk estimate, together with its 95%

TABLE 12-3 Epidemiologic Studies of Lung Cancer and Exposure to Environmental Tobacco Smoke: Methodological Description of Studies Included in Analysis

		Exposure Assessment[a]					
Study	Subjects	Type of Interview	Proxy Informants?	Not Married	Exsmokers[b]	Environments Assessed	Comments
Chan and Fung, 1982	Hong Kong, <39: 84 cases (out of 189); 139 orthopedic controls	Interview, not blind	No criteria given	No criteria given	No criteria given	Home and workplace	Little information on methods or selection of controls; no adjustments of odds ratio; high cancer rate for South China
Trichopoulos, et al., 1983	Greece: 62 cases (out of 102); 190 orthopedic controls (out of 251)	Interview, not blind	No	"Unexposed"	Exclude if smoked within prior 20 yr; "nonsmoker" if no smoking in 20 yr; "ex-smoker" if stopped 5–20 yr before	Spouse (current and former)	Excluded adenocarcinomas and terminal bronchial; original sample similar age and SES, no match on final sample
Correa et al., 1983	Louisiana: 30 (22F, 8M) cases (out of 35) 313 (133F, 180M) hospital controls (diseases not related to smoking)	Interview, blinded	Yes (24% of cases, 11% of controls)	Excluded, include "ever married"	Exclude; used pack yr of husband	Spouse, parents	No adjustment for age, race, or hospital admission; reported odds ratio for older than 40; excluded bronchioalveolar cancer

Kabat and Wynder, 1984	Multicenter USA: 78 (25M, 53F) cases; 78 (25M, 53F) controls (non-tobacco cancers)	Interview, not blind	No	24 cases and 25 controls had no spouse	Only data for 1 yr	Workplace, home	Cases, controls matched for age, sex, race, hospital, and date interviewed
Buffler et al., 1984	Texas: 41 cases (out of 460); 192 population-based controls (out of 482)	Interview	Yes	No criteria given	No criteria given	Spouse	Original population matched age, race, vital status, county; no match on final sample
Garfinkel et al., 1985	NJ, Ohio: 134 cases age 40+; 402 colon cancer	Interview, blinded	Yes	Used data on relative, otherwise "unexposed"	Exclude, exposed	Home, outside home	No dose-response effect; corrected for age, SES, date diagnosed
Pershagen et al., in press	Sweden: 67 registry cases; 347 controls	Mailed	Yes	"Unexposed"	Exclude	Spouse, parents, workplace	Previous interview 1961, 1963 with follow-up 1984; possible interaction with radon; adjusted for occupation, radon, urban; matched for age, vital status
Akiba et al., 1986	Japan: 113 (94F, 19M) cases (out of 164); 380 (270F, 110M) controls (match age, city, vital status)	Interview, not blind	Yes, (90% of cases, 88% of controls)	Excluded	Exclude; spouse "nonsmoker" if no smoking in prior 10 yr	Spouse, parents	Selected from atomic bomb survivors; average age more than 70; no adjustment for radiation dose

TABLE 12-3 *Continued*

		Exposure Assessment[a]					
Study	Subjects	Type of Interview	Proxy Informants?	Not Married	Exsmokers[b]	Environments Assessed	Comments
Koo et al., in press	Hong Kong: 86 cases (out of 200); 136 controls (out of 200)	Interview, not blind	No	Used workplace	Exclude; exposed	Workplace, home, parents	Original sample matched for age, SES; no data on match in final sample; data on former spouses
Lee et al., 1986	England: 47 (32F, 15M) cases (out of 1,863); 96 (66F, 30M) controls	Interview	No	Excluded	Exclude	Home, workplace, leisure, daily travel	Follow-up; original sample matched for age, sex; not matched in final sample
Garfinkel et al., 1981	USA survey: 375,000 women (176,739 married) (total 153 cases)	Mailed	Yes	Used relative	Exclude	Spouse	Interviewed 1959, 1960 followed up 1972; adjusted for age, race, education, occupation, disease
Gillis et al., 1984	Scotland: 4,061 married pairs (total 6 cases)	Interview self-report	No	Excluded	Exclude	Spouse	Survey 1972, 1976 with mortality through 1982; age adjusted
Hirayama, 1981, 1984	Japan: 142,857 women age 40+ (91,450 married) (total 200 cases by death certificates)	Interview, blinded	No	Excluded	Exclude; calculated risk separately	Spouse (current)	Interviewed, follow-up 16 yr later; differences in age, occupation

[a]These columns include the criteria for certain aspects of exposure assessment treated in the data analyses of the study.
[b]Disposition if subject is exsmoker; disposition if husband is exsmoker.

confidence interval, is shown in Figure 12-1 for each of the studies. Also shown in Figure 12-1 is the summary estimate based on the studies combined. The relative risk estimates of lung cancer in nonsmokers in association with ETS exposure, together with the data used for calculating them, are given in Table 12-4. The data given in this table permit readers to combine any subset of the 13 studies which they may wish to consider. A summary estimate of the relative risk for the selected studies can then be calculated using the general method described in Appendix B. The method weights each study by its statistical precision and avoids making inappropriate comparisons across different studies. In the course of examining the data, several such subset analyses were conducted and the results are presented below.

The overall summary relative risk of lung cancer among nonsmokers in association with ETS exposure was 1.34 (95% confidence limits 1.18-1.53). For all *women* the relative risk was 1.32 (1.16-1.51); for *men* it was 1.62 (0.99-2.64). The wide confidence limits for men reflect the fact that most of the data were based on nonsmoking women rather than nonsmoking men. For studies conducted in the United States, the relative risk was 1.14 (0.92-1.40). Considering only the largest studies (those with expected number of lung cancer deaths of 20 or more), the relative risk estimate was 1.32 (1.15-1.52). The confidence limits on each of these estimates all include the overall summary estimate of 1.34.

CORRECTIONS TO ESTIMATES FOR SYSTEMATIC ERRORS

Two alternative explanations can be given for the finding of an increased risk in the epidemiologic studies. The finding may represent a direct and causal effect of ETS exposure on lung cancer in nonsmokers; or it could be due in whole or in part to bias, either in the form of systematic errors in the reporting of information or a confounding factor that is associated both with lung cancer and the fact of living with a spouse who smokes. An important question to answer is "What true risk, modified by a reasonable set of bias-producing factors, could lead to the average risk indicated by the epidemiologic studies?" In the following sections two computations are given that estimate how much the true relative risks might be modified as a result of these possible kinds of misclassification.

TABLE 12-4 Summary of Epidemiologic Studies of Risk Based on Exposure Assessed by Spouse Smoking Habits, When Available, or Smoking by the Household Cohabitants

Study No.	Study Authors	Location	Sex	Lung Cancers in "Exposed" Group: Obs.	Lung Cancers in "Exposed" Group: Exp.	O-E	Var. of (O-E)	Risk[a]	95% Confidence Limits	
Case-Control Studies										
1	Chan and Fung, 1982	Hong Kong	F	34	37.7	−3.7	13.01	0.75	0.44	1.30
2	Trichopoulos et al., 1983	Greece	F	38	29.3	8.7	11.70	2.13	1.18	3.78
3	Correa et al., 1983	U.S.A.	F	14	10.6	3.4	4.75	2.03	0.83	5.03
			M	2	1.2	0.8	0.98	2.29	0.31	16.50
4	Kabat and Wynder, 1984	U.S.A.	F	13	13.7	−0.7	3.06	0.79	0.26	2.43
			M	5	5.0	0.0	1.52	1.00	0.20	4.90
5	Buffler et al., 1984	U.S.A.	F	33	34.1	−1.1	4.78	0.80	0.32	1.99
			M	5	6.6	−1.6	2.37	0.50	0.14	1.79
6	Garfinkel et al., 1985	U.S.A.	F	92	89.5	2.5	22.33	1.12	0.74	1.69
7	Pershagen et al., in press	Sweden	F	33	29.6	3.4	13.88	1.28	0.75	2.16

8	Akiba et al., 1986	Japan	F	73	67.4	5.6	14.19	1.48	0.88	2.50
			M	3	1.8	1.2	1.38	2.45	0.46	13.06
9	Koo et al., in press	Hong Kong	F	51	45.3	5.7	13.19	1.54	0.90	2.64
10	Lee et al., 1986	England	F	22	21.9	0.1	4.71	1.03	0.41	2.47
			M	8	7.3	0.7	2.56	1.30	0.38	4.42
Overall for Case-Control Studies				426	401.0	25.0	114.40	1.24	1.04	1.50
Cohort, Prospective Studies										
11	Garfinkel, 1981	U.S.A.	F	88	81.8	6.2	30.82	1.18[b]	0.90	1.54
12	Gillis et al., 1984	Scotland	F	6	6.0	0.0	1.58	1.00[b]	0.20	4.91
			M	4	2.3	1.7	1.40	3.25[b]	0.60	17.65
13	Hirayama, 1984	Japan	F	146	129.5	16.5	34.83	1.63	1.25	2.11
			M	7	3.3	3.7	3.02	2.25	1.04	4.85
Overall for Prospective Studies				251	222.9	28.1	71.65	1.44	1.20	1.72
Overall for All Studies				692	637.7	53.1	186.0	1.34	1.18	1.53

[a]Risk is given as calculated odds ratios for case-control studies (see Appendix B for calculations) and published relative risk for cohort, prospective studies.

[b]Ratio of age standardized mortality rates.

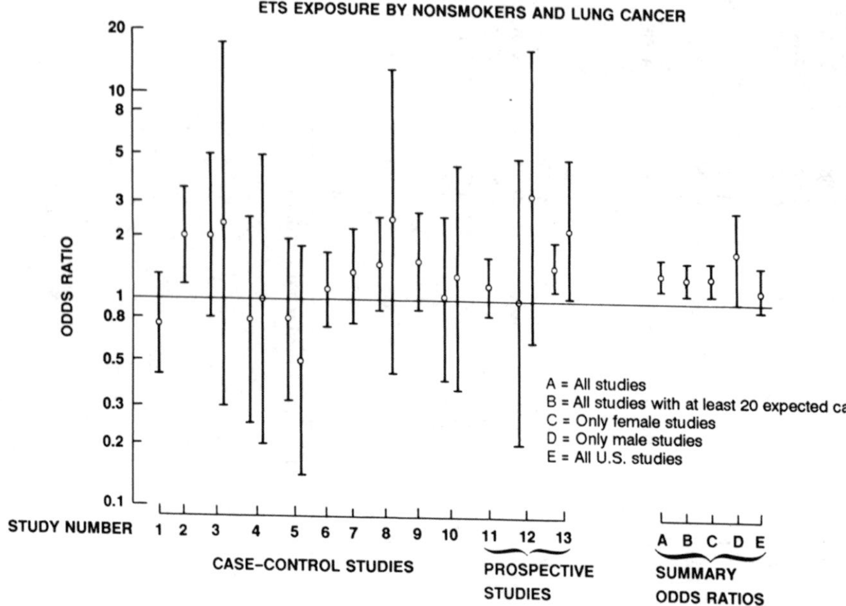

FIGURE 12-1 Passive smoking and lung cancer. The relative risk (point estimate and 95% confidence interval) of lung cancer in nonsmokers whose spouses smoke compared with nonsmokers whose spouses do not smoke for each of the studies given in Table 12-4 and the summary estimate based on all the studies combined. The figures for females are shown first for studies based on male and female subjects. STUDIES: 1. Chan and Fung, 1982; 2. Trichopoulos et al., 1983; 3. Correa et al., 1983; 4. Kabat and Wynder, 1984; 5. Buffler et al., 1984; 6. Garfinkel et al., 1985; 7. Pershagen et al., in press; 8. Akiba et al., 1986; 9. Koo et al., in press; 10. Lee et al., 1986; 11. Garfinkel, 1981; 12. Gillis et al., 1984; 13. Hirayama, 1984.

Misclassified Exsmokers and the Tendency for Spouses to Have Similar Smoking Habits

One source of potential bias that would influence the estimates of relative risk is that some people who occasionally smoke or who have smoked in the past may report that they have never smoked. Having smoked, these people are somewhat more likely to develop lung cancer than would true lifelong nonsmokers. Because smokers tend to marry smokers, they are also more likely to have a spouse who smokes or did smoke in the past. Table 12-5 shows that the bias produced by this misreporting could be serious. The arguments presented in this table are an extension of ideas discussed by Lee (Lehnert et al., 1984). From the table it is apparent that for this misclassification to fully account for the observed excess risk, it would be necessary that 8% or more of smokers and exsmokers report themselves as nonsmokers and that their smoking habits and history be identical with those of the self-reported smokers.

The proportion of people who say that they are nonsmokers, but who in fact do smoke, can be estimated using biochemical markers of tobacco smoke absorption. They appear to constitute about 0.5-3%, depending on the population studied and the questionnaire used (Wald et al., 1981; Saloojee et al., 1982). The proportion of people who smoke or have done so in the past but who say they have never smoked has also been estimated in two cohort studies (see Chapter 6). In one of these studies (N. Britten, England, personal communication University of Bristol, England; see Table 6-4), information on smoking was obtained in detail in a longitudinal study. A proportion (4.9%) of the subjects said they had never smoked as much as one cigarette a day in 1982, when in fact they had previously smoked and reported so in previous interviews. These subjects, however, had smoked at a rate of about half that of the current smokers and nearly all of them (93%) had stopped smoking 10 or more years earlier. Similar, or slightly higher, misreporting has been noted for older persons (see Chapter 6). However, older persons are likely to have smoked less and to have quit longer ago.

Table 12-5 is based on the assumption that people who fail to report that they have been smokers have the same risk of lung cancer as the average current smoker. As indicated in Table 6-4, "misclassified smokers" are more likely to have been exsmokers who failed to record the fact that they had smoked at some time in the past or, if they were current (or recent) smokers, they smoked fewer cigarettes per day than the average smoker (Table 6-4). In either event, their spouses' risk of lung cancer would be lower than for the spouse of a current smoker.

The American Cancer Society's study of smoking (Hammond, 1966) reported that women who smoked 20-30 cigarettes a day had a 4.9-fold increased risk of lung cancer compared with reported nonsmokers. The British Physicians' Study (Doll et al., 1980) yielded an estimate of 6.4. Both studies were conducted a number

TABLE 12-5 Illustration of a Bias Likely to Affect Passive Smoking Studies

ASSUME: (i) proportion of smokers among women = 35%
(ii) proportion of smokers among men = 50%
(iii) aggregation of smokers with smokers and nonsmokers with nonsmokers[a] = 3.5

True Situation

100,000 Women

35% Smokers → 35,000 S → 8% Misclassified as nonsmokers → 2,800 S

65% Nonsmokers → 65,000 NS

	Smokers misclassified as nonsmokers (2,800 S)		Nonsmokers (65,000 NS)	
Odds of having a spouse who smokes	2.28:1		1.3:2	
Spouses	1,947.1 S (a)	852.9 NS (b)	25,660.8 S (c)	39,339.2 NS (d)
Assume true *RR* of lung cancer associated with smoking (8.0) and spouse smoking (1.0)	8.0	8.0	1.0	1.0
Rate/10,000/10 years	40.0	40.0	5.0	5.0
Number of lung cancers	7.79 (e)	3.41 (f)	12.83 (g)	19.67 (h)

Observed Situation

Observed no.	67,800 (65,000 NS + 2,800 smokers misclassified as nonsmokers)	
Observed no. in spouse groups	27,607.9 S (a+c)	40,192.1 NS (b+d)
Observed no. of lung cancers	20.62 (e+g)	23.08 (f+h)
Observed rate/10,000/10 years	7.47	5.74
Observed RR of lung cancer associated with spouse smoking	1.30	

CONCLUSION: Misclassification error would increase the true relative risk of 1.0 to 1.30.

[a]Ratio of cross-products in a 2 × 2 table of smoking status (Yes or No) by spouse smoking status (Yes or No).

ABBREVIATIONS: S = smoker; NS = nonsmoker; RR = relative risk.

of years ago. With the increased duration of smoking in women in recent years, these relative risks also should have increased. The relative risk estimate may be as high as 8.0. To the extent that this may be an overestimate, it will tend to exaggerate the effects of misclassification. The lung cancer relative risk for persons misclassified as nonsmokers is, for the reasons given, probably less than half of that for correctly classified active smokers (relative risk of 4) and probably closer to one-quarter (relative risk of 2).

Applying the same argument illustrated in Table 12-5, the misclassification effect on the relative risk is given in Table 12-6 (N. Wald and K. Nanchahal, personal communication), assuming that the risk of lung cancer of misclassified nonsmokers is half that of current smokers (relative risk = 4.0) or one-quarter (relative risk = 2.0).

Table 12-6 shows the possible effect of a nonrandom marriage (aggregation) pattern. In this table the extent of nonrandom association is described by an "aggregation" factor. The degree of aggregation is estimated by the ratio of the cross-products in a 2 × 2 table of smoking status of study subjects by spouse smoking status. For the computations in Table 12-6, three aggregation factors are assumed, 2.5, 3.5 and 4.5. The smoker aggregation factor (from epidemiologic studies) appears to be about 3 to 4 (see Table 12-7; Wald et al., personal communication).

The overall effect on an assumed true association between passive smoking and lung cancer, i.e., the "true" relative risk, is shown in Table 12-6 for relative risks ranging from 1.0 (i.e., no association) to 1.25 (i.e., 25% increase in lung cancer risk associated with passive smoking). It is assumed that 35% of women smoke and 50% of men smoke. Also, the effects of the misclassification of between 2% and 10% of smokers as nonsmokers is shown. The most plausible assumptions are a relative risk of 2.0 to 4.0, an aggregation factor of 3 to 4, and a misclassification rate of 2 to 7%. To use Table 12-6, locate the rows and columns that correspond the the above most plausible assumptions. The entries in the body of the table that are approximately 1.34, i.e., the observed overall relative risk, correspond to the set of parametric values that, with plausible assumptions of the bias, would inflate a true relative risk to the observed values. Inspection of the data within the body of Table 12-6 shows that an observed relative risk of 1.34, given the range of assumptions specified in the table, could come about if there were a true relative risk of no less than 1.15. That is,

TABLE 12-6 Estimates of the Observed Relative Risk of Lung Cancer from Studies of Married Nonsmokers; Assuming 35% of Women and 50% of Men in the General Population Are Current Smokers

True Relative Risk		Marriage Aggregation Factor[b]	Proportion of Misclassified Smokers				
Passive Smokers	Misclassified Smokers[a]		2%	4%	6%	8%	10%
1.00	2.0	2.5	1.01	1.02	1.03	1.04	1.04
		3.5	1.01	1.03	1.04	1.05	1.06
		4.5	1.02	1.03	1.04	1.06	1.07
	4.0	2.5	1.03	1.05	1.08	1.10	1.12
		3.5	1.04	1.08	1.11	1.14	1.17
		4.5	1.05	1.09	1.13	1.17	1.20
	8.0	2.5	1.06	1.12	1.17	1.21	1.25
		3.5	1.09	1.17	1.24	1.30	1.36
		4.5	1.11	1.20	1.29	1.37	1.43
1.05	2.0	2.5	1.06	1.07	1.08	1.08	1.09
		3.5	1.06	1.08	1.09	1.10	1.11
		4.5	1.07	1.08	1.09	1.11	1.12
	4.0	2.5	1.08	1.10	1.13	1.15	1.17
		3.5	1.09	1.12	1.16	1.19	1.21
		4.5	1.10	1.14	1.18	1.22	1.25
	8.0	2.5	1.11	1.17	1.21	1.26	1.29
		3.5	1.14	1.21	1.28	1.34	1.40
		4.5	1.16	1.25	1.33	1.41	1.48
1.10	2.0	2.5	1.11	1.12	1.13	1.13	1.14
		3.5	1.11	1.12	1.14	1.15	1.16
		4.5	1.12	1.13	1.14	1.16	1.17
	4.0	2.5	1.13	1.15	1.17	1.19	1.21
		3.5	1.14	1.17	1.20	1.23	1.26
		4.5	1.15	1.19	1.23	1.26	1.30
	8.0	2.5	1.16	1.21	1.26	1.30	1.33
		3.5	1.19	1.26	1.33	1.39	1.44
		4.5	1.20	1.30	1.38	1.45	1.52
1.15	2.0	2.5	1.16	1.17	1.17	1.18	1.19
		3.5	1.16	1.17	1.18	1.20	1.20
		4.5	1.17	1.18	1.19	1.21	1.22
	4.0	2.5	1.18	1.20	1.22	1.24	1.26
		3.5	1.19	1.22	1.25	1.28	1.31
		4.5	1.19	1.24	1.27	1.31	1.34
	8.0	2.5	1.21	1.26	1.30	1.34	1.38
		3.5	1.23	1.31	1.37	1.43	1.48
		4.5	1.25	1.34	1.43	1.50	1.56
1.20	2.0	2.5	1.21	1.22	1.22	1.23	1.24
		3.5	1.21	1.22	1.23	1.24	1.25
		4.5	1.21	1.23	1.24	1.25	1.27
	4.0	2.5	1.22	1.25	1.27	1.29	1.30
		3.5	1.24	1.27	1.30	1.33	1.35
		4.5	1.24	1.28	1.32	1.36	1.39

TABLE 12-6 *Continued*

True Relative Risk							
Passive Smokers	Misclassified Smokers[a]	Marriage Aggregation Factor[b]	Proportion of Misclassified Smokers: 2%	4%	6%	8%	10%
	8.0	2.5	1.26	1.30	1.35	1.38	1.42
		3.5	1.28	1.35	1.42	1.47	1.52
		4.5	1.30	1.39	1.47	1.54	1.61
1.25	2.0	2.5	1.26	1.27	1.27	1.28	1.29
		3.5	1.26	1.27	1.28	1.29	1.30
		4.5	1.26	1.28	1.29	1.30	1.31
	4.0	2.5	1.27	1.30	1.31	1.33	1.35
		3.5	1.29	1.32	1.35	1.37	1.40
		4.5	1.29	1.33	1.37	1.40	1.44
	8.0	2.5	1.30	1.35	1.39	1.43	1.46
		3.5	1.33	1.40	1.46	1.52	1.57
		4.5	1.35	1.44	1.52	1.59	1.65

[a]Subjects who have smoked either in the past or currently, but claim to be lifelong nonsmokers.

[b]Marriage aggregation factor defined as ratio of cross-products of 2 × 2 table of smoking status of study subject by smoking status of spouse.

NOTE: The values inside the boxes indicate those situations that are most plausible, based on other sources of data for parameters, and yield observed relative risks of about 1.34.

TABLE 12-7 Number of Smokers and Nonsmokers According to the Smoking Habits of Their Spouses and the Odds Ratio Indicating the Extent of Such Marriage Aggregation[a]

	Females			Males		
Spouse	Smoker	Nonsmoker	Total	Smoker	Nonsmoker	Total
Smoker	53	17	70	20	11	31
Nonsmoker	47	83	130	53	80	133
All	100	100	200	73	91	164
Odds ratio	3.1			2.3		

[a]Based on interviewing 200 women and 164 men attending a health screening center in London or working in the Civil Service in Newcastle in 1985.

SOURCE: Wald et al., personal communication.

a true relative risk of 1.15 or more could, by a reasonable set of misclassification biases, be elevated to 1.30 in an epidemiologic study. Stated differently, this implies that reasonable misclassification does not account for the total increased risks reported by the epidemiologic studies, leaving the conclusion that the risk of lung cancer following exposure to other people's smoke, as judged by whether a nonsmoker has a smoking spouse, would be increased by a minimum of 15%, and most probably increased by 25% (i.e., 1.25). (If the percentage of women smokers were as high as 50%, it would be 1.20.)

The study by Garfinkel et al. (1985) provides data relevant to the misclassification of exsmokers and the tendency for spouses to have similar smoking habits. In this study, subjects were interviewed if the hospital record indicated nonsmoker or made no mention of smoking status. From interviews by the investigators, it was determined that 40% of the women had actually smoked. Among these women who smoked, 81% had husbands who smoked, but only 68% of the women who were in fact nonsmokers had husbands who smoked, yielding an aggregation factor of 2.0.

Effects of Incorrectly Classifying Persons as Unexposed to ETS

In the studies that classify nonsmoker exposure based on whether or not the spouse smokes, some of the "unexposed" nonsmokers, i.e., married to nonsmokers, are likely to be exposed in other settings. For instance, some nonsmokers married to nonsmokers may be exposed to ETS in the workplace. Therefore, some individuals in the baseline, "unexposed," group for these studies must have been exposed, and hence have risks greater than unity if there is an ETS effect. In the studies, which do ask about exposure to ETS in all environments, there still tends to be misclassification of some nonsmokers as "unexposed," because there may be a tendency to overlook episodes of exposure.

The data from urinary cotinine studies and the observed relative risks can be used to estimate this effect. The only known source of cotinine in the body is from nicotine, which is virtually exclusively derived from tobacco, with the exception of nicotine chewing gum and nicotine aerosol rods. Therefore, if people who actively use tobacco or nicotine-containing aids to help stop smoking are excluded, cotinine can be used as an objective measure of (recent) exposure to tobacco smoke in nonsmokers. For the following argument, the cotinine in body fluids is compared for the two groups of nonsmokers, those who reported exposure to ETS and those who reported no exposure. Since both groups are nonsmokers, the concern of whether or not the clearance rates for nicotine or nicotine metabolites differ between smokers and nonsmokers is not germane to these estimates.

In the study by Wald and Ritchie (1984), the urinary cotinine levels among nonsmokers exposed to smoking spouses were 3 times those of nonsmokers married to nonsmokers. Using a linear model of risk and assuming that the 3:1 ratio represents a lifetime difference, the implied relative risk of these two groups would be equal to:

$$RR = \frac{1 + 3\beta d_N}{1 + \beta d_N} = \frac{\text{risk to “exposed” nonsmokers}}{\text{risk to “unexposed” nonsmokers}}, \qquad (12\text{–}1)$$

where d_N is the dose received by nonsmokers who are self-declared "unexposed" and β is the increase in risk per unit dose received (for details, see Appendix C). This equation assumes that the lifetime carcinogenic dose received by nonsmokers who say that they are "exposed" is 3 times that of truly unexposed nonsmokers, assuming cotinine levels to be a proxy for carcinogenic constituents of ETS.

When Equation 12-1 is set equal to the relative risk, one can solve for βd_N. In the previous section, it was noted that the true relative risk is likely to be 1.25 and, as argued above, probably lies between 1.15 and 1.35. Consequently, relative risk values of 1.25, 1.15, and 1.35 will be considered. Using these values, βd_N will be 0.14 ("ranging" 0.08 to 0.21). Therefore, the relative risk of self-identified "unexposed" nonsmokers compared with truly unexposed nonsmokers is:

$$\frac{1 + \beta d_N}{1}, \qquad (12\text{–}2)$$

which would be 1.14 ("ranging" 1.08 to 1.21). The relative risk of "exposed" nonsmokers compared with a truly unexposed nonsmoker is:

$$\frac{1 + 3\beta d_N}{1}, \qquad (12\text{–}3)$$

which would be 1.42 ("ranging" 1.24 to 1.61). That is, the increased risk of lung cancer as a result of chronic exposure to ETS, corrected for the effect of not identifying a truly unexposed reference group of nonsmokers, is likely to be at least as large as the observed risk.

We can say, therefore, that while the epidemiologic studies show a consistent and, in total, a highly significant association between lung cancer and ETS exposure of nonsmokers, the excess might, in principle, possibly be explained by bias. However, detailed consideration of the nature and extent of the bias shows that given some reasonable assumptions the bias would be insufficient to explain the whole effect. In fact, there are some types of bias that lead to underestimates of the effect. It must be concluded, therefore, that some, if not all, of the effect reported in spouse studies is causal.

OTHER CONSIDERATIONS

Some of the spouse-smoking studies show a dose-response effect with rates increasing with increasing exposure as measured by increasing levels of cigarette consumption by the smoking spouse (see Tables 12-8 and 12-9). A dose-response relationship also suggests a causal explanation, although biases could also operate to affect this estimation. It is possible that a person misclassified as a nonsmoker married to a smoker will have a cigarette consumption that is correlated with that of his or her spouse. A misclassified nonsmoker married to a heavy smoker would, therefore, have a higher risk of lung cancer independent of spouse is smoking than a misclassified nonsmoker married to a light smoker, thus giving the appearance of a dose-response relationship between ETS exposure and lung cancer.

This possible pseudo-dose-response effect arises only as a result of misclassifying smokers as nonsmokers. It is of interest, therefore, that one study has reported an effect of passive smoking in smokers as well as nonsmokers (Akiba et al., 1986). However, it does not appear that adjustment has been made for amount smoked. To the extent that smokers married to smokers may smoke more than the smokers married to nonsmokers, this would bias the results.

TABLE 12-8 Risk of Lung Cancer in Nonsmokers According to Cigarette Consumption of Spouse

Authors	Findings	
Case-Control Studies		
Trichopoulos et al., 1983	Exsmoker	1.0
	1-20 cig. per day	2.4
	21+ cig. per day	3.4
Garfinkel et al., 1985	1-19 total cig. per day	0.84
	20-39 total cig. per day	1.08
	40+ total cig. per day	1.99
	Cigar/pipe	1.13
Akiba et al., in press	1-19 cig. per day	1.3
	20-29 cig. per day	1.5
	30+ cig. per day	2.1
Cohort Studies		
Hirayama, 1984	1-19 cig. per day	1.45
	20+ cig. per day	1.91
Garfinkel, 1981	1-19 cig. per day	1.27[a]
	20+ cig. per day	1.10[a]

[a]Mortality ratios, not relative risks.

NOTE: Relative risk for self-reported unexposed is assumed to be 1.0.

Most of the studies considered the histological type of lung cancer. In general they showed a higher proportion of adenocarcinoma in ETS-exposed nonsmokers than would be expected among active smokers. This is to be expected in view of the fact that the proportion of adenocarcinomas is, in general, higher among nonsmokers. Adding some nonadenocarcinoma-type disease, possibly as a result of ETS exposure, would reduce this proportion. It would nonetheless leave the proportion of adenocarcinomas higher than would be found among lung cancer cases among active smokers. If there were a high relative risk of adenocarcinoma associated with ETS exposure of nonsmokers, it would suggest a real effect, but the published data are insufficient or not presented in a way to allow assessing this issue at this time.

Two studies have examined the risk of lung cancer associated with passive smoking using parental smoking as a measure of exposure instead of spouse smoking (Correa et al., 1983; Sandler et al., 1985b). The first found an association with maternal smoking ($RR = 1.66$, $p < 0.05$) but not with paternal smoking ($RR =$

0.83). The second found no significant association with smoking of either parent.

The bias discussed in connection with spouse-smoking studies is likely to apply also to parental-smoking studies. In addition, these two studies included active smokers as well as recorded nonsmokers, and it is likely that the children of smokers start smoking at a younger age and possibly smoke more than do smoking children of nonsmoking parents (U.S. Public Health Service, 1984). This would also be a source of bias.

TABLE 12-9 Risk of Lung Cancer in Nonsmokers According to Duration of Smoking of Spouse or Other Measures of Exposure Not Shown in Table 12-7

Authors	Findings			
Case-Control Studies				
Trichopoulos et al., 1983	Total no. of cig. (in thousands):			
	1-99	1.3		
	100-299	2.5		
	300+	3.0		
Correa et al., 1983	Total pack-years:		*Males*	*Females*
	1-40		—	1.18
	41+		—	3.52
	All		2.0	2.07
Koo et al., 1984	Total hours:			
	1-3,499	1.28		
	3,500+	1.02		
	Any	1.24		
Garfinkel et al., 1985	No. of h/day:		*Last 5 yr*	*Last 25 yr*
	1-2		1.59	0.77
	3-6		1.39	1.34
	>6		0.94	1.14
Pershagen et al., in press			*Kreyburg I*	*Kreyburg II*
	Less than 15 cig./day or 50 g tobacco/wk for less than 30 yr		1.8	0.8
	More than 15 cig./day or 50 g tobacco/wk for more than 30 yr		6.0	2.4
Akiba et al., in press	Pack-days within last 10 yr:			
	<5,000		1.0	
	5,000-9,999		2.8	
	10,000+		1.8	

NOTE: Relative risk for self-reported unexposed is assumed to be 1.0.

Pershagen et al. (in press) reported that the relative risk for lung cancer in women married to smokers *and* living in a home that had measurable radon levels was increased relative to the effects of living with a smoker *or* living in a home with radon. They suggested that this might represent an interaction between exposure to ETS and radon. Research needs to be done that explores this association further in light of recent reports of high radon concentrations in homes (Code of Federal Regulations, 1985).

SUMMARY AND RECOMMENDATIONS

The weight of evidence derived from epidemiologic studies shows an association between ETS exposure of nonsmokers and lung cancer that, taken as a whole, is unlikely to be due to chance or systematic bias. The observed estimate of increased risk is 34%, largely for spouses of smokers compared with spouses of nonsmokers. One must consider the alternative explanations that this excess either reflects bias inherent in most of the studies or that it represents a causal effect. Misclassification can have contributed to the result to some extent. Computations of the effect of two sources of misclassification were presented. Computations taking into account the possible effects of misclassified exsmokers and the tendency for spouses to have similar smoking habits placed the best estimate of increased risk of lung cancer at about 25% in persons exposed to ETS at a level typical of that experienced by nonsmokers married to smokers compared with those married to nonsmokers. Another computation using information from cotinine levels observed in nonsmokers and taking into account the effect of making comparisons with a reference population that is truly unexposed leads to an estimated increased risk of about one-third when exposed spouses were compared with a truly unexposed population. The finding of such an increased risk is biologically plausible, because nonsmokers inhale other people's smoke and, as a result, absorb smoke components containing carcinogens.

What Is Known

1. A summary estimate from epidemiologic studies places the increased risk of lung cancer in nonsmokers married to smokers compared with nonsmokers married to nonsmokers at about 34%.

Assuming linearity at low-to-average doses and a constant proportionality of nicotine and carcinogens in mainstream smoke and ETS, extrapolation from studies of active smokers using relative urinary cotinine places the risk at about 10%.

2. To some extent, misclassification (bias) may have contributed to the results reported in the epidemiologic literature. However, bias is not likely to account for all of the increased risk. The best estimate, allowing for reasonable misclassification, is that the adjusted risk of lung cancer is increased about 25% (i.e., $RR = 1.25$) in nonsmokers married to smokers compared with nonsmokers married to nonsmokers. When one allows for exposure to nonsmokers who report themselves as unexposed, the adjusted increased risk is at least 24%. The adjusted increased risk to a group of nonsmokers married to nonsmokers is at least 8% (i.e., $RR = 1.08$) compared with truly unexposed subjects. This excess risk may come about from exposures in the workplace or other public places.

What Scientific Information Is Missing

1. It would be useful to quantify the dose-response relationship between ETS exposure and lung cancer more precisely using biological markers of exposure. Studies should be done that incorporate these biological markers.

2. Laboratory studies would be important in determining the carcinogenic constituents of ETS and their concentrations in typical daily environments and in facilitating understanding of possible dose-response relationships.

3. The interaction between ETS and radon exposure, which can increase risk of lung cancer, is worth examining further.

REFERENCES

Akiba, S., W.J. Blot, and H. Kato. Passive smoking and lung cancer among Japanese women. Fourth World Conference on Lung Cancer, Toronto, Canada, Aug. 25-30, 1985.

Akiba, S., H. Kato, and W.J. Blot. Passive smoking and lung cancer among Japanese women. Cancer Res. 46:4804-4807, 1986.

Buffler, P.A., L.W. Pickle, T.J. Mason, and C. Contant. The causes of lung cancer in Texas, pp. 83-99. In M. Mizell and P. Correa, Eds. Lung Cancer: Causes and Prevention. New York: Verlag-Chemie International, Inc., 1984.

Chan, W.C., and S.C. Fung. Lung cancer in non-smokers in Hong Kong, pp. 199-202. In E. Grundmann, Ed. Cancer Campaign, Vol. 6. Cancer Epidemiology. Stuttgart: Gustav Fischer Verlag, 1982.

Code of Federal Regulations (CFR). National primary and secondary ambient air quality standards. Code Fed. Regul. 40(Pt. 50):500-573, 1985.

Correa, P., L.W. Pickle, E. Fontham, Y. Lin, and W. Haenszel. Passive smoking and lung cancer. Lancet 2:595-597, 1983.

Doll, R.D., and R. Peto. Cigarette smoking and bronchial carcinoma: Dose and time relationships among regular smokers and lifelong non-smokers. J. Epidemiol. Comm. Health 32:303-313, 1978.

Doll, R., R. Gray, B. Hafner, and R. Peto. Mortality in relation to smoking: 22 years' observations on female British Doctors. Br. Med. J. 967-971, 1980.

Friedman, G.D., D. Pettiti, and R.D. Bawol. Prevalence and correlates of passive smoking. Am. J. Public Health 73:401-405, 1983.

Garfinkel, L. Time trends in lung cancer mortality among nonsmokers and a note on passive smoking. J. Natl. Cancer Inst. 66:1061-1066, 1981.

Garfinkel, L., O. Auerbach, and L. Joubert. Involuntary smoking and lung cancer: A case-control study. J. Natl. Cancer Inst. 75:463-469, 1985.

Gart, J.J., and M.S. Schneiderman. "Low-risk" cigarettes: The debate continues. Science 204:688-690, 1979.

Gillis, C.R., D.J. Hole, V.M. Hawthorne, and P. Boyle. The effect of environmental tobacco smoke in two urban communities in the west of Scotland. Eur. J. Respir. Dis. 133(Suppl.):121-126, 1984.

Haley, N.J. and D. Hoffmann. Analysis for nicotine and cotinine in hair in determination of cigarette smoker status. Clin. Chem. 31:1598-1600, 1985.

Haley, N.J., D. Hoffmann, and E.L. Wynder. Uptake of tobacco smoke components. In D. Hoffmann and C. Harris, Eds. Mechanisms in Tobacco Carcinogenesis (Banbury Report 23). Cold Spring Harbor, New York: Cold Spring Harbor Laboratories, 23:3-19, 1986.

Hammond, E.C. Smoking in relation to the death rates of one million men and women. Natl. Cancer Inst. Monogr. 19:127-204, 1966.

Hirayama, T. Cancer mortality in nonsmoking women with smoking husbands on a large-scale cohort study in Japan. Prev. Med. 13:680-690, 1984.

Hirayama, T. Non-smoking wives of heavy smokers have a higher risk of lung cancer: A study from Japan. Br. Med. J. 282:183-185, 1981.

Hugod, C., L.H. Hawkins, and P. Astrup. Exposure of passive smokers to tobacco smoke constituents. Int. Arch. Occup. Environ. Health 42:21-29, 1978.

Jarvis, M.J., H. Tunstall-Pedoe, C. Feyeraband, C. Vesey, and Y. Saloojee. Biochemical markers of smoke absorption and self reported exposure to passive smoking. J. Epidemiol. Comm. Health 38:355-339, 1984.

Kabat, G.C., and E.L. Wynder. Lung cancer in nonsmokers. Cancer 53:1214-1221, 1984.

Klosterkötter, W., and E. Gono. Zum Problem das Passivrauchens. Zentrabl. Bakteriol. Hyg., I. Abt. 1: Orig. B 162:51-69, 1976.

Knoth, A., H. Bohn, and F. Schmidt. Passive smoking as a causal factor of bronchial carcinoma in female nonsmokers. Medizinisch Klin. 78:66-69, 1983.

Koo, L.C., J.H-C. Ho, and N. Lee. An analysis of some risk factors for lung cancer in Hong Kong. Int. J. Cancer 35:149-155, 1985.

Koo, L.C., J.H-C. Ho, J.F. Fraumeni, W.J. Blot, J. Lubin, and B.J. Stone. Measurements of passive smoking and estimates of risk for lung cancer among non-smoking Chinese females. Fourth World Conference on Lung Cancer, Toronto, Canada, Aug. 25-30, in press.

Kyerematen, G.A., M.D. Damiano, B.H. Dvorchik, and E.S. Vesell. Smoking-induced changes in nicotine disposition: Application of a new HPLC assay for nicotine and its metabolites. Clin. Pharmacol. Ther. 32:769-780, 1982.

Lee, P.N., J. Chamberlain, and M.R. Alderson. Relationship of passive smoking to risk of lung cancer and other smoking-associated diseases. Br. J. Cancer 54:97-105, 1986.

Lehnert, G., L. Garfinkel, T. Kirayama, D. Schmälh, K. Überla, E.L. Wynder, and P. Lee. Rountable discussion. Prev. Med. 13:730-746, 1984.

Matsukura, S., T. Taminato, N. Kitano, Y. Seino, H. Hamada, M. Uchihashi, H. Nakajima, and Y. Hirata. Effects of environmental tobacco smoke on urinary cotinine excretion in nonsmokers. N. Engl. J. Med. 311:828-832, 1984.

Miller, G.H. Cancer, passive smoking and nonemployed and employed wives. West. J. Med. 140:632-635, 1984.

Office of Science and Technology Policy. Chemical carcinogens: A review of the science and its associated principles, Feb. 1985, pp. 10371-10442. Fed. Regist. 50:50(14 Mar. 1985).

Pershagen, G., Z. Hrubec, and C. Svensson. Passive smoking and lung cancer in Swedish women. Am. J. Epidemiol., in press, 1986.

Rylander, R. Environmental tobacco smoke and lung cancer. Eur. J. Respir. Dis. 133(Suppl.):127-133.

Samet, J.M. Relationship between passive exposure to cigarette smoke and cancer, pp. 227-240. In R.B. Gammage, S.V. Kaye, and V.A. Jacobs. Indoor Air and Human Health. Chelsea, Michigan: Lewis Pub., Inc.

Sandler, D.P., R.B. Everson, and A.J. Wilcox. Passive smoking in adulthood and cancer risk. Am. J. Epidemiol. 121:37-48, 1985a.

Sandler, D.P., A.J. Wilcox, and R.B. Everson. Cumulative effects of lifetime passive smoking and cancer risk. Lancet 1:312-315, 1985b.

Saloojee, Y., C.J. Vesey, P.V. Cole, and M.A.H. Russell. Carboxyhemoglobin and plasma thiocyanate: Complementary indicators of smoking behavior? Thorax 37:521-525, 1982.

Sepkovic, D.W., W.J. Haley, and D. Hoffmann. Elimination from the body of tobacco products by smokers and passive smokers. JAMA 256:863, 1986 (letter).

Trichopoulos, D., A. Kalandidi, and L. Sparros. Lung cancer and passive smoking: Conclusion of Greek study. Lancet 2:677-678, 1983.

U.S. Public Health Service. The Health Consequences of Smoking: Chronic Obstructive Lung Disease. A Report of the Surgeon General. DHHS (PHS) Publ. No. 84-50205. Rockville, Maryland: U.S. Department of Health and Human Services, Public Health Service, Office on Smoking and Health, 1984. 545 pp.

Vutuc, C. Quantitative aspects of passive smoking and lung cancer. Prev. Med. 13:698-704, 1984.

Wald, N.J. Validation of studies on lung cancer in nonsmokers married to smokes. Lancet 1:1067, 1984 (letter).

Wald, N.J., and C. Ritchie. Validation of studies on lung cancer in nonsmokers married to smokers. Lancet 1:1067, 1984.

Wald, N.J., M. Idle, J. Boreham, and A. Bailey. Carbon monoxide in breath in relation to smoking and carboxyhemoglobin levels. Thorax 36:366-369, 1981.

Wald, N.J., J. Boreham, A. Bailey, C. Ritchie, J.E. Haddow, and G. Knight. Urinary cotinine as marker of breathing other people's tobacco smoke. Lancet 1:230-231, 1984.

Wu, A.H., B.E. Henderson, M.C. Pike, and M.C. Yu. Smoking and other risk factors for lung cancer in women. J. Natl. Cancer Inst. 74:747-751, 1985.

13
Cancers Other Than Lung Cancer

The association of lung cancer with exposure to ETS has yielded relative risks of 2 or less for nonsmokers. As cancer of the lung is the cancer most strongly associated with active smoking, weaker effects would be expected for cancers that are less closely related to smoking. The first emphasis in this chapter is on smoking-related cancers, because these might be more plausibly associated with exposure to ETS. However, exposure to ETS occurs at earlier ages than active smoking; thus, there may be effects of ETS exposure on risk for other cancers.

SMOKING-RELATED CANCERS

Active tobacco smoking is an important cause not only of lung cancer, but also of bladder cancer, cancers of the pancreas and renal pelvis, and probably of the nasal sinus and kidneys. Oral, oropharyngeal, hypopharyngeal, laryngeal, and oesophageal cancers are also strongly associated with active smoking, especially in conjunction with the use of alcohol. Primary cigar and pipe smokers face a somewhat lower risk for cancer of the lung than cigarette smokers, but their risk for cancer of the larynx, pharynx, oral cavity, and esophagus is similar if not greater than that of cigarette smokers (U.S. Department of Health and Human Services, 1982). Also, lip cancer is associated with tobacco smoking, as well as pancreatic cancer and, perhaps, renal adenocarcinoma. An increased risk of cervical cancer has been observed in tobacco smokers, but

TABLE 13-1 Studies of Passive Smoking and Cancers Other Than Lung Cancer with Significantly Increased Risks

Author	Study Design	Size (Cases and Population or Controls)	Tumor Outcome Studied	Odds Ratios[a]
Hirayama, 1984	Cohort	34/91,540	Brain	3.0;6.3;4.3
		28/91,540	Nasal sinus	1.7;2.0;2.6
Miller, 1984	Case-Control	123/537	All sites	1.40
Gillis, 1984	Cohort	Male: 8/827 Female: 43/1917	Sites other than lung	0.5 (M) 1.26 (F)
Sandler et al., 1985a (adulthood exposure)	Case-Control (total) includes smokers	518/518	All sites	1.6
			Breast	1.8
			Cervix	1.8
			Endocrine glands	3.2
Sandler et al., 1985b (lifetime exposure)	Case-control (subset) includes smokers	869/409	All sites	1.4;2.3;2.6
			Breast	2.0;2.4;3.3
			Cervix	1.6;3.6;3.4
			Leukemia and lymphoma	2.5;5.1;6.8
Sandler et al., 1985c (early life exposure)	Case-control (subset) includes smokers	438/470	All sites	1.5
			Cervix	1.7
			Hematopoetic tissue	2.4

[a]Given with increasing dose, if available.

the causal relationship is unclear (International Agency for Research on Cancer, 1986). The risk for these cancers to nonsmokers exposed to ETS has been the subject of a few studies.

Hirayama (1984; see Chapter 12 and Table 13-1) examined cancers of the mouth, pharynx, oesophagus, bladder, pancreas, and cervix. The relative risks were not given, but they were reported to be insignificant. However, a relationship between ETS exposure in nonsmokers and nasal sinus cancer was noted, with rate ratios for the aforementioned exposure categories of 1.7, 2.0, and 2.6, respectively (see Table 13-1).

Sandler et al. (1985a; described in more detail below and in Table 13-1) also did not find a significant odds ratio for any of the smoking-related cancers (including lung cancer), except for cervical cancer ($p < 0.05$). The odds ratios given for these cancers included smokers as well as nonsmokers. Therefore, since the odds ratios were not significant for the combined group, they would not be expected to be significant for the nonsmokers analyzed separately.

CANCERS NOT RELATED TO SMOKING

Hirayama's (1984) study, based on a cohort of 91,450 nonsmoking Japanese women, suggested an increased mortality from brain tumors among women whose husbands smoked. The rate ratios were 3.0, 6.3, and 4.3 for exposure to husbands smoking 1-14, 15-19, or 20 or more cigarettes per day, as compared with nonsmoking wives of nonsmoking husbands as the reference group. A trend was noted for all cancer sites, but the risk elevation became insignificant when lung, nasal sinus, brain, and breast cancers were excluded. No significant associations were found for cancers of the stomach, colon, rectum, liver, peritoneum, ovary, skin, or bone, or for malignant lymphoma or leukemia.

Sandler et al. (1985a,b,c), reporting on a case-control study from North Carolina, suggested an association of exposure to ETS at different periods during a lifetime with various types of cancer. People with cancer at any site, except basal cell cancer of the skin, were included in this study. The cases were drawn from a hospital-based tumor registry, irrespective of personal histories of smoking. Mailed questionnaires were used for collecting data on exposure, preceded by a telephone call for the control subjects, but not for the cases.

Many of the odds ratios reported in these articles are for the combined group, as briefly reported in Table 13-1. However, some results were reported separately for nonsmoking cases (No. = 231) and controls (No. = 235). The results discussed below are based on the latter group and thus reflect only 31% of the total eligible patient group.

The overall crude cancer risk among individuals who were ever married to smokers was 2.1 times that of those never married to smokers. Significantly elevated risks ($p < 0.05$) were seen also for cancer of the cervix (odds ratio 2.1) and endocrine glands (odds ratio 4.4) (Sandler et al., 1985a). A nonsignificant odds ratio of 2.0 was obtained for cancer of the breast.

A subset of this study involved subjects who had lived with both natural parents for most of the first 10 years of life and had information on the smoking habits of both parents and spouses.

Overall cancer risks were found to increase steadily and significantly with each additional household member who smoked (Sandler et al., 1985b). The overall risk was significant only for adulthood exposure, either alone or in addition to childhood exposure (Sandler et al., 1985d). This trend appeared both for cancers traditionally associated with smoking and for other sites, with the strongest trend for the smoking-related cancers.

The transplacental and childhood exposures to ETS were specifically studied in another subset of the same study; however, the data were not adjusted for prenatal exposure (Sandler et al., 1985c). There were no significantly increased risks indicated for all sites or for specific cancers. Hematopoietic-tissue-cancer risk had an odds ratio of 2.3 when maternal smoking was considered and 2.4 when paternal smoking was considered (significance not given).

Cancers of hematopoietic tissues have been reported as increased in children whose mothers smoked during and after pregnancy. Neutel and Buck (1971) studied 65 cancer deaths among 89,302 children and found that the rate of leukemia among children of smokers was about twofold that of nonsmokers, but without a dose-response trend. The total number of leukemia cases in this study was 22. Manning and Carroll (1957) studied 187 cases of leukemia, 42 cases of lymphoma, and 93 other cancers among children, but found no effect of mothers' smoking habits. Neither of these studies separated the effects of in utero exposure from the exposure to ETS after birth.

Two studies have evaluated all sites of cancer as a group. Miller (1984) questioned relatives of women who died between 1972 and 1976 in Erie County, Pennsylvania. He found a nonsignificant increased risk (1.40) of any cancer among women whose husbands smoked. In another study (Gillis et al., 1984), a population in Scotland was followed up 10 years after an initial screening survey for cardiovascular disease. The West of Scotland Cancer Registry was screened for subsequent incidence of cancer. Among the nonsmoking males, there were 8 cases of cancer other than lung cancer. The standardized mortality rates were actually decreased among men whose wives smoked (ratio = 0.50). Among the nonsmoking women, there were 43 cases of cancer other than lung cancer, and the ratio of standardized mortality rates was nonsignificantly increased (1.26).

In the study by Preston-Martin et al. (1982) of childhood brain tumors, case and control mothers were similar in use of cigarettes during pregnancy. This is in contrast to the finding that significantly more case mothers than control mothers lived in a household with a smoker. The lack of an association of risk with maternal smoking, the association of smoking behavior with other lifestyle-related exposures, and the lack of apparent adjustment for smoking status of the mother make these uncorroborated results difficult to interpret.

INTERPRETATION

Interpretation of these observations regarding a possible association of ETS exposure and cancers with or without previously found associations with smoking is difficult. Only a few studies have been reported, on cancer and ETS exposure other than lung cancer.

The Sandler et al. (1985a,b,c) reports have been criticized for not maintaining matching (Higgins, 1985), for recruiting controls through two separate mechanisms, for conducting interviews in two different ways (telephone interviews or mailed questionnaires), and for insufficient information on other variables known to be risk factors for the various cancers that have been studied in these reports (Burch, 1985; Friedman, 1986; Mantel, 1986). The criticism of the lack of information on other known risk factors is of special concern and is also pertinent to the Hirayama study. For instance, alcohol use, reproductive and sexual histories, and occupational exposures are important risk factors for several of the cancers studied.

Considering increased risks for hematological malignancies, leukemia has not been thought to be smoking-related even though there have been reports of higher leukemia risks among smokers. However, there is a possibility that inhaled lead-210, originating from the tobacco or from radon daughters attaching to ETS, could end up in the skeleton, especially in young individuals who are building up their skeletons, and would result in irradiation of the bone marrow. Such an explanation is presently highly speculative, but increased concentrations of lead-210 have been found in the skeletons of adult smokers (Holtzman and Ilcewicz, 1966; Blanchard, 1967). Adults would be less sensitive to radiation than children. Austin and Cole (1986) suggest that, in addition to the possible influence of radioactive elements, benzene, urethane, and nitrosamines may be contributing factors. All of these chemicals are found in cigarettes and ETS, and they have been shown to be leukemogenic in experimental animals, or in humans.

The findings of increased brain cancer associated with ETS exposure in the Hirayama (1984) study, and possibly in the Preston-Martin et al. (1982) study, are of note. *N*-nitroso compounds are potent nervous system carcinogens in animals (Magee et al., 1976; Preussman, 1984, 1986).

SUMMARY AND RECOMMENDATIONS

These recent observations on a possible connection between ETS and various forms of cancer have created much discussion and some confusion. The lack of consistency with other data on tumors among children of smoking mothers and the appearance of tumors that are not clearly smoking-related call for further epidemiologic research. Any new studies in this area will, hopefully, have a very careful, rigorous design, so that more definitive evaluation of this possible health hazard from ETS exposure is possible.

What Is Known

1. There is no consistent evidence at this time of any increased risk of ETS exposure for cancers other than lung cancer.

What Scientific Information Is Missing

1. Smoking-related cancers other than lung cancer need to be studied with adequate numbers and good exposure data and with consideration of the potential confounding effects from other known risk factors for these cancers.
2. Some cancers not related to active smoking, especially lymphohematopoietic neoplasms, should be studied in relation to ETS exposure, particularly in childhood. Then the possibility of a etiologic role of inhaled decay products of radon (like bone-seeking lead-210) should be considered.

REFERENCES

Austin, H., and P. Cole. Cigarette smoking and leukemia. J. Chronic Dis. 39:417-421, 1986.

Blanchard, R.L. Concentration of ^{210}Pb and ^{210}Po in human soft tissues. Health Phys. 13:625-632, 1967.

Burch, P.R.J. Lifetime passive smoking and cancer risk. Lancet 1:866, 1985 (letter).

Friedman, G.D. Passive smoking in adulthood and cancer risk. Am. J. Epidemiol. 123:367, 1986 (letter).

Gillis, C.R., D.J. Hole, V.M. Hawthorne, and P. Boyle. The effect of environmental tobacco smoke in two urban communities in the west of Scotland. Eur. J. Respir. Dis. 33:S121-S126, 1984.

Higgins, I. Lifetime passive smoking and cancer risk. Lancet 2:867, 1985.

Hirayama, T. Cancer mortality in nonsmoking women with smoking husbands based on a large scale cohort study in Japan. Prev. Med. 13:680-690, 1984.

Holtzman, R.B., and F.H. Ilcewicz. Lead-210 and polonium-210 in tissues of cigarette smokers. Science 153:1259-1260, 1966.

International Agency for Research on Cancer (IARC) Monograph. Evaluation of Carcinogenic Risk of Chemicals to Humans, Vol. 38, pp. 163-314. Tobacco Smoking. Lyon: IARC, 1986. 421 pp.

Magee, P.N., R. Montesano, and R. Preussman. N-Nitroso compounds and related carcinogens. In: C.E. Searle, Ed. Chemical Carcinogens. Washington, D.C.: ACS Monogr. 173:491-625, 1976.

Manning, M.D., and B.E. Carroll. Some epidemiological aspects of leukemia in children. J. Natl. Cancer Inst. 19:1087-1094, 1957.

Mantel, N. Passive smoking in adulthood and cancer risk. Am. J. Epidemiol. 123:367-368, 1986 (letter).

Miller, G.H. Cancer, passive smoking and nonemployed and employed wives. West. J. Med. 140:632-635, 1984.

Neutel, C.I., and C. Buck. Effect on smoking during pregnancy on the risk of cancer in children. J. Natl. Cancer Inst. 47:59-63, 1971.

Preston-Martin, S., M.C. Yu, B. Benton, and B.E. Henderson. N-nitroso compounds and childhood brain tumors: A case-control study. Cancer Res. 42:5240-5245, 1982.

Preussman, R. Carcinogenic N-nitroso compounds and their environmental significance. Naturwissenchaften 71:25-30, 1984.

Preussman, R., and B.W. Stewart. Carcinogenic N-nitroso compounds and related carcinogens. In C.E. Searle, Ed. Chemical Carcinogens. 2nd Ed. Washington, D.C.: American Chemical Society 182:643-828, 1984.

Sandler, D.P., R.B. Everson, and A.J. Wilcox. Passive smoking in adulthood and cancer risk. Am. J Epidemiol 121:37-48, 1985a.

Sandler, D.P., A.J. Wilcox, and R.B. Everson. Cumulative effects of lifetime passive smoking on cancer risk. Lancet 1:312-315, 1985b.

Sandler, D.P., R.B. Everson, A.J. Wilcox, and J.P. Browder. Cancer risk in adulthood from early life exposure to parents' smoking. Am. J. Public Health 75:487-492, 1985c.

Sandler, D.P., R.B. Everson, and A.J. Wilcox. The authors reply. Am. J. Epidemiol. 123:369-370, 1986 (letter).

U.S. Department of Health and Human Services. The Consequence of Smoking. Cancer. A Report of the Surgeon General. DHSS (PHS) Publ. No. 82-50179. Rockville, Maryland: U.S. Department of Health and Human Services, Public Health Service, Office on Smoking and Health, 1982. 302 pp.

14
Cardiovascular System

The effects of active smoking on exercise tolerance, blood pressure, and the risk of developing cardiovascular disease have been reviewed elsewhere (U.S. Public Health Service, 1983). This chapter discusses studies of ETS exposure to nonsmokers and subsequent possible cardiovascular effects. The constituents that are thought to have the greatest effect on the cardiovascular system are carbon monoxide (CO) and nicotine. The possibility exists that the mechanisms, as well as the magnitude of the effects, for acute and chronic cardiovascular effects may be different for exposure to whole smoke and to ETS.

ACUTE CARDIOVASCULAR EFFECTS OF ENVIRONMENTAL TOBACCO SMOKE EXPOSURE

Administration of nicotine at level similar to those induced by active cigarette smoking is shortly followed by increases in heart rate and blood pressure (U.S. Public Health Service, 1983). Platelet aggregation has been shown to be increased in in vitro studies. CO rapidly combines with hemoglobin in the blood to form carboxyhemoglobin (COHb), thereby leading to some degree of tissue hypoxia. CO combines with muscle myoglobin, which is followed by some muscle hypoxia. The level of exposure of the nonsmoker to these cigarette smoke constituents, however, is less than that of the active smoker, and the effects are expected to be less.

TABLE 14-1 Carbon Monoxide and Carboxyhemoglobin Levels in Nonsmoking Individuals

Experimental Studies (Controlled Chambers)

Study	No. of Cigarettes/h/10 m^3	No. of Subjects	CO, ppm[a]	Carboxyhemoglobin Control	Carboxyhemoglobin Change
Anderson and Dalhamm, 1973	3.1	—	4.5	0.3	0
Dahms et al., 1981	—	10	15-20	0.6	+0.4
Harke, 1970	3.9	7	30	0.9	+1.2
Huch et al., 1980	2.3	12	—	1.3	+0.5
Hugod et al., 1978	2.5	10	20	0.7	+0.9
Pimm et al., 1978	2.4	10	24	0.5	+0.3
	2.4	10	24	0.7	+0.2
Polak, 1977	6.7	15	23	2.0	+0.3
Russell et al., 1973	15.1	12	38	1.6	+1.0
Seppänen and Uusitalo, 1977	3.8	28	16	1.6	+0.4
Srch, 1967	50	—	90	2	+3

Observational Studies

Study	Subjects/Exposure	No. of Subjects	Nonexposed: Exposed Carboxy-hemoglobin, %	Nonexposed: Exposed CO Expired, ppm
Foliart et al., 1982	Flight attendants/8 h	6	1.0:0.7	
Jarvis et al., 1983	Normal/public house for 2 h	7		4.7:10.6
Lightfoot, 1972	Normal/submarine		—:1.0	
Wald et al., 1981	Participants in health screening program	6,641		
Jarvis et al., 1984	Normal/self report	10	0.9:0.8	5.7:5.5
Seppänen and Uusitalo, 1977	Restaurant for 5 h (CO:2.5-15 ppm)	47	2.1:2.1	
	Office for 8 h (CO:2.5 ppm)	15	2.3:2.3	

[a] Carbon monoxide (CO) measured as a proxy to indicate the concentration of ETS in the chamber.

COHb commonly observed in active smokers are higher, ranging between 4 to 6 percent, rarely greater than 12 percent (Schievelbein and Richter, 1984). Because exposure of the nonsmoker is qualitatively different than exposure to smokers, a simple scaling down of effects observed in active smokers does not appear to be fully appropriate. Therefore, the effects of exposure to nicotine,

TABLE 14-2 Resting Acute Cardiovascular Effects in Nondiseased Humans of Exposure to Environmental Tobacco Smoke

Authors	Study Population	Conditions	Results: Measured Variable	Before	After
Luguette et al., 1970	40 children	Room: 9 m^3	Heart rate	89	97
		No. cig.: 6	Blood pressure	116/67	120/72
		Time: 15 min			
Harke and Bleichert, 1972	10	Room: n.g.	Heart rate	72 ± 8	74 ± 12
		No. cig.: 150	Blood pressure	123/84	121/84
		Time: 20 min	Skin temperature (−°C/min)	0	0.0273
Rummel et al., 1975	56	Room: 30 m^3	Heart rate	72 ± 10	71 ± 11
		No. cig.: 6–8	Blood pressure	117/71	117/71
		Time: 20 min			
Hurshman et al., 1978	8	Room: n.g.	Heart rate	73	79
		No. cig.: 2–6	Blood pressure	107/67	114/68
		Time: 10 min			
Pimm et al., 1978	10 males	Room: 14.6 m^3	Heart rate	84(F)	80(F)
	10 females	No. cig.: 7		77(M)	70(M)
	Age = 22.3	Time: 2 h			

CO, or ETS need to be separately studied. In addition, consideration needs to be given to persons of different sensitivity or vulnerability.

Healthy Subjects

Table 14-2 lists studies that report on the consequences of exposure of nondiseased individuals to ETS for periods up to 2 hours under experimental, resting conditions. There were no significant changes noted in heart rate or blood pressure in school-aged children or in adult men and women.

Two studies evaluated the physiologic responses to exercise with and without exposure to ETS. In the first, Pimm et al. (1978) (see also Table 14-2) had subjects perform a 7-minute progressive exercise test on an electronic bicycle ergometer. During exercise, the women had higher heart rates after exposure to ETS when compared with control conditions (differences of 6.3 beats per minute at 2 minutes and 4.5 beats per minute at 7 minutes, $p < 0.01$). The recovery heart rates were not significantly different. The men, however, showed little difference between test and control conditions (differences of -0.1 beats per minute at 2 minutes and 1.5 beats per minute at 7 minutes). In the second study, Sheppard and colleagues (1979b) tested 11 males and 12 females at two different levels of ETS (i.e., 7 cigarettes over 2 hours, CO = 20 ppm, or 9 cigarettes over 2 hours, CO = 31 ppm). Under both exposure conditions, contrary to expectations, both the increment in heart rate and average heart rate were less with ETS exposure.

In summary, for normal young adult males and females, no significant acute effects of ETS exposure on heart rate or blood pressure have been reported, either under resting or aerobic conditions.

There have been several studies of exposure of normal subjects under resting and aerobic conditions to low levels of CO but higher than those found with ETS exposure (reviewed in Environmental Protection Agency, 1984). No significant effects were found in healthy, exercising subjects during short-term exposure (e.g., Drinkwater et al., 1974; Raven et al., 1974a,b; DeLucia et al., 1983).

Angina Patients

Angina pectoris is a symptom complex involving feelings of pressure and pain in the chest, which is produced by mild exercise or excitement, presumably because of insufficient oxygen supply to the heart muscle. Under conditions of ETS exposure, the CO levels are increased, thus possibly placing individuals with angina at an increased risk of recurrent episodes.

Anderson et al. (1973) and Aronow and his colleagues, in a series of experiments (1973, 1974, 1978, 1981) (Table 14-3), studied angina patients under aerobic conditions with exposures to low levels of CO and to ETS. Ten patients with diagnosed angina pectoris, of whom two were smokers and eight exsmokers, were tested (Aronow et al., 1978). Significant increases in systolic blood pressure and heart rate, and decreases in time to onset of angina, were noted when the subjects were exposed to smoke in either ventilated or unventilated rooms (the actual levels of CO under these conditions were not noted). There were some subjective elements in the evaluation of these patients, and the physician conducting these tests was aware of the test conditions, i.e., smoking or not and ventilated or not. Consequently, the findings of this study, in

TABLE 14-3 Acute Cardiovascular Effects of Exposure to CO or Environmental Tobacco Smoke by Nonsmoking Angina Patients

Study	Design	No.	Conditions	Results
Anderson et al., 1973	Double-blind, Cross-over	10[a]	CO: 50 ppm or 100 ppm Time: 4 h for 5 days	Mean duration before onset of pain shortened (50 ppm and 100 ppm); duration of pain longer (100 ppm only)
Aronow and Isbell, 1973	Double blind, Cross-over	10[b]	CO: 50 ppm Time: 2 h	Times until onset decreased; decrease in BP and heart rate at angina
Aronow, 1978	Not blinded	10[c]	No. cig.: 15 Time: 2 h Room: 30.28 m^3	Earlier onset of angina; increased systolic BP and heart rate at angina
Aronow et al., 1979	Double-blind, Cross-over	20	COHb: 4%	Impairment in visualization test
Aronow, 1981	Double-blind, Cross-over	15	CO: 50 ppm Time: 1 h COHb: 2%	Time until onset decreased; decreased systolic BP and heart rate at angina

[a]Includes five smokers and five nonsmokers.
[b]Not current smokers.
[c]Includes eight exsmokers and two current smokers.

the absence of a true double-blind approach, require verification by other research workers.

The effects of rapid angina onset would be expected to be due to increased COHb levels. Anderson et al. (1973) and Aronow et al. (1973, 1981) exposed angina patients to low levels of CO. In these studies, angina pain appeared when COHb levels of patients were measured at 2 and 4%. These studies have been reviewed extensively as part of the Environmental Protection Agency's (1984) activity in establishing air quality criteria for carbon monoxide. The review group found that the results were suggestive for effects at COHb levels above 3%, based on animal and theoretical models. There is concern that elevated levels of CO exposure may affect the electrical stability of the heart in previously compromised heart muscle, thus possibly leading to sudden death. The levels reviewed in Table 14-1 are close to the 3% level. This suggests that there is reason to be concerned with possible effects of exposure. However, a firm quantitative estimate of the risk to nonsmoking persons, under conditions of ETS exposure, cannot be made from the literature at this time.

CARDIOVASCULAR DISEASE MORBIDITY AND MORTALITY

Possible pathophysiologic mechanisms for the atherogenic influence of cigarette smoking were reviewed in the 1983 Report of the Surgeon General. Experimental studies of subcutaneous or intravenous administration of nicotine in rabbits (Schievelbein et al., 1970; Schievelbein and Richter, 1984) and monkeys (Liu et al., 1979) have demonstrated that long-term exposure leads to arteriosclerotic lesions. Exposure to carbon monoxide also leads to atherosclerosis in rabbits, pigeons, and other animals (Astrup and Kjeldsen, 1979). Studies of whole tobacco smoke indicate that total serum cholesterol concentrations are increased and the ratios of the various lipoprotein fractions are changed (McGill, 1979). The contribution of whole tobacco smoke to modifying the lipoprotein fractions is not conclusive. However, there have not been experimental studies of the effects of ETS exposure or administration of ETS extracts.

Smoking and Cardiovascular Disease

The effects of active smoking on human health are summarized in the Surgeon General's report *The Health Consequences of Smoking: Cardiovascular Disease* (U.S. Public Health Service, 1983). The principal conclusions are that cigarette smokers experience a 70% greater coronary heart disease (CHD) death rate than do nonsmokers and that smokers of more than two packs per day have 2 to 3 times greater CHD death rates than nonsmokers. The incidence of CHD in smokers is twice that of nonsmokers. Heavy smokers (more than two packs per day) have an almost fourfold increase. The relative risk in smokers for sudden death is greater than that for all deaths from CHD. The relative risk in young smokers is greater than that in older smokers. The relative risk for young women smokers, especially those who use oral contraceptives, is greater than 5.

The excess relative risk associated with smoking declines rapidly upon cessation of smoking, in some studies as much as 50% in 1 year. For exsmokers who previously smoked more than one pack per day, the residual excess risk also declines, but never completely disappears. The decline in risk on cessation of smoking cannot be explained by differences in known cardiac risk factors between individuals who continue smoking and individuals who have quit. Smokers who have used only pipes or cigars did not appear to experience a substantially greater CHD risk than nonsmokers.

The rapid decline in risk associated with smoking cessation and the greater relative risk for sudden death suggest that active smoking can precipitate cardiac events in individuals with preexisting coronary artery disease. Autopsy evidence of increased arteriosclerosis in smokers, coupled with the fact that risk of exsmokers never returns to the levels found in nonsmokers, suggests that cigarette smoking is also implicated in the development of arteriosclerotic cardiovascular disease (ASCVD). The mechanism by which cigarette smoke may lead to the development of chronic ASCVD, sudden death, or acute myocardial infarction is unknown. There appears, however, to be no threshold in the number of cigarettes smoked below which there is no increase in risk.

Data on uptake of cotinine by nonsmokers exposed to ETS indicate that the exposure in nonsmokers chronically exposed to ETS is approximately 1% that of an active smoker (who smokes one pack per day) (see Chapters 8 and 12). If the excess relative risk for CHD mortality or morbidity is a linear, nonthreshold function of dose and, further, if the excess risk of CHD in a one-pack-a-day smoker is twofold, then the relative risk from CHD in nonsmokers exposed to ETS (compared to true nonsmokers) would be approximately 1.02. Such relative risks would be difficult to detect or estimate reliably in nonexperimental studies. Such small increases in relative risk are of the same order of magnitude as what might arise from expected residual confounding due to unmeasured covariates. Nonetheless, because of the large number of cardiovascular deaths each year, these possibilities deserve close attention and further study that could lead to firmer estimates of excess risk.

Studies of Environmental Tobacco Smoke Exposure and Mortality from Cardiovascular Disease

Garland et al. (1985) have reported that, in a prospective study of the effect of passive smoking, the age-adjusted rates of cardiac disease deaths in nonsmoking women whose husbands were former or current smokers were significantly elevated. It is not certain, however, that the report is correct, because of a possible miscalculation or misuse of the Mantel-Haenszel statistic and some other methodologic problems. Data for the wives of former smokers were grouped with wives of current smokers. If this grouping were made after examining the data, which indicated that the risk was greater among the women whose husbands were former smokers, then this combination would be suspect. The p values based on the Mantel-Haenszel test may be inappropriate in view of the small sample sizes. The authors employ the Cox Proportional Hazard analysis to control for other factors associated with cardiovascular risk, such as age, blood pressure, cholesterol, obesity, years of marriage, etc. They report a relative risk for women married to current or former smokers compared with women married to never-smokers of 2.7 (Garland, 1985, corrected from an earlier report). The p value (< 0.10) associated with this estimate is based on the asymptotic assumptions that are implicit in likelihood-based inference from the Cox model. These assumptions may not hold for small sample sizes. In summary, because of the small sample sizes, the significance calculations arising from this study must be looked upon as approximations.

Gillis et al. (1984) reported the results of a follow-up study of residents of two urban communities in Scotland. Nonsmokers exposed to cigarette smoke in their homes had a slightly higher rate of myocardial infarction than those unexposed. The sample size was small, so that few of the results were statistically significant, and other risk factors for myocardial infarction were not controlled for.

Hirayama (1984) reported the results of a 15-year prospective study of nonsmoking Japanese women classified at start of follow-up by the smoking status of their husbands. A relative risk from ischemic heart disease of 1.3 was found for nonsmoking women whose husbands smoked more than 19 cigarettes per day compared with nonsmoking women whose husbands did not smoke. A Mantel-Haenszel test for a linear trend was significant at the $p < 0.01$ level.

It is unlikely that Hirayama's results can be explained by chance. The potential biases inherent in this study (see Chapter 12) limit the weight that can be placed on these results. The observed relative risk of 1.3 is at the upper limit of the expectations derived from extrapolations from active smokers, unless the uptake of the active component of cigarette smoke to which passive smokers are exposed is of the order of 10% of that of active smokers. Matsukura et al. (1984) have suggested that such high levels of uptake in passive smokers may be seen in Japan. If there were independent evidence that nonsmokers exposed to other people's cigarette smoke do not differ on known risk factors for CHD from unexposed nonsmokers, more reliance could be placed on Hirayama's results.

Svendsen et al. (1985) reported on the effect of cigarette smoke exposure to smoking wives among men participating in the Multiple Risk Factor Intervention Trial (MRFIT). MRFIT, which began in the mid-1970s, was a randomized primary prevention trial designed to test the effect of a multifactor intervention program on mortality from coronary heart disease in men with previous cardiac episodes. The men were chosen for participation if they had at least two of three risk factors for heart disease, including smoking, high cholesterol levels, or high blood pressure. The results reported by Svendsen et al. (1985), based on the group of men who never smoked but whose wives may or may not have been smokers, indicate no difference between exposed (i.e., smoking wives) and nonexposed (i.e., nonsmoking wives) of nonsmoking men for blood pressure or serum cholesterol. The MRFIT study demonstrates a roughly twofold increase in the risk of CHD mortality and morbidity among nonsmokers exposed to ETS. The sample size was small, and the results were not statistically significant. Adjustment for other risk factors for CHD did not change the estimates of effect.

SUMMARY AND RECOMMENDATIONS

What Is Known

1. No statistically significant effects of ETS exposure on heart rate or blood pressure were found in healthy men, women, and school-aged children during resting conditions. During exercise there is no difference in the cardiovascular changes for men and women between conditions of exposure to ETS and control conditions.

2. With respect to chronic cardiovascular morbidity and mortality, although biologically plausible, there is no evidence of statistically significant effects due to ETS exposure, apart from the study by Hirayama in Japan.

What Scientific Information Is Missing

1. Experimental studies with animal models need to be performed with ETS to determine whether the cardiovascular changes seen following exposure to whole smoke also occur following exposure to ETS.

2. Existing studies have not provided evidence of serious harm in people with heart disease. With regard to angina onset, the findings are uncertain and need to be repeated.

REFERENCES

Anderson, G., and T. Dalhamn. Health risks due to passive smoking (in Swedish). Läkartidningen 70:2833-2836, 1973.

Anderson, E.W., R.J. Andelman, J.M. Strauch, N.J. Fortuin, and J.H. Knelson. Effect of low-level carbon monoxide exposure on onset and duration of angina pectoris. Ann. Intern. Med. 79:46-50, 1973.

Aronow, W.S. Effect of passive smoking on angina pectoris. N. Engl. J. Med. 299:21-24, 1978.

Aronow, W.S. Aggravation of angina pectoris by two percent carboxyhemoglobin. Am. Heart. J. 101:154-157, 1981.

Aronow, W.S., and M.W. Isbell. Carbon monoxide effect on exercise-induced angina pectoris. Ann. Intern. Med. 79:392-395, 1973.

Aronow, W.S., J. Cassidy, J.S. Vangrow, H. March, J.C. Kern, J.R. Goldsmith, M. Khemka, J. Pagano and M. Vawter. Effect of cigarette smosking and breathing carbon monoxide on cardiovascular hemodynamics on anginal patients. Circulation 50:340-347, 1974.

Aronow, W.S., R. Charter, and G. Seacat. Effect of 4% carboxyhemoglobin on human performance in cardiac patients. Prev. Med. 8:562-566, 1979.

Astrup, P., and K. Kjeldsen. Model studies linking carbon monoxide and/or nicotine to arteriosclerosis and cardiovascular disease. Prev. Med. 8:295-302, 1979.

Bridge, D.P., and M. Corn. Contribution to the assessment of nonsmokers to air pollution from cigarette and cigar smoke in occupied spaces. Environ. Res. 5:192-209, 1972.

Dahms, T.E. J.F. Bolin, and R.G. Slavin. Passive smoking: Effects on bronchial asthma. Chest 80:530-534, 1981.

DeLucia, A.J., J.H. Whitaker, and L.R. Byrant. Effects of combined exposure to ozone and carbon monoxide (CO) in humans, pp. 145-159. In S.D. Lee, M.G. Mustafa, and M.A. Mehlman, Eds. Advances in Modern Environmental Toxicology, Vol. V. International Symposium on the Biomedical Effects of Ozone and Related Photochemical Oxidants. Princeton, New Jersey: Princeton Scientific Publishers, 1983.

Drinkwater, B.L., P.B. Raven, S.M. Horvath, J.A. Gliner, R.O. Ruhling, and N.W. Bolduan, and S. Taguchi. Air pollution, exercise and heat stress. Arch. Environ. Health 28:277-282, 1974.

Environmental Protection Agency. Revised Evaluation of Health Effects Associated with Carbon Monoxide Exposure: An Addendum to the 1979 EPA Air Quality Criteria Document for Carbon Monoxide. Publ. No. EPA-600/8-83-033F. Washington, D.C.: U.S. Government Printing Office, 1984.

Foliart, D., N.L. Benowitz, and C.E. Becker. Passive absorption of nicotine in airline flight attendants. N. Engl. J. Med. 308:1105, 1982.

Garland, C., E. Barrett-Connor, L. Suarez, M. Criqui, and D. Wingard. Effects of passive smoking on ischemic heart disease mortality of nonsmokers. Am. J. Epidemiol. 121:645-650, 1985.

Gillis, C.R., D.J. Hole, V.M. Hawthorne, and P. Boyle. The effect of environmental tobacco smoke in two urban communities in the west of Scotland. Eur. J. Respir. Dis. 65(S133):121-126, 1984.

Harke, H.-P. Zum Problem des "Passiv-Rauchens." Münch Med Wochenschr. 51:2328-2334, 1970.

Harke, H.-P., and A. Bleichert. Zum Problem des Passivrauchens. Int. Arch. Arbeitsmed. 29:312-322, 1972.

Hirayama, T. Lung cancer in Japan: Effects of nutrition and passive smoking, pp. 175-195. In M. Mizell and P. Correa Eds. Lung Cancer: Causes and Prevention. New York: Verlag Chemie, International, Inc., 1984.

Huch, R., J. Danko, L. Spatling, and R. Huch. Risks the passive smoker runs. Lancet 2:1376, 1980.

Hugod, C., L.H. Hawkins, and P. Astrup. Exposure of passive smokers to tobacco smoke constituents. Int. Arch. Occup. Environ. Health 42:21-29, 1978.

Hurshman, L.G., B.S. Brown, and R.G. Guyton. The implications of sidestream cigarette smoke for cardiovascular health. J. Environ. Health 41:145-149, 1978.

Jarvis, M.J., M.A.H. Russell, and C. Feyerabend. Absorption of nicotine and carbon monoxide from passive smoking under natural conditions of exposure. Thorax 38:829-833, 1983.

Lawther, P.J., and B.T. Commins. Cigarette smoking and exposure to carbon monoxide. Ann. N.Y. Acad. Sci. 174:135-147, 1970.

Lightfoot, N.F. Chronic carbon monoxide exposure. Proc. R. Soc. Med. 65:798-799, 1972.

Liu, L.B., C.B. Taylor, S.K. Peng, and B. Mikkelson. Experimental arteriosclerosis in Rhesus monkeys induced by multiple risk factors: Cholesterol, vitamin D and nicotine. Arterial Wall 5:25-38, 1979.

Luquette, A.J., C.W. Landess, and D.J. Merki. Some immediate effects of a smoking environment on children of elementary school age. J. Sch. Health 40:533-535, 1970.

Matsukura, S., T. Taminato, N. Kitano, Y. Seino, H. Hamada, M. Uchihashi, H. Nakajima, and Y. Hirata. Effects of environmental tobacco smoke on urinary cotinine excretion in nonsmokers: Evidence for passive smoking. N. Engl. J. Med. 311:828-832, 1984.

McGill, H.C. Jr. Potential mechanisms for the augmentation of atherosclerosis and astherosclerotic disease by cigarette smoking. Prev. Med. 8:390-403, 1979.

Pimm, P.E., F. Silverman, and R.J. Shephard. Physiological effects of acute passive exposure to cigarette smoke. Arch. Environ. Health 33:201-213, 1978.

Polak, E. Le papier à cigarette. Son rôle dans la pollution des lieux habites. Tabagisme passif: Notion nouvellee precise. Brux. Med. 57:335-340, 1977.

Raven, P.B., B.L. Drinkwater, R.O. Ruhling, N.W. Bolduan, S. Taguchi, J. Gliner, and S.M. Horvath. Effect of carbon monoxide and peroxyacetyl nitrate on man's maximal aerobic capacity. J. Appl. Physiol. 36:288-293, 1974a.

Raven, P.B., B.L. Drinkwater, S.M. Horvath, R.O. Ruhling, J.A. Gliner, J.C. Sutton, and N.W. Bolduan. Age, smoking habits, heat stress, and their interactive effects with carbon monoxide and peroxyacetylnitrate on man's aerobic power. Int. J. Brometeor. 18:222-232, 1974b.

Rummel, R.M., M. Crawford, and P. Bruce. The physiological effects of inhaling exhaled cigarette smoke in relation to attitude of the nonsmoker. J. Sch. Health 45:524-529, 1975.

Russell, M.A.H., P.V. Cole, and E. Brown. Absorption by nonsmokers of carbon monoxide from room air polluted by tobacco smoke. Lancet 1:576-579, 1973.

Schievelbein, H., and F. Richter. The influence of passive smoking on the cardiovascular system. Prev. Med. 13:626-644, 1984.

Schievelbein, H., V. Londong, W. Londong, H. Grumbach, V. Remplik, A. Schauer, and H. Immich. Nicotine and arterioscherosis. An experimental contribution to the influence of nicotine on fat metabolism. Z. Klin. Chem. Klin. Biochem. 8:190-196, 1970.

Seppänen, A., and A.J. Uusitalo. Carboxyhemoglobin saturation in relation to smoking and various occupational conditions. Ann. Clin. Res. 9:261-268, 1977.

Shephard, R.J., R. Collins, and F. Silverman. "Passive" exposure of asthmatic subjects to cigarette smoke. Environ. Res. 20:392-402, 1979a.

Shephard, R.J., R. Collins, and F. Silverman. Responses of exercising subjects to acute "passive" cigarette smoke exposure. Environ. Res. 19:279-291, 1979b.

Srch M. On the significance of carbon monoxide in cigarette smoking in an automobile. Dtsch. Z. Gesamte. Gerichtl. 60:80-89, 1967.

Svendsen, K.H., L.H. Kuller, and J.D. Neaton. Effects of passive smoking in the Multiple Risk Factor Intervention Trial (MRFIT). AHA Circ. Monogr. 114(Suppl.):III-53, 1985. (Abstract 210)

U.S. Public Health Service. The Health Consequences of Smoking: Cardiovascular Disease. A Report of the Surgeon General. DHHS(PHS) Publ. No. 84-50204. Washington, D.C.: U.S. Department of Health and Human Services, Public Health Service, Office on Smoking and Health, 1983. 384 pp.

Wald, N.J., M. Idle, J. Boreham, and A. Bailey. Carbon monoxide in breath in relation to smoking and carboxyhemoglobin levels. Thorax 36:366-369, 1981.

15
Other Health Considerations in Children

Several other health outcomes have been studied that relate to the growth and health of children. This chapter discusses studies of the influence of ETS exposure on birthweight of the offspring of nonsmoking pregnant women and its influence on childhood growth and ear infections. For all postnatal outcomes, it is often not possible to differentiate effects of in utero exposure to tobacco smoke constituent from subsequent childhood exposures to ETS.

ENVIRONMENTAL TOBACCO SMOKE EXPOSURE BY NONSMOKING PREGNANT WOMEN

The fetus of a smoking mother is exposed in a unique way to the chemicals produced in cigarette smoke. Many studies have documented the adverse effect this relationship has on intrauterine fetal growth, especially during the third trimester of pregnancy (U.S. Department of Health and Human Services, 1976). Maternal cigarette smoking apparently affects fetal oxygenation, due to high levels of carboxyhemoglobin in the blood of both mother and child (Abel, 1980). However, the effects on the fetus of a nonsmoking mother chronically exposed to ETS are not well documented. Some studies have indirectly approached this problem by evaluating paternal cigarette smoking and birth outcomes in nonsmoking pregnant women.

Some early studies of paternal smoking and birthweight demonstrated a dose-response relationship that was discounted as "not easily acceptable as meaningful in terms of cause and effect" (Yerushalmy, 1962). An interview survey of 982 pregnancies indicated a strong dose-response association between paternal cigarette smoking and the percent of infants weighing less than 5 pounds, 8 ounces (Yerushalmy, 1962). In a later prospective study of nearly 13,000 births, Yerushalmy (1971) reported that paternal smoking was more strongly associated with low birthweight than was maternal smoking. The healthiest low-birthweight infants were found for couples where the wife smoked and her husband did not; the highest mortality rate was found among infants produced by couples where the husband smoked and the wife did not. These latter couples also had increased risks of producing premature offspring. The possibility that these differences in smoking were associated with differences in social class was not explored. On the bases of these data, Yerushalmy (1971) inferred that paternal smoking may be incidental to birthweight. When the mother's smoking was considered, the importance of paternal smoking disappeared.

In a study of 12,192 births, MacMahon et al. (1966) confirmed the negative association between maternal smoking and birthweight of offspring and also found that infants of fathers who smoked weighed about 3 ounces less than those of fathers who did not smoke. They attributed this finding to the correlation between husbands' and wives' smoking habits, or to chance. MacMahon et al. (1966) referred to Yerushalmy's (1962) observation of an association of father's smoking habits with infant weight as "biologically nonsensical."

In a study of 175 normal neonates and 202 neonates with congenital malformations, Borlee et al. (1978) found that paternal smoking was independently and significantly associated with reduced birthweight and higher perinatal mortality. They speculated that the effect occurred through its association with another factor. Gibel and Blumberg (1973) reported on a study of 5,000 children in which children of nonsmoking mothers whose fathers smoked more than 10 cigarettes per day had higher perinatal mortality than children whose parents were both nonsmokers. The incidence of severe malformations in children of fathers who were heavy smokers was double that of children of nonsmoking fathers, independent of parental age and social class.

Using code sheets prepared at birth of 48,505 women in worldwide naval installations, Underwood et al. (1967) found that fathers' smoking habits influenced pregnancy outcome. However, this was attributed to the increased numbers of wives who smoked when husbands smoked. For paternal smoking in the absence of maternal smoking, no association was found. Holmberg and Nurminen (1980) and Hughes et al. (1982) also reported no association of paternal smoking with low birthweight in cross-sectional reviews of several thousand births.

Rubin et al. (1986) provide a recent contribution to this subject based on a survey of 500 consecutive births. About two-fifths of the women reported smoking during pregnancy; 70 percent reported drinking. Paternal smoking was evaluated in terms of frequency and quantity of substance smoked, as reported in standardized interviews. They found that birthweight was reduced an average of 120 g per pack of cigarettes smoked per day by the father. This relationship remained statistically significant after controlling for relevant variables, including mother's age, parity, maternal smoking, and alcohol and tobacco consumption during pregnancy. The effect was greatest in the lower social classes.

In a prospective study, Martin and Bracken (1986) studied 3,891 antenatal patients, 2,613 of whom did not smoke during pregnancy. One-third of the nonsmoking mothers (i.e., 906) were exposed to ETS for at least 2 hours per day. ETS exposure was related to lower birthweight in full-term babies (23.5 g, not significant). A logistic regression to control for gestational age, parity, ethnicity, and maternal age produced a significantly increased risk of delivering a low-birthweight baby, i.e., less than 2,500 g at birth for ETS-exposed mothers (relative risk = 2.17, $p < 0.05$). The retardation in fetal growth rate is small but appears to be clinically meaningful at the low end of the birthweight distribution. That is, exposure to ETS increases the risk that the infant will weigh less than 2,500 g and, therefore, will have a higher perinatal mortality.

GROWTH IN CHILDREN

A few studies have examined possible relationships between chronic exposure to ETS by children and parameters of growth and development. Many studies have demonstrated that smoking during pregnancy results in newborns who are lighter and shorter than other infants, even when gestational age has been taken into account (Meredith, 1975; U.S. Department of Health and Human Services, 1976). This deficit in height and weight appears to persist into infancy and childhood (Goldstein, 1971; Butler and Goldstein, 1973; Dunn et al., 1976; Miller et al., 1976; Rantakallio, 1983).

Current smoking status of the mother also has been associated with decreased attained height (Rona et al., 1981; Berkey et al., 1984), although growth rate was not slower among these children (Berkey et al., 1984). These studies, however, did not differentiate between smoking during pregnancy and subsequent exposures during infancy and preschool years.

Rona and colleagues (1985) reanalyzed data from the National Study of Health and Growth (England) for a sample of 5,903 children aged 5 to 11 years, separating the effects of smoking during pregnancy from those of later smoking. After adjusting the data for social class and other social factors, they found that reduced height was associated with increasing numbers of cigarettes smoked in the home, regardless of whether the mother smoked during pregnancy and regardless of which parent smoked. There remained a small but significant effect on height—a reduction of approximately 0.05 standard deviations of height (approximately 0.3 cm) for each 20 cigarettes consumed daily in the home.

To verify this small change in height, other studies of comparable magnitude are needed. Growth is an especially difficult phenomenon to study. Many factors, such as genetics, nutrition, social class, and ethnicity play important roles, and it is difficult to assign proportionate causality to each factor. Recall bias in the mothers of school-age children regarding their smoking habits during the pregnancy may produce unreliable results, especially in light of the increasing publicity regarding ill effects on the fetus of maternal smoking during pregnancy. Moreover, height and weight ratios and other growth measures are not reliably obtained in standard pediatric surveys.

CHRONIC EAR INFECTIONS

A number of studies have linked household exposure to ETS with increased rates of chronic ear infections and effusions in children. Chronic ear infections or effusions in young children can lead to hearing loss and consequent speech pathology. Kraemer and colleagues (1983) conducted a hospital-based case-control study of 76 children with persistent middle-ear effusions contrasted with 76 children admitted for other types of surgery who were matched for age, sex, season, and surgical ward. They found that the daily exposure to ETS was greater among cases. They also reported that middle-ear effusions clear less readily in children heavily exposed to ETS. They concluded that a combination of several factors increased the risk of persistent middle-ear effusions, including recurrent otitis media, nasal catarrh, cigarette smoke exposure, and nasal allergies that chronically inflame the nasal and middle-ear cavities, causing persistent eustachian tube dysfunction. For children with regular exposure to ETS, atopy, and congestion, the relative risk for PPME was 6.3 (95% confidence interval, 1.9-21.1).

In another case-control study of 150 children hospitalized for chronic middle-ear effusions and 150 children hospitalized for other reasons (Black, 1985), the odds ratio for parental smoking was found to be significantly elevated (1.6). This effect was consistent across age groups, and became more evident in older children where effusions are less common. Pukander et al. (1985) reported that ETS was a significant risk factor for acute otitis media in 2- and 3-year-old children. They evaluated a number of important indoor environmental conditions, including relative humidity, carbon dioxide, and temperature. In this study, children of smoking parents also had 60% more middle-ear effusions than children of nonsmoking parents.

SUMMARY AND RECOMMENDATIONS

For all postnatal outcomes among children, it is difficult to differentiate effects of in utero exposure to tobacco smoke constituents from subsequent childhood exposures to ETS. However, for the above outcomes, there are indications that exposures to ETS may have effects on the fetus or child.

What Is Known

1. Evidence has accumulated indicating that nonsmoking pregnant women exposed to ETS on a daily basis for several hours are at increased risk for producing low-birthweight babies, through mechanisms which are, as yet, unknown. Recent studies show a dose-response relationship between the number of cigarettes smoked by the father and birthweight of the children of nonsmoking pregnant women.

2. A few studies have reported that children of smokers have reduced growth and development. These require further corroboration to differentiate in utero exposure from subsequent childhood exposures.

3. Household exposure to ETS is linked with increased rates of chronic ear infections and middle-ear effusions in young children. For children with nasal allergies and recurrent otitis media, ETS exposure may synergistically increase their risk of persistent middle-ear effusions.

What Scientific Information Is Missing

1. Experimental studies should be developed to articulate possible mechanisms through which paternal smoking adversely effects fetal growth in nonsmoking pregnant women. Special emphasis should be placed on identifying relevant effects of pregnancy on excretion and absorption of ETS, including transplacental metabolism.

2. Additional study is needed to corroborate one finding of a dose-response relationship between reduced height of children and increasing numbers of cigarettes smoked in the home, regardless of whether the mother smoked during pregnancy and regardless of which parent smoked.

3. Research should be conducted to explore the mechanisms by which exposure to ETS might adversely affect the functioning of the ear and to study possible long-term consequences of ETS exposure for the auditory apparatus.

REFERENCES

Abel, E.L. Smoking during pregnancy: A review of effects on growth and development of offspring. Hum. Biol. 52:593-625, 1980.

Berkey C.S., J.H. Ware, F.E. Speizer, and B.G. Ferris, Jr. Passive smoking and height growth of preadolescent children. Int. J. Epidemiol. 13:454-458, 1984.

Black, N. The aetiology of glue ear—A case-control study. Int. J. Pediatr. Otorhinolaryngol. 9:121-133, 1985.

Borlee, I., A. Bouckaert, M.F. Lechat, and C.B. Mission. Smoking patterns during and before pregnancy: Weight, length and head circumference of progeny. Eur. J. Obstet. Gynecol Reprod. Biol. 8:171-177, 1978.

Butler, N.R., and H. Goldstein. Smoking in pregnancy and subsequent child development. Br. Med. J. 4:573-575, 1973.

Dunn, H.G., A.K. McBurney, S. Ingram, and C.M. Hunter. Maternal cigarette smoking during pregnancy and child's subsequent development. I. Physical growth to the age of 6 1/2 years. Can J. Public Health 67:499-505, 1976.

Gibel, W., and H.-H. Blumberg. Die Auswirkungen der Rauchgewohnheiten von Eltern auf das ungeborene und neugeborene Kind. Z. Ärztl. Fortbild. 73:341-342, 1973.

Goldstein, H. Factors influencing the height of seven year old children—Results from the National Child Development Study. Hum. Biol. 43:92-111, 1971.

Hughes, J.R., L.H. Epstein, F. Andrasik, D.F. Neff, and D.S. Thompson. Smoking and carbon monoxide levels during pregnancy. Addict. Behav. 7:271-276, 1982.

Holmberg, P.C., and M. Nurminen. Congenial defects of the central nervous system and occupational factors during pregnancy. A case-referrent study. Am. J. Ind. Med. 1:167-176, 1980.

Kraemer, M.J., M.A. Richardson, N.S. Weiss, C.T. Furukawa, G.G. Shapiro, W.E. Pierson, and W. Bierman. Risk factors for persistent middle-ear effusions. Otitis media, catarrh, cigarette smoke exposure and atopy. JAMA 249:1022-1025, 1983.

MacMahon, B., M. Alpert, and E.J. Salber. Infant weight and parental smoking habits. Am. J. Epidemiol. 82:247-261, 1966.

Martin, T.R., and M.B. Bracken. Association of low birth weight with passive smoke exposure in pregnancy. Am. J. Epidemiol. 124:633-642,1986.

Meredith, H.V. Relation between tobacco smoking of pregnant women and body size of their progeny: A compilation of published studies. Hum. Biol. 47:451-472, 1975.

Miller, H.C., K. Hassanein, and P.A. Hensleigh. Fetal growth retardation in relation to maternal smoking and weight gain in pregnancy. Am J. Obstet. Gynecol. 125:55-60, 1976.

Pukander, J., J. Lustonen, M. Timore, and P. Karma. Risk factors affecting the occurrence of acute otitis media among two and three year old urban children. Acta Otolaryngol. 100:260-265, 1985.

Rantakallio, P. A follow-up study up to the age of 14 of children whose mothers smoked during pregnancy. Acta Paediatr. Scand. 72:747-753, 1983.

Rona, R.J., C. Du Ve Florey, G.C. Clarke, and S. Chinn. Parental smoking at home and height of children. Br. Med. J. 283:1363, 1981.

Rona, R.J., S. Chinn, and C. Du Ve Florey. Exposure to cigarette smoking and children's growth. Int. J. Epidemiol. 14:402-409, 1985.

Rubin, D.H., P.A. Krasilnikoff, J.M. Leventhol, B. Weile, and A. Berget. Effect of passive smoking on birth-weight. Lancet 2:415-417, 1986.

Underwood, P.B., K.F. Kesler, J.M. O'Lane, and D.A. Collagan. Parental smoking empirically related to pregnancy outcome. Obstet. Gynecol. 29:1-8, 1967.

U.S. Department of Health and Human Services. The Health Consequences of Smoking. Selected Chapters from the 1971-1975 Report. Report of the Surgeon General Publ. No. CDC 78-8357. Washington, D.C.: U.S. Department of Health, Education, and Welfare, Public Health Service, Office on Smoking and Health, 1976. 657 pp.

Yerushalmy, J. Statistical considerations and evaluation of epidemiological evidence. In G. James, Ed. Tobacco and Health. Springfield, Illinois: Charles C Thomas, 1962.

Yerushalmy, J. The relationship of parents' cigarette smoking to outcome of pregnancy—Implications as to the problem of inferring causation from observed associations. Am. J. Epidemiol. 93:443-456, 1971.

APPENDIXES

Appendix A: Guidelines for Public and Occupational Chemical Exposures to Materials That Are Also Found in Environmental Tobacco Smoke

Table A-1 gives a series of guidelines for public and industrial populations regarding exposure to chemicals that are also constituents in environmental tobacco smoke (ETS). Not all of the constituents of ETS thought to be toxic or carcinogenic have had guideline levels established. The values in the table are taken from the fourth edition of the *Documentation of the Threshold Limit Values*, published by the American Conference of Governmental and Industrial Hygienists (1986). The NIOSH recommendations and OSHA standards can be found in the NIOSH *Pocket Guide to Chemical Hazards*, published by the U.S. Department of Health and Human Services (National Institute for Occupational Safety and Health, 1981).

Each of these guidelines and standards has been established with different considerations in mind. The EPA standards, which apply to outdoor environments, have been established by law to protect the most susceptible individuals. The OSHA standards and ACGIH, NIOSH, and European guidelines have been established for the normal, healthy adult working populations. These guidelines accept some level of risk to some people. They do not consider children, the elderly, or populations with preexisting health conditions who may be at greater risk for health effects of exposure. The appropriate guidelines for susceptible populations probably would be lower. These industrial guidelines also differ from the environmental standards in that they assume that the exposure is limited to a workday period or a time-limited emergency.

TABLE A-1 Some Occupational and Public Standards for Materials That Are Also in Environmental Tobacco Smoke

	Public	Industrial			
	EPA	ACGIH[a]	NIOSH[b]	OSHA[c]	European Standards[d]
Vapor Phase					
Carbon monoxide	1 mg/m^3—max. 8-h 40 mg/m^3—max. 1-h Neither to be exceeded more than once per year	TLV[e]—50 ppm STEL[f]—400 ppm	35 ppm—8 h TWA[g] 200 ppm ceil[h] (no min time)	50 ppm	West Germany—50 ppm Sweden—35 ppm
Carbon dioxide	None	TLV—5,000 ppm STEL—30,000 ppm	10,000 ppm—10-h TWA 30,000 ppm—10-min ceil.	5,000 ppm	—
Benzene	None	TLV—10 ppm A2	1 ppm—60-min ceil.	10 ppm 50 ppm—10-min ceil.	Sweden—10 ppm West Germany—0 ppm
Toluene	None	TLV—100 ppm STEL—150 ppm	100 ppm—10-h TWA 200 ppm—10-min ceil.	200 ppm 300 ppm ceil. 500 ppm—10-min peak	West Germany—200 ppm Sweden—100 ppm
Formaldehyde	None	TLV—1 ppm A2	Lowest feasible limit	3 ppm 5 ppm ceil. 10 ppm—30-min ceil.	Sweden—2 ppm West Germany—1 ppm
Acrolein	None	TLV—0.1 ppm STEL—0.3 ppm	None	0.1 ppm	—
Acetone	None	TLV—750 ppm STEL—1,000 ppm	250 ppm—10-h TWA	1,000 ppm	Sweden—500 ppm Germany—1,000 ppm
Pyridine	None	TLV—5 ppm STEL—10 ppm	None	5 ppm	West Germany, Sweden—5 ppm
Hydrogen cyanide	None	Ceiling limit[i]—10 ppm	4.7 ppm—10-min ceil.	4.7 ppm	West Germany, Great Britain—10 ppm

Hydrazine	None	TLV—0.1 ppm A2	0.04 mg/m^3— 120-min ceil.	1 ppm	—
Ammonia	None	TLV—25 ppm STEL—35 ppm	50 ppm—5-min ceil.	50 ppm	West Germany—50 ppm Sweden—25 ppm
Methylamine	None	TLV—10 ppm	None	10 ppm	—
Dimethylamine	None	TLV—10 ppm	None	10 ppm	—
Nitrogen oxide	None	TLV—25 ppm	25 ppm	25 ppm— 10-h TWA	—
Nitrogen dioxide	0.053 ppm—annual arithmetic mean	TLV—3 ppm STEL—5 ppm	1 ppm—15 min ceil.	5 ppm ceil.	West Germany—5 ppm Sweden—2 ppm
N-Nitroso-dimethylamine	None	A2	None	Listed as a cancer-suspect agent	—
Formic acid	None	TLV—5 ppm	None	5 ppm	—
Acetic acid	None	TLV—10 ppm STEL—15 ppm	None	10 ppm	—
Particulate phase					
Particulate matter	75 μg/m^3—annual geometric mean 260 μg/m^3/24-h max Not to be exceeded more than once per year	TLV—10 mg/m^3	None	15 mg/m^3	—
Nicotine	None	TLV—0.5 mg/m^3	None	0.5 mg/m^3	—
Phenol	None	TLV—19 mg/m^3	20 mg/m^3—10-h TWA 60 mg/m^3—15-min ceil.	19 mg/m^3	West Germany— 19 mg/m^3
Catechol	None	TLV—5 ppm	None	None	—
Hydroquinone	None	TLV—2 mg/m^3	2 mg/m^3—15-min ceil.	2 mg/m^3	—
Aniline	None	TLV—2 ppm	None	5 ppm	—
2-Toluidine	None	TLV—2 ppm A2	None	5 ppm	West Germany—5 ppm

TABLE A-1 *Continued*

	Public	Industrial			
	EPA	ACGIH[a]	NIOSH[b]	OSHA[c]	European Standards[d]
2-Naphthylamine	None	A1b	None	Listed as a cancer-suspect agent	—
4-Aminobiphenyl	None	A1b	None	Listed as a cancer-suspect agent	—

[a]American Conference of Governmental and Industrial Hygienists.
[b]National Institute for Occupational Safety and Health.
[c]Occupational Safety and Health Administration.
[d]Includes standards set in Sweden, Great Britain, and West Germany as examples.
[e]TLV = threshold limit value—time-weighted average concentration for a normal 8-hour workday, 40-hour week.
[f]STEL = short-term exposure limit—15-minute time-weighted average exposure that should not be exceeded.
[g]TWA = time-weighted average.
[h]Ceil. = ceiling.
[i]Ceiling Limit—concentration that should not be exceeded during any part of the working exposure.

A2—Industrial substance suspect of carcinogenic potential for man; exposure should be avoided.

A1b—Human carcinogen. Substance associated with industrial processes, recognized to have carcinogenic potential without an assigned TLV. For substances of this designation, no exposure or contact by any route—respiratory, skin, or oral, as detected by the most sensitive methods—should be permitted.

NOTE: Materials in ETS for which there are no standards: carbonyl sulfide, 3-methylpyridine, 3-vinylpyridine, anatabine, benz(*a*)anthracene, benzo(*a*)pyrene, cholesterol, y-butyrolactone, quinoline, harman, N-nitrosonornicotine, NNK, N-nitrosodiethanolamine, zinc, polonium-210.

The guidelines are given in terms of cumulative exposure over a period of time or in terms of maximal concentrations. The Threshold Limit Value (TLV) is the time-weighted average concentration of a normal 8-hour workday or 40-hour work week. The Short-Term Exposure Limit (STEL) is defined as a 15-minute time-weighted average exposure that should not be exceeded at any time during a workday, even if the 8-hour time-weighted average is within the TLV. Exposures at the STEL should not be repeated more than four times per day, with at least 60 minutes between successive exposures at the STEL. The ceiling limit is the concentration that should never be exceeded.

Finally, it should be noted that the guidelines are established for individual chemicals, without consideration of complex mixtures that may contain these chemicals. The behavior of the chemicals in a complex mixture over time is likely to be complicated. In summary, the direct comparisons of these guidelines with ambient levels measured in natural or experimental conditions should be made with caution. In some cases, the comparison may be inappropriate.

REFERENCES

American Conference of Governmental Industrial Hygienists (ACGIH). Documentation of the Threshold Limit Values and Biological Exposure Indices, fifth ed. Cincinnati, Ohio: ACGIH, 1986. 743 pp.

National Institute for Occupational Safety and Health (NIOSH). NIOSH/OSHA Pocket Guide to Chemical Hazards. DHEW Publ. No. 85-14. Cincinnati, Ohio: National Institute for Occupational Safety and Health, 1985. 241 pp.

Swedish Board of Occupational Safety and Health (Arbetarksyddsstyrelsens). Hygieniska Gransvarden. Stockholm, Sweden: Liber Distribution, 1984. 60 pp.

Appendix B: Method of Combining Data from Studies of Environmental Tobacco Smoke Exposure and Lung Cancer

Consider the following kinds of data that might be reported in an epidemiological study of chronic exposure to environmental tobacco smoke (ETS) and lung cancer:

		Lung Cancer		
		Yes	No	Total
Exposure to ETS	Yes	a	b	m_1
	No	c	d	m_2
Total:		m_3	m_4	T

Therefore, T is the total number of people in the study, a is the number of people chronically exposed to ETS who also have lung cancer, b is the number of people chronically exposed to ETS who do not have lung cancer, c is the number of people not chronically exposed to ETS who have lung cancer, and d is the number of people not chronically exposed to ETS who do not have lung cancer. The marginal totals are $m_1 = a + b$, $m_2 = c + d$, $m_3 = a + c$, and $m_4 = b + d$. The data that correspond to these variables from all of the studies examined in Chapter 12 are shown in Table B-1.

CASE-CONTROL STUDIES

In a case-control design, the subjects are chosen on the basis of the health outcome, and their exposure history is assessed.

TABLE B-1 Passive Smoking and Lung Cancer: Observed Numbers Used to Calculate Values in Table 12-4[a]

Type of Study	Study Authors	Sex	Spouse Smoker Cases (a)	Spouse Smoker Controls (b)	Spouse Nonsmoker Cases (c)	Spouse Nonsmoker Controls (d)	Risks Computed	Risks Published
CC	Chan and Fung, 1982	F	34	66	50	73	0.75	—
CC	Trichopoulos et al., 1983	F	38	81	24	109	2.13	2.4, 3.4
CC	Correa et al., 1983	F	14	61	8	72	2.03	2.00
		M	2	26	6	154	2.29	2.07
CC	Kabat and Wynder, 1984	F	13	15	11	10	0.79	—
		M	5	5	7	7	1.00	—
CC	Buffler et al., 1984	F	33	164	8	32	0.80	0.78
		M	5	56	6	34	0.50	0.52
CC	Garfinkel et al., 1985	F	92	266	42	136	1.12	1.12
CC	Pershagen et al., in press	F	33	150	34	197	1.28	1.2
CC	Akiba et al., 1986	F	73	188	21	82	1.48	1.5
		M	3	9	16	101	2.45	1.8
CC	Koo et al., 1985	F	51	66	35	70	1.54	1.64
CC	Lee et al., 1986	F	22	45	10	21	1.03	1.00
		M	8	14	7	16	1.30	1.30
PRO	Garfinkel, 1981	F	88	127,164	65	49,422	—	1.27, 1.10
PRO	Gillis et al., 1984	F	6	1,388	2	521	—	1.00
		M	4	306	2	515	—	3.25
PRO	Hirayama, 1984	F	146	69,287	37	21,858	—	1.45, 1.91
		M	7	1,003	57	19,222	—	2.25

ABBREVIATIONS: CC = Case-Control
PRO = Prospective

[a]For the calculations, (a) through (d) are used for case-control studies and published RR are used for prospective studies.

The expected number of people who are exposed to environmental tobacco smoke and develop lung cancer is given by:

$$\frac{m_1 \times m_3}{T}.$$

Expected numbers for each of the studies are shown in Table 12-4. The difference between observed and expected numbers of people with lung cancer who are exposed to ETS can be calculated, and the variance of this difference is given by:

$$\frac{m_1 \times m_2 \times m_3 \times m_4}{T \times T \times (T-1)}.$$

Therefore, the natural logarithm of the odds ratio (ψ) can be estimated by:

$$\psi = \frac{\text{Observed} - \text{Expected}}{\text{Variance(Observed} - \text{Expected)}}$$

and the variance of this estimate is given by:

$$\text{Variance of } \psi = [(\text{Variance(Observed} - \text{Expected)}]^{-1}$$

(Yusuf et al., 1985).

The odds ratio is estimated by $\exp[\psi]$ and is shown in Tables 12-4 (and B-1) with its 95% confidence intervals for each of the studies.

PROSPECTIVE (OR COHORT) STUDIES

In prospective studies, also known as cohort studies, the subjects are classified (or chosen) on the basis of exposure and the health endpoint is then assessed.

In all of the articles the authors have estimated the relative risk, adjusting for such variables as age. Therefore, the published relative risk values were used in the following calculations rather than the estimates of the crude relative risk that could be calculated from the data given in the text. For those studies where a relative risk estimate was given for different levels of smoking by the spouse (Garfinkel et al, 1981; Hirayama, 1984), a combined estimate of the relative risk was calculated using the method given below for combining the prospective studies.

The number of people who are exposed to ETS who are expected, under the null hypothesis of no effect, to develop lung cancer is:

$$m_3 - (m_3/E) \times c,$$

where E is the expected number for m_3, based on the published relative risk (RR), that is:

$$E = c + (a/RR).$$

The approximate variance of the observed minus expected numbers of people with lung cancer who are exposed to environmental tobacco smoke is:

$$\frac{m_1 \times m_2 \times m_3 \times m_4}{T \times T \times (T - 1)}.$$

The variance of the natural logarithm of the relative risk was calculated using the published confidence limits for the estimate of the relative risk, except for one study (Gillis et al., 1984), where the method given above for the case-control studies use used since no confidence limits were available.

SUMMING OVER STUDIES

The overall values for the case-control studies were calculated by adding the values of Observed − Expected (i.e., $O - E$) and their variance for the individual studies as follows:

$$\ln OR = \frac{\sum (O - E)_i}{\sum \mathrm{Var}(O - E)_i}$$

and for the variance:

$$\mathrm{Variance}(\ln OR) = \sum \frac{1}{\mathrm{Var}(O - E)_i}$$

(Yusuf et al., 1985).

For the prospective studies, the overall value for the ln RR was calculated as:

$$\ln RR = \sum \frac{(\ln RR)_i}{\mathrm{Var}(\ln RR)_i} \Big/ \sum \frac{1}{\mathrm{Var}(\ln RR)_i}$$

and for the variance:

$$\mathrm{Var}(\ln RR) = \frac{1}{\sum \mathrm{Var}(\ln RR)_i}$$

(Kleinbaum et al., 1982).

The overall value, for all of the studies combined, was obtained using the same method as was used to pool results from the prospective studies using the overall values for the case-control and prospective studies in the above equations.

REFERENCES

Akiba, S., W.J. Blot, and H. Kato. Passive smoking and lung cancer among Japanese women. Fourth World Conference on Lung Cancer, Toronto, Canada, Aug. 25-30, 1985.

Buffler, P.A., L.W. Pickle, T.J. Mason, and C. Contant. The causes of lung cancer in Texas, pp. 83-99. In M. Mizell and P. Correa, Eds. Lung Cancer: Causes and Prevention. New York: Verlag Chemie International, Inc., 1984.

Chan, W.C., and S.C. Fung. Lung cancer in nonsmokers in Hong Kong, pp. 199-202. In E. Grundmann, Ed. Cancer Campaign, Vol. 6. Cancer Epidemiology. Stuttgart: Gustav Fischer Verlag, 1982.

Corea, P., L.W. Pickle, E. Fontham, Y. Lin, and W. Haenszel. Passive smoking and lung cancer. Lancet 2:596-597, 1983.

Garfinkel, L. Time trends in lung cancer mortality among nonsmokers and a note on passive smoking. J. Natl. Cancer Inst. 66:1061-1066, 1981.

Garfinkel, L., O. Auerback, and L. Joubert. Involuntary smoking and lung cancer: A case-control study. J. Natl. Cancer Inst. 75:463-469, 1985.

Gillis, C.R., D.J. Hole, V.M. Hawthorne, and P. Boyle. The effect of environmental tobacco smoke in two urban communities in the west of Scotland. Eur. J. Respir. Dis. 133(Suppl.):121-126, 1984.

Hirayama, T. Cancer mortality in nonsmoking women with smoking husbands on a large-scale cohort study in Japan. Prev. Med. 13:680-690, 1984.

Kabat, G.C., and E.L. Wynder. Lung cancer in nonsmokers. Cancer 53:1214-1221, 1984.

Kleinbaum, D.G., Kupper, L.L., and H. Morgenstern. Epidemiologic Research: Methods and Application. New York: Nordstrum Reinhold, 1982. 341 pp.

Koo, L.C., J.H-C. Ho, and N. Lee. An analysis of some risk factors for lung cancer in Hong Kong. Int. J. Cancer 35:149-155, 1985.

Lee, P.N., J. Chamberlin, and M.R. Alderson. Relationship of passive smoking to risk of lung cancer and other smoking-associated disease. Br. J. Cancer. 54:97-105, 1986.

Miettenen, O.S. Estimability and estimation in case-referrent studies. Am. J. Epidemiol. 103:226-235, 1976.

Pershagen, G., Z. Hrubec, and C. Svensson. Passive smoking and lung cancer in Swedish women. Am. J. Epidemiol., in press.

Trichopoulous, P., A. Kalandidi, and L. Sparros. Lung cancer and passive smoking: Conclusion of Greek study. Lancet 2:677-678, 1983.

Wu, A.H., B.E. Henderson, M.C. Pike, and M.C. Yu. Smoking and other risk factors for lung cancer in women. J. Natl. Cancer Inst. 74:747-751, 1985.

Yusuf, S. R. Peto, J. Lewis, R. Collins and P. Sleight. Beta blockade during and after myocardial infarction: An overview of the randomized trials. J. Prog. Cardiovasc. Dis. 27:335-371, 1985.

Appendix C: Adjustments to Epidemiologic Estimates of Excess Lung Cancer in Persons Exposed to Environmental Tobacco Smoke

Chapter 12 describes 13 epidemiologic studies that estimate the relative risks of lung cancer in nonsmoking spouses of smokers compared with nonsmoking spouses of nonsmokers. A weighted average of the relative risks of "exposed" to "unexposed" persons is 1.34, i.e., a 34% increase in lung cancer risk as a consequence of environmental tobacco smoke (ETS) exposure. On the other hand, one can extrapolate in a linear fashion from the relative levels of cotinine that had been measured in active smokers and exposed nonsmokers. The expected relative risk for exposed nonsmokers would range from about 1.03 to 1.10. Neither of these estimates has been corrected for possible misclassification of subjects in the epidemiologic studies. The latter risk assumes that the one-time measure is a satisfactory surrogate for lifetime exposure. Misclassification problems and problems in estimating actual carcinogen exposure make it very difficult to provide an estimate of the numbers of cancer cases both in smokers and nonsmokers that might be attributable to ETS.

In this section we combine information from several sources to generate crude estimates of the relative risk to nonsmokers as a consequence of chronic exposure to ETS. The computations reported here are highly simplified and should be looked on as providing only a first approach to risk evaluation. A more detailed approach, including a more explicit statement of the assumptions involved, is given in Appendix D. A major concern is that persons who have been identified as "unexposed" to ETS may have really been exposed. If this were true, then the risks relative to truly unexposed persons would be underestimated. To estimate this possible effect, the results from studies of urinary cotinine are used here to adjust for the proportion of self-reported "unexposed" nonsmokers who, in fact, may have been exposed to ETS.

USING COTININE MEASUREMENTS TO CORRECT MISREPORTING

The only source of cotinine or nicotine in body fluids is tobacco smoke exposure. Therefore, urinary cotinine provides an objective measure of (recent) exposure. It has been reported (Jarvis et al., 1984; Wald et al., 1984) that urinary nicotine and cotinine are 3 times as high in "exposed" nonsmoking spouses of current smokers than in "unexposed" nonsmoking spouses of current nonsmokers. For example, Wald and Ritchie (1984) report urinary cotinine in the ratio 1:3:215 for "unexposed" nonsmokers, ETS-exposed nonsmokers, and regular smokers, respectively.

Several assumptions need to be made to permit the use of these data before any quantitative risk computation can be made:

- Current smoking patterns reflect past patterns.
- Cotinine or nicotine concentrations in the urine are linearly related to recent exposures to ETS and to the carcinogens in ETS among nonsmokers.
- All subjects in the various studies began to be exposed to ETS at the same age and have continued to be exposed at the same rate throughout the follow-up period.
- The excess relative risk for lung cancer in nonsmokers is proportional to the dose (in cigarette equivalents) of ETS absorbed.

An assumption of a linear dose-response relationship implies that if the risk (i.e., mortality rate) at a given age (t) for a specific calendar period (s), given some absorbed dose (d), then $\gamma(t,s|d)$ is:

$$\gamma(t, s|d) = \gamma_0(t, s)(1 + \beta d). \quad (1)$$

This equation expresses the risk as equal to the base mortality risk, $\gamma_0(t,s)$, for a truly unexposed person for the same age and calendar period, multiplied by an excess relative risk that increases linearly with dose, i.e. $(1 + \beta d)$, where β is the amount of increase per unit dose.* Further, the risk for a truly unexposed nonsmoker, i.e., $\gamma_0(t,s)$, is assumed to be the same for men and women. This assumption is supported, in part, by the results given in Chapter 12 and, in part, by earlier studies of Garfinkel (1981) and Friedman et al. (1984). Doll (1984), however, gives different risks for men and women of lung cancer mortality in nonsmokers.

If d_E is actual dose in the "exposed" persons and d_N is the actual dose in persons who believe themselves to be "unexposed," then we have, from Equation 1:

$$\gamma(t, s|d_E) = \gamma_0(t, s)(1 + \beta d_E), \tag{2A}$$

and

$$\gamma(t, s|d_N) = \gamma_0(t, s)(1 + \beta d_N), \tag{2B}$$

The relative risk for a person identified as "exposed" compared to a person identified as "unexposed" $[RR(d_E)]$ is given by Equation 2A divided by 2B:

$$RR(d_E) = \frac{1 + \beta d_E}{1 + \beta d_N}, \tag{3}$$

which, from Chapter 12, is 1.34, the relative risk estimated from the epidemiologic studies.

From the studies that measured cotinine in "exposed" and "unexposed" persons, we assume that the operative dose level, d_E, among "exposed" individuals is 3 times as high as the dose level in the self-reported "unexposed" persons, d_N, and that the ratio of 3:1 is proportional to a lifetime dose difference. Therefore, Equation 3 may be rewritten as:

$$RR(d_E) = \frac{1 + 3\beta d_N}{1 + \beta d_N} = 1.34. \tag{4}$$

Equation 4 can be solved for βd_N, which is the increase in risk for persons called "unexposed," but who, in fact, have been exposed

---

* Work by Doll and Peto (1978) shows that the relative risk for direct smokers increases as a linear-quadratic function of dose, rather than the simple linear form shown here. A more sophisticated model would take into account the several stages at which cigarette smoke operates in the multistage development of cancer. At low doses the linear-quadratic is well approximated by the linear, i.e., $1 + \beta_1 d + \beta_2 d^2$ is close to $1 + \beta d$ because the d^2 term approaches zero.

to some recent ETS, as indicated by their non-zero levels of urinary cotinine or nicotine. Solving Equation 4 gives:

$$\beta d_N = 0.20.$$

Thus, the relative risk for a self-identified "unexposed" person compared with a truly unexposed person is:

$$1 + 0.20 = 1.20,$$

and the relative risk for an "exposed" person compared with a truly unexposed person is:

$$1 + 3(0.20) = 1.60.$$

To see what possible effect these relative risk estimates would have on the population-attributable risk, i.e., the fraction of lung cancer in nonsmoking individuals attributable to ETS, the proportion of the population that is exposed to ETS needs to be estimated. Wald and colleagues (1984) have reported that 17% of nonsmoking women and 12% of nonsmoking men fall into the category of "exposed," i.e., nonsmoking spouses of smokers. By subtraction, this means that 83% of nonsmoking women and 88% of nonsmoking men would consider themselves "unexposed." Given this, we can estimate the population-attributable risk, which is given in general form as:

$$\frac{p_1(RR_1 - 1) + (1 - p_1)(RR_2 - 1)}{p_1(RR_1) + (1 - p_1)(RR_2)} = PAR, \tag{5}$$

where p_1 is the proportion of people who call themselves "exposed," RR_1 is the relative risk of self-reported "exposed" persons, and RR_2 is the relative risk of self-reported "unexposed" persons. Thus, for men:

$$PAR_{\text{men}} = \frac{0.12(0.60) + 0.88(0.20)}{0.12(1.60) + 0.88(1.20)} = 0.20.$$

and for women:

$$PAR_{\text{women}} = \frac{0.17(0.60) + 0.83(0.20)}{0.17(1.60) + 0.83(1.20)} = 0.21.$$

That is, about 21% of the lung cancers in *nonsmoking* women and 20% in *nonsmoking* men may be attributable to exposure to ETS.

REFERENCES

Doll, R.D. Epidemiological discovery of occupational cancers. Ann. Acad. Med. Singapore 13(Suppl.):331-339, 1984.

Doll, R.D., and R. Peto. Cigarette smoking and bronchial carcinogenic: Dose and time relationships among regular smokers and lifelong nonsmokers. J. Epidemiol. Comm. Health 32:303-313, 1978.

Friedman, G.D., R.D. Bawol, and D.B. Pettiti. Prevalence and correlates of passive smoking. Am. J. Public Health 73:401-405, 1983.

Garfinkel, L. Time trends in lung cancer mortality among nonsmokers and a note on passive smoking. J. Natl. Cancer Inst. 66:1061-1066, 1981.

Jarvis, M., H. Tunstall-Pedoe, C. Feyerabend, C, Vesey, and Y. Salloyee. Biochemical markers of smoke absorption and self reported exposure to passive smoking. J. Epidemiol. Comm. Health 38:335-339, 1984.

Wald, N.J., A. Boreham, A. Bailey, C. Ritche, J.E. Haddow, and G. Knight. Urinary cotinine as a marker of breathing other people's smoke. Lancet 1:230-231, 1984.

Wald, N.J., and C. Ritchie. Validation of studies on lung cancer in non-smokers married to smokers. Lancet 1:1067, 1984.

Appendix D: Risk Assessment—Exposure to Environmental Tobacco Smoke and Lung Cancer

James Robins

This authored appendix was prepared by Dr. James Robins of the Harvard University School of Public Health. The material was not considered by the committee largely because of lack of time, nor was it reviewed by the National Research Council. It gives an approach to risk assessment that considers both the epidemiologic data and some measures of exposure to the constituents of ETS. It is included as an addendum of this report and is presented here as one possible way to integrate the data contained in the remainder of the report.

INTRODUCTION

In Chapter 12, the results of 13 epidemiologic studies are summarized. Each study provided an estimate of the ratio of the lung cancer mortality rate among nonsmokers who answered "yes" to a question like "Is your spouse a smoker?" (hereafter called "exposed" individuals) to the mortality rate among nonsmokers who answered "no" to that question (hereafter called "unexposed" individuals). A weighted average of the 13 study-specific rate ratios is roughly 1.3. In this appendix, we assume that a weighted average of 1.3 is causally related to differences in environmental tobacco smoke (ETS) exposure between "exposed" and "unexposed" individuals and not to bias (e.g., misclassification of smokers as nonsmokers—see Chapter 12).

Wald and Ritchie (1984) have shown that "unexposed" individuals have, on average, 8.5 ng/ml of cotinine in their urine. Since virtually the only source of cotinine or nicotine in body fluids is tobacco products, primarily through tobacco smoke exposures, it follows that "unexposed" individuals are exposed to ETS. For this reason, whenever we refer to such "unexposed" subjects, we place the word "unexposed" in quotation marks. If the "unexposed" subjects have, in fact, been exposed to ETS, the observed relative risk of 1.3 would be an underestimate of the true adverse effect of ETS on "exposed" individuals. The correct measure of the adverse effect of ETS on "exposed" individuals would be the ratio of the lung cancer mortality rate in "exposed" individuals to the rate in truly unexposed individuals (which we shall call the true relative risk in the "exposed").

In Section D-1, we use the data collected by Wald and Ritchie (1984) on levels of urinary cotinine in "exposed" and "unexposed" individuals to estimate this true relative risk by two different methods.

In Section D-2, we combine the existing epidemiologic data on active smokers with data on nonsmokers exposed to ETS to estimate the ETS exposure of an average nonsmoker in cigarette-equivalents per day. Additionally, we compare this estimate to independent estimates of ETS exposure based on (1) levels of respirable suspended particulates (RSP), benzo[*a*]pyrene (B*a*P), and *N*-nitrosodimethylamine (NDMA) in ETS and in mainstream smoke and (2) levels of urinary cotinine and nicotine in active smokers and nonsmokers.

In Section D-3, we compute how many of the lung cancer deaths estimated to occur among (lifelong) nonsmoking persons in 1985 might be attributable to ETS. The estimate is made separately for women and for men.

Many environmental exposures are regulated to a level where the anticipated lifetime risk of death attributable to exposure is less than 1 in 100,000 or 1 in 1,000,000. In Section D-4, we consider whether the lifetime risk of death (from lung cancer) attributable to ETS among nonsmokers with moderate ETS exposure is in excess of 1 in 100,000. (Although we do not estimate the lifetime risk of death attributable to ETS from causes other than lung cancer, this does not imply that we believe that lung cancer is the only cause of mortality influenced by ETS exposure. The decision to restrict the analysis to lung cancer mortality reflects the fact that the data necessary to perform an adequate quantitative risk assessment for causes of death other than lung cancer do not exist.)

In discussions of the health effects of ETS exposure, one should consider the effect on exsmokers of breathing other people's cigarette smoke, since exsmokers have given up smoking, presumably to protect their health. Therefore, in Section D-4 we estimate, for exsmokers, the lifetime risk of death from lung cancer attributable to breathing other people's cigarette smoke.

The sections D-1 to D-4 give nontechnical expositions of the issues. A separate Technical Discussion Section provides additional technical support and mathematical background.

In order to make quantitative estimates of the lung cancer risk attributable to ETS, numerical values must be chosen for a large number of parameters. When there are either no data or inconsistent data as to the magnitude of an important parameter, results are reported for a range of plausible values (i.e., a sensitivity analysis is performed).

Summary of Main Results Under the Assumption That the Summary Rate Ratio of 1.3 Is Causal

We summarize our main results. We caution the reader that the proper interpretation of these results requires that one read Section D-1 to D-4 and the discussion section that follows.

The estimated true relative risk for "exposed" individuals lies between 1.41 and 1.87. For "unexposed" individuals, the estimated true relative risk lies between 1.09 and 1.45. The number of (actively smoked) cigarettes effectively inhaled by a nonsmoker living with a smoking spouse lies in the range of 0.36-2.79 cigarettes/day. If the spouse is a nonsmoker, however, the estimated number lies between 0.12 and 0.93 cigarettes/day.

Of the roughly 7,000 lung cancer deaths estimated to have occurred among lifelong nonsmoking women in 1985, between 1,770 and 3,220 may be attributable to ETS. Of the roughly 5,200 lung cancer deaths estimated to have occurred among lifelong nonsmoking males in 1985, between 720 and 1,940 may be attributable to ETS.

The estimated lifetime risk of lung cancer attributable to ETS in a nonsmoker with moderate ETS exposure lies between 390 and 990 in 100,000. The estimated lifetime risk of lung cancer attributable to other people's cigarette smoke for an exsmoker who smoked one pack per day from age 18 to 45 and was moderately exposed to other people's cigarette smoke lies between 520 and 2,030 per 100,000.

D-1 ESTIMATION OF THE TRUE RELATIVE RISK

Method 1

The first method for estimating the true relative risk relies on two assumptions:

- The excess relative risk in a nonsmoker is proportional to the lifetime dose of ETS. That is, if an individual's dose of ETS (at all ages) were doubled, his excess relative risk would be doubled.
- At every age, "exposed" subjects have been exposed to ETS at a rate 3 times that of "unexposed" subjects. A factor of 3 was selected to reflect the empirical observation that the concentration of cotinine in the urine of nonsmokers with smoking spouses is about 3 times that of nonsmokers without smoking spouses (Wald and Ritchie, 1984).

These two assumptions imply that the excess (true) relative risk in "exposed" individuals is 3 times that of "unexposed" individuals. Hence, in the absence of bias, the summary rate ratio of 1.3 equals the ratio of the true relative risk in "exposed" individuals to that in "unexposed" individuals. Therefore,

$$1.3 = \frac{1 + 3x}{1 + x},$$

where x and $3x$ are the excess true relative risks in "unexposed" and "exposed" individuals, respectively. Solving for x gives $x = 0.18$ and, thus, the true relative risk in "exposed" and "unexposed" individuals of 1.54 and 1.18, respectively. If we used the summary rate ratio of 1.14 from only the U.S. studies (see Chapter 12), we estimate the true relative risk in "exposed" and "unexposed" individuals to be 1.23 and 1.08, respectively.

It is likely that the second assumption above may be inappropriate (see Remark 4 in the Technical Discussion). For instance, it is unlikely that the ETS exposure in childhood is 3 times greater in subjects who later married smokers, i.e., "exposed" subjects, than in subjects who later married nonsmokers, i.e., "unexposed" subjects. If it is not appropriate, then another approach is necessary. This approach is outlined in Method 2, which follows.

Method 2

Method 2 relies on the following two assumptions:

- Assume that (a) cigarette smoke influences the rates of the first- and fourth-stage cellular events in a five-stage multistage cancer process (Day and Brown, 1980; Brown and Chu, in press); (b) ETS affects the same two stages; and (c) the ratio of the relative magnitude of the effect (on a multiplicative scale) on stage 4 to that on stage 1 is the same for ETS and mainstream smoke. If we let β_1 and β_4 represent the magnitude of the effect on the first and fourth stages, respectively, then (c) implies that β_4/β_1 is the same for ETS and mainstream smoke.
- Assume the observed overall summary rate ratio of 1.3 is the ratio of the true relative risk in "exposed" subjects to that in "unexposed" subjects at age 70 (see Remark 3 in the Technical Discussion).

It is possible to estimate the true relative risk in "exposed" and "unexposed" study subjects, given two additional pieces of information (see Remark 8 in the Technical Discussion).

First, we require an estimate of the ratio β_4/β_1. An estimate of β_4/β_1 can be obtained by fitting the above multistage cancer model to data on the lung cancer experience of active smokers. In particular, an estimate of 0.0124 is obtained by fitting the multistage model to the continuing smoker data among British physicians given by Doll and Peto (1978). Brown and Chu (in press) obtained an estimate of 1.8, derived by fitting the multistage model to data from a large European case-control study of lung cancer. These two estimates of β_4/β_1, however, differ from one another by 150-fold. A third estimate of β_4/β_1 was computed, based on the following considerations. The estimate of β_4/β_1 from Doll and Peto (1976) fails to adequately account for the rapid fall off in relative risk in British physicians upon cessation of smoking. Since a larger ratio of β_4/β_1 will be associated with a more rapid fall off of risk when smoking is stopped (especially among smokers of relatively few cigarettes a day), we computed the maximum estimate of β_4/β_1 that was statistically consistent (at the 5% level) with the continuing smoker data in Doll and Peto (1978). This estimate was 0.225. Rather than choose among these estimates, we performed a sensitivity analysis using the three estimates of

β_4/β_1 of 0.0124, 1.8, and 0.225 (see Remark 5 in the Technical Discussion).

Second, we require, at each age, an estimate of the age-specific ETS exposure of "exposed" and "unexposed" study subjects relative to the current ETS exposure of an average adult nonsmoker whose spouse is a nonsmoker. Information does not exist to answer questions such as "How many times greater (or less) was the past ETS exposure in average "exposed" subjects from age 0 to 20 than the current ETS exposure of an average adult nonsmoker with a nonsmoking spouse?" Therefore, a sensitivity analysis was performed using 30 different choices for the lifetime exposure histories of "exposed" and "unexposed" subjects (relative to the current ETS exposure of an adult nonsmoker without a smoking spouse). The choice of exposure histories was influenced by the following general considerations. Smaller differences postulated between the lifetime ETS exposures of "exposed" and "unexposed" individuals will be associated with larger estimates of the true relative risk. (Having an observed rate ratio as large as 1.3 when there is truly only a small difference in dose between the "exposed" and "unexposed" subjects would imply that ETS is a potent carcinogen.) Therefore, we tried to select some exposure histories that would modestly underestimate the true difference in exposures between the "exposed" and "unexposed" study subjects and others that would modestly overestimate this difference. The rationale for our particular choices of the 30 exposure histories is given in Remark 7.

Thirty possible exposure histories are given in Table D-1. Remark 6 in the technical discussion describes how to read the exposure histories from this table.

Table D-2 gives the maximum and minimum estimates of the true relative risk among the "exposed" and "unexposed" for each choice of β_4/β_1, over the 30 exposure histories. The column denoted "all" gives the overall maximum and minimum as the choice of both β_4/β_1 and exposure history varies.

The most striking finding is that the estimate of the excess (true) relative risk for "exposed" individuals varies only twofold, from 0.41 to 0.87, and includes the estimate, 0.54, obtained with Method 1. All estimates exceed the uncorrected value of 0.30. Estimates of the excess true relative risk in the "unexposed" range from 0.09 to 0.45. Because of the possibility that the 30 exposure histories are not representative of those in Japan and Greece, two

TABLE D-1 Thirty Population Exposure Histories in Various Age Groups[a]

Value of a, b, or c	Population Subgroup	Age 0–20 yr			Age 20–55 yr			Age 55–70 yr		
		p_a	f_{1a}	f_{2a}	p_b	f_{1b}	f_{2b}	p_c	f_{1c}	f_{2c}
1	E	0.39	1.53[a]	0.3	1.0	3.0	—	0.5	3.0	3.0
	$\bar{E}$	0.25	1.53	0.3	1.0	1.0	—	1.0	1.0	—
2	E	0.44	1.53	0.3	1.0	1.5	—	0.5	3.0	2.0
	$\bar{E}$	0.18	1.53	0.3	1.0	0.15	—	1.0	1.0	—
3	E	0.44	1.53	0.3				0.5	3.0	1.0
	$\bar{E}$	0.18	0.75	0.15				1.0	1.0	—
4	E	0.44	0.75	0.15						
	$\bar{E}$	0.18	0.75	0.15						
5	E	0.44	1.0	0.6						
	$\bar{E}$	0.18	0.5	0.3						

[a]In units of d_0.

NOTATION: E = "Exposed"; $\bar{E}$ = "Unexposed". Population Exposure History $(a, b, c) = (1, 2, 3)$, has $p_{aE} = 0.39$, $p_{a\bar{E}} = 0.25$, $f_{1aE} = f_{1a\bar{E}} = 1.53$, $f_{2aE} = f_{2a\bar{E}} = 0.3$, $p_{bE} = p_{b\bar{E}} = 1.0$, $f_{1bE} = 1.5$, $f_{1b\bar{E}} = 0.15$, $p_{cE} = 0.5$, $p_{c\bar{E}} = 1.0$, $f_{1cE} = 3$, $f_{2cE} = 1$, $f_{1c\bar{E}} = 1$. The interpretation follows.

INTERPRETATION: 39% of E-individuals were exposed to ETS dose rate 1.53 d_0 and 61% to 0.3 d_0 from ages 0–20. 25% of $\bar{E}$ subjects were exposed to 1.53 d_0 and 75% to 0.3 d_0. From 20–55, all E-subjects were exposed to 1.5 d_0, all $\bar{E}$ subjects to 0.15 d_0. From 55–70, 50% of E-subjects were exposed to 3 d_0 and 50% to 1 d_0. All $\bar{E}$-subjects were exposed to 1 d_0.

TABLE D-2 Estimated Ranges for the True Relative Risks (*RR*) in "Exposed" and "Unexposed" Subjects

Rate Ratio[a]	Group	β_4/β_1 All	0.0124	0.225	1.8
1.3	"Exposed"	1.41-1.87[b] (321)-(113)[d]	1.41-1.87[c] (321)-(113)	1.43-1.72 (321)-(113)	1.43-1.64 (321)-(113)
	"Unexposed"	1.09-1.45 (321)-(113)	1.09-1.45 (321)-(113)	1.10-1.34 (321)-(113)	1.11-1.27 (321)-(113)
1.14	"Exposed"	1.19-1.35 (321)-(113)	—	—	—
	"Unexposed"	1.04-1.18 (321)-(113)	—	—	—

[a]Assume causal summary rate ratio.

[b]Range of *RR* over 30 exposure histories and three values of β_4/β_1.

[c]Range of *RR* over 30 exposure histories.

[d]Exposure histories (*a, b, c*) at which minimum and maximum, respectively, occur [see Table D-1 for definition of exposure histories (*a, b, c*)].

of the countries in which epidemiologic studies were conducted, we repeated the analysis using the overall summary rate ratio of 1.14 from the U.S. studies. In this case the overall range in the estimates of the true relative risk was 1.19 to 1.35 in the "exposed" and 1.04 to 1.18 in the "unexposed."

D-2 THE CARCINOGEN-EQUIVALENT NUMBER OF ACTIVELY SMOKED CIGARETTES INHALED DAILY BY PASSIVE SMOKERS: COMPARISONS OF EPIDEMIOLOGIC WITH DOSIMETRIC ESTIMATES

In this section we attempt to estimate the number of cigarettes, d_0, that would have to be actively smoked to deliver to the lung of the smoker a dose of active carcinogen equal to the daily pulmonary dose of carcinogen (attributable to ETS) of an average adult nonsmoker with a nonsmoking spouse. Roughly speaking, d_0 is the (lung) carcinogen-equivalent number of (actively smoked) cigarettes inhaled daily by an average adult nonsmoker with a nonsmoking spouse.

Under the assumptions of Method 2, we saw that knowledge of β_4/β_1 and of the relative exposure histories of "exposed" and "unexposed" study subjects was sufficient to estimate the true relative risks. If we also have an independent estimate of β_1, we can estimate d_0 as well (see Remark 8). Each of our three methods of deriving an estimate for β_4/β_1 from data on active smokers also produces an estimate of β_1. In particular, estimates of β_1 of 2.93, 0.803, and 0.14 are associated with β_4/β_1 of 0.0124, 0.225, and 1.8, respectively.

Some conflicting results need to be resolved, however. For any given level of smoking, the relative risk estimated from the British physicians data (Doll and Peto, 1978) is greater than that estimated from the American Cancer Society's follow-up data on a million Americans (Hammond, 1966) or from the multicenter European case-control lung cancer data (Lubin et al., 1984; Brown and Chu, in press). The relative risks in these latter two studies are consistent with one another and will here be treated as identical. Doll and Peto (1981) suggest that these differences in relative risk may be real differences, attributable in part to the different way cigarettes are smoked in Britain and other countries. To bring the British data in line with the other data, we adjusted our estimates of β_1 from the Doll and Peto data as follows. Separately, for the β_4/β_1 of 0.0124 and 0.225 (both based on the British physicians data), we computed the value of β_1 that would be necessary for an individual smoking 25 cigarettes per day since age twenty to have the same lung cancer incidence at age 65 as would follow if $\beta_4/\beta_1 = 1.8$, $\beta_1 = 0.14$ (based on the European case-control data). This gives adjusted estimates of 1.41 and 0.46 for β_1, corresponding to values for β_4/β_1 of 0.0124 and 0.225, respectively. These values are approximately half those previously estimated from the British physicians data. In our sensitivity analysis we use both the adjusted and unadjusted estimates of β_1 (see Remark 9).

Estimates of d_0 are given in Table D-3. Under the assumption that the summary rate ratio of 1.3 is causal, estimates of d_0 vary about eightfold from 0.12 to 0.93 cigarettes per day. For a given pair of values of β_1 and β_4/β_1, the variation in d_0 over the 30 exposure histories is only about twofold. When we use the summary estimate of 1.14 from the U.S. studies in lieu of the summary estimate of 1.3, our estimates of d_0 are diminished accordingly.

We next compare the above estimates of d_0, which are based on the epidemiologic data, with estimates based on the dosimetric measurements reported in Chapters 2 and 7. Estimates of d_0 based on dosimetric calculations are given in Table D-4. In Table D-4 we

TABLE D-3 Estimated Range for d_0, the Carcinogen-Equivalent Number of (Actively Smoked) Cigarettes Inhaled Daily by Subjects *Without* a Smoking Spouse

β_4/β_1:	All	0.0124		1.8	0.225	
β_1:	All	2.93	1.41	0.14	0.803	0.46
Rate ratio						
1.3[a]	0.12–0.93[b] (311)–(123)[c]	0.12–0.27[d] (311)–(123)	0.24–0.57 (311)–(123)	0.48–0.89 (311)–(423)	0.26–0.53 (311)–(123)	0.46–0.93 (311)–(123)
1.14	0.05–0.47 (311)–(123)					

[a]Assured causal rate ratio.
[b]Range of d_0 in cigarettes/day over 30 exposure histories and all $(\beta_4/\beta_1, \beta_1)$.
[c]Exposure history where maximum and minimum occurred.
[d]Range of d_0 over 30 exposure histories.

TABLE D-4 Estimates of d_0 Based on Various Constituents of ETS in Cigarettes/Day

Constituent	Range
NDMA	0.17–3.75
BaP	0.0084–1.89
RSP	0.0001–0.005

give an estimated range for d_0 under the assumptions that the ratio of the pulmonary (tissue) dose of active carcinogen in nonsmokers without smoking spouses to the pulmonary dose in active smokers is equal to the ratio of the pulmonary dose of B*a*P, NDMA, or RSP in the same populations. The estimates in Table D-4 are based on (1) the dosimetric measurements given in Table 2-10 and Chapter 7 and (2) the daily number of hours of self-reported ETS exposure among nonsmokers without smoking spouses (Wald and Ritchie, 1984; Friedman et al., 1983). Details of the calculations used to produce Table D-4 are given in Remark 11 of the Technical Discussion. The dosimetry of the biomarkers nicotine and cotinine is more complicated and is discussed in Remark 12.

There is a serious problem in reconciling the estimate of d_0 (Table D-4) based on B*a*P with that based on RSP, since RSP is often assumed to be a good surrogate for polycyclic hydrocarbons such as B*a*P. The estimate derived from the B*a*P measurements is several orders of magnitude higher. A possible, although unlikely, explanation is that the measurements of B*a*P levels in ETS (summarized in Table 2-10) inappropriately reflect total environmental B*a*P, which includes contributions from cooking, coal burning, and other sources, and that the contribution of B*a*P from ETS to total B*a*P is of the order of 2% or less.

The large uncertainty in d_0 seen in Table D-4 restricts the utility of these dosimetric calculations, especially given the lack of knowledge concerning the identity of the active carcinogens in ETS and mainstream smoke. In fact, the limitations of our dosimetric data may be even more serious than Table D-4 would lead one to believe. Specifically:

- the range of values entered in Table D-4 for NDMA could actually be orders of magnitude too high (see step 4 of Remark 11),
- the range of values for RSP and B*a*P do not reflect differences between the particulate phase of ETS and that of mainstream smoke with regard to deposition sites, clearance rates, and particle size,
- the range of values given for B*a*P in Table D-4 could be orders of magnitude too high if, as discussed above, the B*a*P entries in Table 2-10 represent the total environmental B*a*P inhaled by a nonsmoker, and
- the ratio of urinary nicotine (or cotinine) in nonsmokers to that in active smokers may not reflect, even qualitatively, the ratio of the biologically effective dose of active lung carcinogen absorbed by nonsmokers to the dose absorbed by active smokers (see Remark 12).

D-3 ESTIMATING THE NUMBER OF LUNG CANCER DEATHS IN NONSMOKERS IN 1985 ATTRIBUTABLE TO ETS

An estimate of the total number of lung cancer deaths among lifelong nonsmoking women in 1985 is $\sum_t I_0(t)N(t)$, where $N(t)$ is the number of nonsmoking women at risk at age t in 1985 and $I_0(t)$ is the age-specific lung cancer death rate among nonsmoking women in 1985. Data on $I_0(t)$ are given in Garfinkel (1981) for 1972; thus, this may be somewhat inaccurate for 1985. National Health Interview Survey data on N(t) were made available from

R. Wilson of the National Center for Health Statistics. Using these data, the number of lung cancer deaths was estimated to be 7,000, similar to the estimate obtained by Seidman (personal communication) using a related approach.

The total number of lung cancer deaths among nonsmoking women attributable to ETS in 1985 is

$$AN = \sum_{t} AF(t) I_o(t) N(t), \tag{11}$$

where $AF(t)$ is the age-specific fraction of lung cancer deaths due to ETS exposure in nonsmoking women. That is, $AF(t)$ is the age-specific average excess true relative risk (i.e., the average relative risk minus 1) divided by the age-specific average relative risk. In order to estimate the age-specific average relative risk among nonsmoking women, we require age-specific estimates of the probability of being married to a smoker (i.e., the probability of being "exposed") and of the true relative risk in "exposed" and "unexposed" subjects. We obtained age-specific estimates of the probability of being "exposed" from the Garfinkel et al. (1985) control population (Garfinkel, personal communication).

We estimated the true relative risk in three different ways. First, we use the estimates derived using Method 1 in Section D-1. Second, we use the estimates based on Method 2 of Section D-1. Third, we completely ignore the epidemiologic data on passive smoking and estimate the true relative risk by combining estimates of β_1 and β_4/β_1 extrapolated from data on active smokers, and estimates of d_0 based on dosimetry (Method 3). In a sensitivity analysis, we allow d_0 to equal 0.01, 0.2, and 2 to crudely represent (approximate) exposures to RSP, BaP, and NDMA, respectively (see Table D-4). The estimates of the attributable number based on Methods 1 and 2 are valid whenever the assumptions justifying those methods hold. For a given choice of d_0, the estimates of the attributable number based on the third method are valid when the first assumption under Method 2 holds and the choice of d_0 is correct (see Remark 13).

Using the relative risk estimates based on Method 1, we obtained an attributable number of 2,010.

In Table D-5, estimated ranges for the attributable number are reported. AN(EP) represents the estimates based on Method 2. $AN(0.01)$, $AN(0.2)$, and $AN(2)$ represent estimates based on the dosimetry estimates of 0.01, 0.2, and 2. (Since the estimate of the true relative risk based on Method 2 depends only on β_4/β_1 (and not on β_1), the estimate of $AN(EP)$ also depends only on β_4/β_1.) Estimates of the attributable number of lung cancer deaths based on Method 2 lie between 1,768 and 3,220. (These estimates are approximately halved when the summary rate ratio of 1.14, from the U.S. studies is used in place of the overall summary rate ratio of 1.3.) If the true value of d_0 were 0.01 cigarettes per day, then 259 lung cancer deaths in nonsmoking women would be attributable to ETS. On the other hand, the maximum estimate of the attributable number based on Method 3 with $d_0 = 0.2$ (3,170 deaths) is in agreement with that based on Method 2 (3,220 deaths). The minimum estimates, however, differ by approximately threefold.

The calculation of the number of lung cancers attributable to ETS in 1985 in nonsmoking males is similar. Garfinkel (1981) and Wilson (personal communication), respectively, give data on $I_0(t)$ and $N(t)$ for nonsmoking males. Since estimates of $I_0(t)$ in males and females are nearly equal and the estimates for females are more stable (Garfinkel, 1981), we use the same estimates of $I_0(t)$ for males as for females. Using these data, the estimated number of lung cancers which occurred in lifelong nonsmoking males in 1985 is 5200. For males, the fraction "exposed" is taken to be 14% (based on the control series from the Correa et al. (1983) study of males). Using relative risk estimates based on Method 1, it is estimated that 820 of the 5,200 lung cancer deaths are attributable to ETS. Estimates of the attributable number in males based on Methods 2 and 3 are given in Table D-5. Overall, the results for men are similar to those for women.

D-4 LIFETIME RISK OF DEATH FROM LUNG CANCER ATTRIBUTABLE TO ETS

Among Lifelong Nonsmokers

Permissible exposure limits to environmental agents are often set at levels low enough to reduce the lifetime risk of death attributable to the agent to 1 in 10^5 or 10^6. For purposes of comparison with other environmental and occupational standards, we have attempted to estimate the fractions of all deaths among nonsmoking men and women who survive past age 45 that are attributable to ETS-induced lung cancer. (This fraction is precisely the lifetime risk of lung cancer attributable to ETS exposure among persons surviving to age 45.) Since the risk of lung cancer is nearly 0 before age 45, we have chosen to condition this estimate on survival until that age. (Although years of life lost due to ETS exposure would be more preferable as a public health measure than the attributable fraction of deaths, we restrict our analysis to this latter measure in order to help determine whether, for regulatory purposes, ETS is being treated differently than other environmental exposures.) Because environmental regulations are generally set with the intention of protecting all (or at least almost all) individuals, we chose to estimate the attributable fraction for a representative subject with ETS exposure history of $2d_0$ for ages 0-18 and $4d_0$ for ages greater than 18. Based on data from Wald and Ritchie (1984) and Jarvis et al. (1984), this exposure history represents an exposure to ETS that is slightly greater than the average exposure of a nonsmoker exposed as a child to a smoking mother and as an adult to a smoking spouse. We label this exposure history as M, since it represents a moderately high lifetime exposure to ETS.

The fraction of all deaths subsequent to age t_0 (in our case age 45) attributable to exposure-induced lung cancer is, by definition,

$$AF(M) = \sum_{t>t_o} \gamma_{\text{EXCESS}}(t) S(t|t_o),$$

where $\gamma_{\text{EXCESS}}(t)$ is the excess lung cancer death rate at age t due to exposure history M and $S(t|t_0)$ is the overall probability of surviving to age t, given one has survived to t_0. Given that the assumptions of Method 2 hold, we can obtain an estimate of $AF(M)$ for each value of β_4/β_1 and each of the 30 exposure histories for the "exposed" and "unexposed" study subjects, provided we have data on the age-specific lung cancer rates in nonsmoking women, $I_0(t)$, and data on the all-cause age-specific mortality rates among nonsmoking women (which we estimated from data given in Hammond (1966) (see Remark 14).

The maximum and minimum of the $AF(M)$ across all exposure histories for each β_4/β_1 are given in Table D-6 in the "never-smoked" rows for males and females. $AF(M)$ is estimated to be between 390 and 990 in 100,000. A similar calculation, using the

TABLE D-5 Estimates of ETS-Attributable Lung Cancer Deaths Among U.S. Nonsmokers in 1985 (by Sex)

β_4/β_1:	All	0.0124	0.225	0.0124	0.225	1.80
β_1: Sex	All	2.93	0.803	1.41	0.461	0.140
Rate Ratio = 1.3						
AN (EP)[a]						
F	1768–3220[b] (323)–(113)[d]	1768–3220 (323)–(113)	1820–2800[c] (321)–(113)	1768–3220 (323)–(113)	1820–2800 (321)–(113)	1939–2492 (323)–(113)
M	721–1942 (321)–(113)	721–1942 (321)–(113)	751–1611 (321)–(113)	721–1942 (321)–(113)	750–1611 (321)–(113)	850–1390 (321)–(113)
AN (0.01)						
F	31–259 (423)–(211)	125–259 (423)–(211)	54–102 (423)–(211)	61–127 (423)–(211)	31–59 (423)–(211)	34–55 (423)–(211)
M	14–137 (423)–(111)	53–137 (423)–(111)	24–50 (423)–(111)	26–67 (423)–(111)	14–29 (423)–(111)	16–25 (423)–(111)

AN (0.2)						
F	585-3174 (423)-(211)	1921-3174 (423)-(211)	978-1695 (423)-(211)	1059-1939 (423)-(211)	585-1052 (423)-(211)	634-988 (423)-(211)
M	265-1890 (423)-(111)	908-1890 (423)-(111)	450-891 (423)-(111)	425-1094 (423)-(111)	265-540 (423)-(111)	305-465 (423)-(111)
AN (2)						
F	3793-6778 (423)-(211)	5992-6778 (423)-(211)	5039-6198 (423)-(211)	4702-5973 (423)-(211)	3793-5163 (423)-(211)	3854-4955 (423)-(211)
M	2016-4803 (423)-(111)	3812-4803 (423)-(111)	2904-4060 (423)-(111)	2758-4057 (423)-(111)	2016-3170 (423)-(111)	2151-2908 (423)-(111)
Rate Ratio = 1.14						
AN (EP)						
F	935-1730 (323)-(113)					
M	360-980 (321)-(113)					

[a] *AN (EP)* is based on epidemiologic data in nonsmokers exposed to ETS.
[b] Range of attributable number of lung cancers over 30 exposure histories and five choices of $(\beta_1, \beta_4/\beta_1)$.
[c] Range of AN of lung cancers over 30 exposure histories in nonsmoking females for $\beta_4/\beta_1 = 0.225$, $\beta_1 = 0.803$.
[d] Exposure history where minimum and maximum occurs.

TABLE D-6 Range of Estimated Lung Cancer Deaths Attributable to Breathing Other People's Cigarette Smoke per 10,000 Deaths (All Causes)

		Smoking	β_4/β_1: All	0.0124		1.8	0.225	
Rate	Sex	Status[a]	β_1: All	2.93	1.41	0.14	0.803	0.46
1.3[b]	M	N	39–99	48–99	45–95[d]	48–99	45–95	39–77
		Ex	52–197	62–126	74–149	52–106	100–197	62–115
		C	58–307[c]	78–157	107–209	58–117	159–307	86–158
	F	N	40–99	49–99	45–96	49–99	45–96	40–78
		Ex	54–203	64–130	77–154	54–110	103–203	64–120
		C	62–331	84–169	115–225	62–125	171–331	92–170
1.14	M	N	19–49					
		Ex	26–99					
		C	29–159					
	F	N	21–52					
		Ex	29–109					
		C	33–182					

[a]Smoking Status: N = never; Ex = smoked 1 pack per day, age 18–45; C = continuing smoker, 1 pack per day from age 18.

[b]Assumed causal rate ratio.

[c]Range over 30 exposure histories, 5 values of (β_1, β_4/β_1).

[d]Range over 30 exposure histories.

NOTE: All maxima were associated with exposure history (423); all minima with history (311).

summary risk of 1.14 from the U.S. studies (instead of 1.3), halves our estimates for $AF(M)$.

Among Current and Exsmokers

We now estimate $AF(M)$ for $t_0 = 45$ for current and exsmokers of 20 cigarettes per day. To clarify the approach, consider a female exsmoker (or continuing smoker) who was exposed to exposure history M of ETS from other people's cigarette smoke. (The subject's total ETS exposure is even greater, since it consists of contributions from her own cigarette smoke, as well.) Then $\gamma_{\text{EXCESS}}(t)$ necessary for the calculation of $AF(M)$ is the difference between the lung cancer mortality rate at age t, given her total smoke exposure, and her lung cancer mortality rate at age t, had she had the same active smoking history without exposure to other people's cigarette smoke. We require the same assumptions and information to estimate $AF(M)$ for exsmokers and continuing smokers as we did for nonsmokers, plus an estimate of β_1. Estimates of $S(t|t_0)$ are obtained as before, except the exsmoker and continuing smoker all-cause mortality rates given in Hammond (1966) are used (see Remark 15).

In Table D-6 the maximum and minimum of $AF(M)$ for each of five combinations of $(\beta_1, \beta_4/\beta_1)$ and all 30 exposure histories for the "exposed" and "unexposed" are given for continuing smokers and exsmokers of 20 cigarettes per day starting at age 18 and, in the case of exsmokers, stopping at age 45. For exsmokers, the estimate lies between 520 and 2,030 per 100,000. For continuing smokers, it lies between 580 and 3,310 per 100,000. A similar calculation, using the summary rate ratio of 1.14 from the U.S. studies, halves our estimates.

DISCUSSION

Exercises in quantitative risk assessment serve several useful purposes. First, public health decisions must often be made without certainty as to the magnitude of the likely health benefits that would result from implementing the various policy options. Quantitative risk assessment can aid in the decision-making process by quantifying this uncertainty. Second, difficulties encountered in providing precise estimates in quantitative risk assessment highlight areas where scientific knowledge is inadequate. Thus, exercises in risk assessment can serve to help focus future research.

All quantitative assessments of risk rely on assumptions. Interval estimates of quantitative risk are reliable only insofar as (1) the assumptions under which they were derived are valid and (2) the range of parameter values used in the estimation process includes the true value. It follows that no quantitative risk estimates can be guaranteed to be reliable. Nonetheless, some risk estimates are more (or less) reliable than others.

With regard to point (2) above, it should be noted that, in performing the risk assessment presented here, a sensitivity analysis was performed only over those parameters for which there were either inadequate empirical estimates (e.g., the lifetime ETS exposure history of "exposed" and "unexposed" subjects) or grossly inconsistent estimates (e.g., the estimates of β_4/β_1). Thus, the analyses did not account for other sources of uncertainty, such as statistical uncertainty, in estimates of other parameters. If they had, the width of the interval risk estimates may have increased severalfold. Generally, the more parameters that are varied in a sensitivity analysis, the more information that analysis provides; nonetheless, for simplicity, we chose to vary only those parameters with inadequate or inconsistent estimates. It is inevitable that some readers, often with good justification, will feel that we should have used different values for the parameters we treated as fixed or different ranges for the parameters we varied. (Computer programs are available from Dr. Robins.)

In our risk assessment, the most important assumption was that the observed summary rate ratio of 1.3 was causal. If this assumption is correct (below we discuss the possibility that it is not), we believe that the estimate of the lifetime risk of lung cancer among lifelong nonsmokers attributable to moderate ETS exposure $[AF(M)]$ will be accurate to within a factor of 2 to 6. This belief depends on the fact that if the rate ratio of 1.3 is causal, we are not extrapolating outside the range of the data (for example, from high to low dose) in estimating $AF(M)$. (Even though our reported uncertainty in estimating $AF(M)$ in never-smokers (Table D-6) is only twofold, nonetheless, as discussed above, our estimate of overall uncertainty would likely be larger; we have guessed twofold to sixfold). For any reasonably flexible model, such as the multistage model, the data (when ample) will drive the risk estimates provided one does not extrapolate outside the range of the data. For instance, even though our estimates of β_4/β_1 used in the sensitivity analysis differed by 150-fold, the overall variation in the lifetime risk of lung cancer due to ETS in nonsmokers varied only twofold (Table D-6). In contrast, in estimating the lifetime risk of lung cancer due to ETS in exsmokers we were forced to extrapolate outside the range of the data. To do this we used statistical models. We found an uncertainty factor of about fourfold (Table D-6) because of the sensitivity of this extrapolation to the particular coefficients assumed for the multistage model. But even this range of four underestimates the true uncertainty, because we have little assurance that it is appropriate to use the multistage model to extrapolate.

Given that we can know the lifetime risk of ETS-caused lung cancer in nonsmokers within a factor of 2 to 6, is this degree of accuracy sufficient for our purposes? Obviously, it depends on the purpose. If there were a regulatory process through which we wished to ensure that the lifetime risk of lung cancer attributable to ETS among nonsmokers would be no greater than 1 in 100,000 (or even 1 in 1,000), by limiting, if necessary, exposure to environmental tobacco smoke, our risk analysis would appear to be sufficient to drive that process. This is true because, even if the lower estimate of risk of 390 per 100,000 were reduced by factor of 2 or 3 (to take into account additional sources of uncertainty), it would still greatly exceed 1 per 100,000.

In this appendix, we confined our risk estimates to those arising under the assumptions that the causal summary rate ratio from the various epidemiologic studies was either 1.3 or 1.14 (the summary rate ratio from the U.S. studies). In Chapter 12 it was concluded that, considering the evidence as a whole, exposure to ETS increases the rate of lung cancer among nonsmokers. Furthermore, it was concluded that our best overall estimate of the causal summary rate ratio from the 13 studies was about 1.3. In light of this conclusion about causation, for purposes of making public health decisions for the United States, it would seem prudent to operate under the assumption that the true summary rate ratio was most likely 1.3 and at least 1.14 (even though values less than 1.14 cannot be excluded). We therefore did not prepare estimates for values less than 1.14.

We also did not make risk estimates under the assumption that the causal summary rate ratio was greater than 1.3, largely because the estimated lifetime risk of lung cancer at this rate ratio of 1.3 was sufficiently large that it did not seem important to quantify how large the lifetime risk might be if the true causal rate ratio were 1.48 (the 95% upper confidence limit for the summary rate ratio of 1.3). Finally, it would have been helpful to be able to compare estimates of risk derived from the 13 epidemiologic studies of nonsmokers exposed to ETS with independent estimates based on dosimetric measurements made in active and passive smokers. Unfortunately, as discussed in Section D-2, uncertainties in the identity and dose of the active carcinogens in ETS and mainstream smoke effectively preclude this possibility at this time.

TECHNICAL DISCUSSIONS

Estimation of the True Relative Risk

Method 1

The assumptions presented in Section D-1 above are replaced by more formal assumptions:

Assumption 1a We assume that, in the "low-dose" range represented by ETS exposure, the increment in the mortality rate at age t due to an increment of ETS exposure experienced at age u ($u < t$) is uninfluenced by any other increment of ETS exposure (whether received at time u or at any other time u').

The mathematical formulation of Assumption 1a is

$$\gamma(t|\{d(u); u \leq t\}) = \gamma_0(t)[1 + \beta(t) \int_0^t f(t,u)d(u)du], \qquad \text{(D-1)}$$

where $\gamma_0(t)$ is the mortality rate at t in the absence of exposure to ETS, $d(u)$ is the dose at age u of the active carcinogen in ETS, $\gamma(t|\{d(u); u \leq t\})$ is the mortality rate at t given a history of exposure to ETS represented by the curve $\{d(u); u \leq t\}$, $\int_0^t f(t,u)d(u)du$ may be interpreted as a weighted average of an individual's past exposure, and $\beta(t)$ is an age-specific measure of the magnitude (on a ratio scale) of the ETS effect. (For example, if there were a 5-year biologic latency period, $f(t,u) = 0$ for $t - u < 5$).

Remark 1 In the above description of Equation D-1, we have implicitly assumed that $\int_0^t f(t,u)du = 1$ so that $\int_0^t f(t,u)d(u)du$ is a weighted average and $\beta(t)$ is an effect measure. In fact, the restriction

$$\int_0^t f(t,u)du = 1 \qquad \text{(D-2)}$$

is not in general necessary for Equation D-1 to be meaningful, although some restriction is necessary to identify $\beta(t)$. Nonetheless, Equation D-1 can always be "reparameterized" so that Equation D-2 holds. If, in Equation D-1, $\beta(t) = \beta$ independent of t, we say that we have a linear excess relative risk model. If in Equation D-1, $\beta(t)\gamma_0(t) = \beta'$, independent of t, we have a linear excess absolute risk model. If there exists a function $f(t,u)$ for which Equation D-1 is a linear excess relative (or absolute) risk model, then Equation D-1 generally cannot be "reparameterized" so that simultaneously Equation D-2 holds and $\beta(t) = \beta$ or $\beta(t)\gamma_0(t) = \beta'$.

Remark 2 By extending the argument given by Crump et al. (1976), one can show that sufficient (but not necessary) conditions for Assumption 1a to hold are (1) the dose of ETS to passive smokers at any time u has a very small influence on risk at t and

(2) other risk factors for lung cancer operate through the same mechanism as ETS. Since the true relative risk associated with passive smoking exceeds 1.3, Crump et al.'s argument may not be relevant. In Remark 18, we empirically assess the validity of Assumption 1a under the further assumption that cigarette smoke affects two stages of a five-stage multistage cancer process.

Consider now the subset of the source population of an epidemiologic study that includes "exposed" individuals at risk at age t. Clearly, the exposure at any time $u, u < t$, to ETS, say $d(u)$, will vary among persons in this subset. Let $d_E(u|t)$ be the average pulmonary dose at age u among "exposed" individuals at risk at age t.

In a follow-up study in which the data collected includes age, cause of death, and "exposure" status, we can empirically estimate the age-specific (average) mortality rate among "exposed" individuals, $\gamma(t|E)$, and unexposed individuals, $\gamma(t|\bar{E})$. Furthermore, it follows from the linearity of Equation D-1 that

$$
\begin{aligned}
RR(t|E) &\equiv \gamma(t|E)/\gamma_0(t) \\
&= 1 + \beta(t)\int_0^t f(t,u)d_E(u|t)du,
\end{aligned}
\tag{D-3}
$$

where $RR(t|E)$ is the true relative risk (i.e., the ratio of the mortality rate among "exposed" individuals to that of truly unexposed individuals). Unfortunately, we cannot estimate $\gamma_0(t)$ [and thus $RR(t|E)$] without further assumptions. Similarly, we are unable to estimate $RR(t|\bar{E})$, the true relative risk due to ETS in "unexposed" individuals. (Remember, "unexposed" individuals are truly exposed.) But, in the absence of bias, from either prospective or case-control data we can empirically estimate

$$
\frac{\gamma(t|E)}{\gamma(t|\bar{E})} = \frac{1 + \beta(t)\int_0^t f(t,u)d_E(u|t)du}{1 + \beta(t)\int_0^t f(t,u)d_{\bar{E}}(u|t)du} = \frac{RR(t|E)}{RR(t|\bar{E})}.
\tag{D-4}
$$

(In a case-control study the left side of Equation D-4 is the age-specific odds ratio comparing "exposed" to "unexposed" individuals.)

Assumption 1b

$$
\frac{d_E(u|t)}{d_{\bar{E}}(u|t)} \equiv c(u|t) = c(t),
\tag{D-5}
$$

where $c(t)$ is a known constant independent of u. Note $c(u|t)$ is a ratio of the average exposure at age u of "exposed" subjects at risk at age t to that of "unexposed" subjects at risk at t. Our main result is:

Lemma 1: If Assumptions 1a and 1b hold then $RR(t|E) = 1 + c(t)x$ and $RR(t|\bar{E}) = 1 + x$ where

$$x = \frac{\frac{\gamma(t|E)}{\gamma(t|\bar{E})} - 1}{c(t) - \frac{\gamma(t|E)}{\gamma(t|\bar{E})}}.$$

Proof: Let $\beta(t) \int_0^t f(t,u) d_{\bar{E}}(u|t) du = RR(t|\bar{E}) - 1 \equiv x$. Then $RR(t|E) = 1 + c(t)x$ and $RR(t|\bar{E}) = 1 + x$. Thus, substituting in Equation D-4,

$$\frac{\gamma(t|E)}{\gamma(t|\bar{E})} = \frac{1 + c(t)x}{1 + x}$$

implies:

$$x = \frac{\frac{\gamma(t|E)}{\gamma(t|\bar{E})} - 1}{c(t) - \frac{\gamma(t|E)}{\gamma(t|\bar{E})}}. \quad \text{(D-6)}$$

Example: Suppose $c(70) = 3$ and $\gamma(70|E)/\gamma(70|\bar{E}) = 1.3$, then $x = 0.18$, $RR(70|\bar{E}) = 1.18$, $RR(70|E) = 1.54$.

We now show that, under Assumption 1a, if $c(u|t) < 3$ for all u, the previous estimates of $RR(t|E)$ and $RR(t|\bar{E})$ must, in fact, be underestimates (although the magnitude of the underestimation cannot itself be assessed without further assumptions such as those given under Method 2). First note that even when Equation D-5 is false, it is still true that, under Assumption 1a, with $x \equiv RR(t|\bar{E}) - 1$, Equation D-6 holds provided $c(t)$ is replaced by $c^*(t)$, where

$$c^*(t) = \frac{\int_0^t f(t,u) d_E(u) du}{\int_0^t f(t,u) d_{\bar{E}}(u) du}.$$

[Note that $c^*(t) > \gamma(t|E)/\gamma(t|\bar{E})$.] Furthermore, $RR(t|\bar{E})$ is still $1+x$ (by definition) and $RR(t|E) = 1 + c^*(t)x$.

Now it is straightforward to check that $RR(t|\bar{E})$ and $RR(t|E)$ are decreasing functions of $c^*(t)$ reaching respective minima of 1 and $\gamma(t|E)/\gamma(t|\bar{E})$ when $c^*(t) \to \infty$ and maxima of ∞ when

$c^*(t) = \gamma(t|E)/\gamma(t|\bar{E})$ is greater than 1. $c^*(t) = \gamma(t|E)/\gamma(t|\bar{E})$ is the condition of maximum misclassification between "exposed" and "unexposed" groups in terms of exposure to ETS. On the other hand, when $c^*(t) = \infty$ no "unexposed" individual is exposed to ETS.

Furthermore, it is easy to check that if

$$d_E(u|70)/d_{\bar{E}}(u|70) = c(u|70) \leq 3 \tag{D-7}$$

for all $u \leq 70$, then $c^*(t) \leq 3$. It follows that in our previous example, $RR(t|\bar{E}) = 1.18$ and $RR(t|E) = 1.54$ would, in general, be underestimates of the true $RR(t|\bar{E})$ and $RR(t|E)$ if Equation D-7 holds.

Remark 3 Note that the investigators of the 13 epidemiologic studies analyze their results as if their observed rate ratios were not dependent on age, as evidenced by the fact that none of the authors reported age-specific rate ratios. But if the rate ratio varies with age, then the observed rate ratio reported in each study will be a weighted average of varying age-specific rate ratios. Since Garfinkel et al. (1985) found the median age of lung cancer in nonsmoking women in his population was approximately 70 (Garfinkel, personal communication), we would expect that this weighted average approximates the rate ratio at 70. This implies that the second assumption under Method 2 in section D-1 is probably close to correct. To be precise, if, in a case-control study, one-to-one matching on age is employed and a matched pair analysis is performed, the matched pair odds ratio estimator will estimate the following weighted average of the age-specific rate ratios, $\gamma(t|E)/\gamma(t|\bar{E})$. The large sample expected value of the odds ratio estimator $(\widetilde{OR})$ is $E[\widetilde{OR}] = \int[\gamma(t|E)/\gamma(t|\bar{E})]f(t)dt$ where

$$f(t) = \frac{h(t)f_D(t)}{\int h(t')f_D(t')dt'},$$

$$h(t) = \frac{p(E|t)p(\bar{E}|t)}{[\gamma(t|E)/\gamma(t|\bar{E})]p(E|t) + p(\bar{E}|t)},$$

$f_D(t)$ is the fraction of all lung cancers in nonsmoking women that occur at age t, and $p(\bar{E}|t)$ is the fraction of nonsmokers in the study source population of age t who are "unexposed."

Remark 4 We now examine the conditions under which Assumption 1b holds with $c(70) = 3$. We conclude from the following examination that it is unlikely that Assumption 1b is true, even as an approximation.

Wald and Ritchie (1984) estimate that, in 1982 in England, the urinary cotinine concentration of an average nonsmoking male with a smoking spouse is 3 times that of the average nonsmoking male without a smoking spouse. Urinary nicotine data from Jarvis et al. (1984) and interview data from Friedman et al. (1983) suggest that similar results would be obtained in women. Given these observations, the following six conditions must, in general, be met in order for Assumption 1b to hold with $c(70) = 3$.

Condition 1 The ratio of 3 also applies to exposure to the biologically relevant carcinogen or carcinogens in ETS.

Condition 1 is likely to hold, at least in our approximate sense, in the United States and England. [Olav Axelson has pointed out a situation in which it would not hold. Suppose that the carcinogenic effect of ETS is largely due to the adsorption of environmental radon onto ETS particles. Then, home exposure to ETS would be of greater importance if, in general, only home ventilation rates are low enough to allow significant accumulation of environmental radon onto ETS particles. Friedman et al. (Table 6, 1983) showed that the number of hours currently-"exposed" women are exposed to ETS at home is 12.7 times the number of hours that currently-"unexposed" individuals are exposed at home. On the other hand, the total number of hours of ETS exposure in currently-"exposed" women is only 3 times that of currently-"unexposed" individuals. Thus, if radon uptake rather than urinary cotinine had been measured, Wald and Ritchie may have found a ratio nearer 12 than 3.]

On the other hand, in Japan and Greece the ratio of urinary cotinine in nonsmoking women with a smoking spouse to that in nonsmoking women without a smoking spouse probably exceeds the value of 3 measured by Wald and Ritchie (1984) in England, since women in those countries are likely to spend less time in contact with cigarette smokers outside the home. It follows that one might expect the observed rate ratio in the Hirayama (1984) and Trichopoulos et al. (1983) studies in Japan and Greece, respectively, to exceed that found in studies in the United States. Table 12-4 bears out this expectation. Thus, we might want to exclude Hirayama's and Trichopoulos et al.'s studies in calculating the overall summary rate ratio. We have seen that the U.S.

studies have an overall summary relative risk of 1.14. Assuming Assumption 1b with $c(70) = 3$ holds for the United States, we would estimate the true relative risk in "exposed" and "unexposed" study subjects in the United States to be 1.225 and 1.075. Nonetheless, since 1.225 is less than the observed rate ratios of 1.45 and 2.01 in the Hirayama and Trichopoulos et al. studies, we must also assume that the ETS exposure of nonsmoking women with smoking spouses in Japan and Greece exceeds that in the United States (if we ignore sampling variability and other sources of bias and interaction). Matsukura et al.'s (1984) data on urinary cotinine suggests this may be the case for spouse-exposed Japanese nonsmokers.

Because 10 of the 13 epidemiologic studies were case-control studies, we concentrate on case-control studies in the following. (Most of our remarks would have to be only slightly modified in order to apply to prospective studies such as Garfinkel (1981) and Hirayama (1981), in which the follow-up is only 10 to 15 years.) To characterize further conditions sufficient to imply that $c(70) = 3$, we shall need to be more precise in our definition of "exposed" and "unexposed" subjects. We define an ever-"exposed" (never-"exposed") subject to be a nonsmoker who, when queried in a case-control study in approximately 1982, answered "yes" ("no") to the question "Did you ever live with a smoking spouse?" We define a currently-"exposed" (currently-"unexposed") subject to be a nonsmoker who, in an epidemiologic study in 1982, answered "yes" ("no") to the question "Do you currently live with a smoking spouse?" Some of the case-control studies compared ever-"exposed" and never-"exposed" individuals (for example, Garfinkel et al., 1985). Approximately half of Garfinkel's ever-"exposed" subjects were currently-"unexposed," with the median time since their spouse stopped smoking of 15 years (Garfinkel, personal communication). Other studies compared currently-"exposed" subjects to never-"exposed" subjects.

Condition 2 Wald and Ritchie's (1984) ratio of 3 is independent of age and thus applicable to 70-year-olds. Sufficient urinary cotinine measurements have not been made on 70-year-olds to provide empirical evidence as to whether this condition holds.

Condition 3 Nearly all 70-year-old currently-"exposed" individuals married smokers at about age 20 in approximately 1932. This is probably a reasonable approximation, assuming little divorce and remarriage in this population.

Condition 4 If the study compares ever-"exposed" to never-"exposed" subjects, the magnitude of the ETS exposure in the years preceeding the study date of ever-"exposed" individuals who are currently-"unexposed" (because their spouses either died or quit smoking on average 15 years ago) is the same as that of currently-"exposed" individuals. For this latter condition to hold (even as an approximation), it is necessary either that only a small proportion of the total ETS exposure in currently-"exposed" individuals is directly from their spouses or that, when the smoking spouse of a nonsmoker either dies or quits smoking, the amount of time the nonsmoker spends with other smokers increases. Our guess, based on Table 6 of Friedman et al. (1983), is that the ETS exposure of an average ever-"exposed" female diminishes by a half or more when her husband either dies or quits. Thus, it is unlikely that Condition 4 holds.

Condition 5 The ratio of 3 applies to the ETS exposure of "exposed" and "unexposed" subjects even during childhood. It seems unlikely that children who grew up to marry smoking spouses would have 3 times the ETS exposure in childhood as children who grew up to marry nonsmoking spouses, although in Remark 7 we consider empirical evidence which suggests it is conceivable that Condition 5 might approximately hold.

Condition 6 Wald and Ritchie (1984) would have found the same ratio of 3 if their study had been performed in any year from 1932 to 1982. Even in those case-control studies that compared currently-"exposed" subjects to never-"exposed" subjects, Condition 6 may well be false. For example, in the 1930s and 1940s, nonsmoking women study subjects (who were then 20 to 30 years old) were presumably less often in contact with smokers outside the home. This would suggest that in the 1930s and 1940s the ratio of ETS exposure in nonsmoking women with smoking spouses compared to nonsmoking women without smoking spouses was closer to 12 than to 3 (provided the results of Friedman et al. (1983) mentioned in the discussion under Condition 1 can be extrapolated to the 1930s).

Remark 5: Estimates of β_4/β_1 We used three different estimates for β_4/β_1 in our sensitivity analysis. All were obtained from data on active smokers. To obtain the first, we fit by the method of maximum likelihood a five-stage multistage model, with the first and fourth stages affected, to the data on continuing smokers given in Doll and Peto (1978) (excluding, as did Doll and Peto, the subgroup who smoked more than 40 cigarettes per day). This gave $\beta_4/\beta_1 = 0.0124$ (and $\beta_1 = 2.93$). To be precise, we fit, as did Doll and Peto, the data enclosed in rectangles in their Tables 2 and 3. We used the mean number of cigarettes for each "cigarette-per-day" group given in their Table 2 and assumed, for each "cigarette-per-day" group, a variance that was half the maximum possible variance. We then fit the data in three different ways. First, we used the reported actual mean age of onset of cigarette smoking (19.2 years) as date of onset and the means of the age groups defining the rows in Tables 2 and 3 as the age of the event. Secondly, we used age 22.5 years as date of onset. Thirdly, we used age 19.2 years as date of onset, but subtracted 3.3 years from the means of the age groups defining the age of the event. The first and third methods both gave essentially the estimates reported above, while the second method gave $\beta_4/\beta_1 = 0.014, \beta 1 = 3.42$. The estimates based on the second method are not used in this appendix.

For our second estimate we used an estimate of $\beta_4/\beta_1 = 1.8$, given by Brown and Chu (in press), based on fitting this same multistage model to data from a large European case-control study. Brown and Chu found that $\beta_4/\beta_1 = 1.8$ (and $\beta_1 = 0.14$) for individuals who smoked 21-30 cigarettes per day (see Table 3 of Brown and Chu). (Brown and Chu find a ratio of 4 for β_4/β_1 for smokers of 1-10 cigarettes per day. We did not use this estimate due to its presumed lack of stability.) Note that the ratio of 1.8 found by Brown and Chu was 150 times that of Doll and Peto. The low β_4/β_1 ratio in the Doll and Peto continuing smoker data does not appear to adequately account for the rapid decline in risk associated with cessation of cigarette smoking as given in Doll and Peto (1976). This implied that the estimate of 0.0124 was probably too low. Furthermore, the estimate of β_4/β_1 from the Doll and Peto continuing-smoker data was quite imprecise, since the correlation between the estimates of β_1 and β_4 was -0.93. Based on these considerations, we computed a revised estimate of β_4/β_1 from the Doll and Peto continuing-smoker data by finding the maximum value of β_4/β_1 associated with a point on the 2 log likelihood surface that lay 3.87 (chi-squared units) below the value of the 2 log likelihood surface at its maximum above. At this point, the ratio of β_4/β_1 had increased 20-fold to 0.225 (and $\beta_1 = 0.803$). In our sensitivity analysis, therefore, we used ratios of β_4/β_1 equal to 0.0124, 0.225, and 1.8.

(One might believe that if the estimate of β_4/β_1, which one would hope to be a biological constant, can differ by 150-fold across data sets, Method 2 is useless. We actually are not so skeptical. If the sensitivity analysis shows that such large differences in estimates of β_4/β_1 have little influence on our estimate of the true relative risk in "exposed" and "unexposed" study subjects, this will indicate a high degree of robustness (insensitivity) to the actual model for lung cancer risk. Therefore, our confidence in the estimates of the true relative risk may therefore be enhanced. As we shall see, we do indeed find such robustness.)

Remark 6: Reading the Exposure Histories from Table D-1 Each of our exposure histories can be represented by a vector (a, b, c), where the value of a characterizes five possible population-exposure histories from age 0-20 ($a = 1, ..., 5$), b characterizes two possible exposure histories from age 20-55 ($b = 1, 2$) and c characterizes three possible exposure histories from ages 55-70 (c = 1,2,3). Since we can select any of five exposure histories between ages 0 and 20, any of two between ages 20 and 55 and any of three between 55 and 70, we have $5 \times 3 \times 2 = 30$ exposure histories. Each value of c gives an exposure history for "exposed" and "unexposed" subjects between the ages of 55 and 70. The population-exposure history between ages 55 and 70 represented by a particular value of c is described by the (up to) six values entered in Table D-1. As an example of how to read Table D-1, consider the case $c = 3$. Reading Table D-1, we see that $p_{cE} = 0.5$, $f_{1cE} = 3d_0$, $f_{2cE} = 2d_0, p_{c\bar{E}} = 1.0$, $f_{1c\bar{E}} = 1d_0$, and $f_{2c\bar{E}}$ is undefined. By definition, p_{cE} gives the fraction of "exposed" individuals exposed at rate f_{1cE} between ages 55 and 70. $1 - p_{cE}$ is the fraction of "exposed" individuals exposed at rate f_{2cE}. Therefore, 50% of "exposed" individuals receive a dose of ETS of $3d_0$ from 55 to 70 and 50% receive $1d_0$. Similarly, 100% of "unexposed" individuals receive a dose of $1d_0$ between ages 55 and 70. (Therefore, $f_{2c\bar{E}}$ need not be defined.)

Remark 7: Choice of 30 Exposure Histories In choosing the exposure histories, we rely heavily on data from the control series in Garfinkel et al. (1985), because similar detailed information is not available for any other study. We made the following assumptions.

1. All study subjects were age 70 at the time of the study. (In the Garfinkel et al. study (1985), the average age of cases and controls was approximately 70.) The choice of 55 as the upper age cutoff reflects the fact that among controls in Garfinkel et al. who were ever-"exposed" but not currently-"exposed," the median time since their smoking spouses either died or quit was roughly 15 years. Thus, we chose $70 - 15 = 55$ as the age at which ever-"exposed" individuals who are currently-"unexposed" ceased to be exposed to their spouses' cigarette smoke. The choice $c = 2$ represents our best guess as to the actual ETS exposure in the Garfinkel et al. study population between ages 55 and 70. The choice $c = 3$ assumes the ever-"exposed" subjects who are currently "unexposed" receive the same ETS dose, d_0, from age 55 to 70 as never-"exposed" subjects. Note that $c = 1$ represents a study in which all exposed individuals are currently-"exposed."

2. For exposure histories between ages 20 and 55, we assume that all subjects were married at age 20. $b = 1$ represents a population in which Wald and Ritchie (1984) would have obtained the same urinary cotinine measurements had they performed their study in any year from 1932 to 1982. In contrast, $b = 2$ represents a situation in which from 1932 to 1967 never-"exposed" individuals were exposed to ETS at a rate only 15% of that of currently-"unexposed" individuals in 1982 and ever-"exposed" individuals were exposed at a rate half that of a currently-"exposed" individual in 1982. Thus, $b = 2$ represents an extreme example of the situation discussed under Condition 6 of Remark 4 with $c(30|70) = 10$. The true exposure rates between ages 20 and 55 presumably lie between those represented by $b = 2$ and $b = 1$.

3. We next consider ETS exposures between the ages of 0 and 20. 39% (25%) of "exposed" ("unexposed") individuals in the control series in Garfinkel et al. (1985) reported that they were regularly exposed to ETS in their homes during childhood (presumably because, in the large majority of cases, at least one of their parents was a smoker). These controls, who are on average age 70, had to remember their parents' smoking habits over more than 50 years. Therefore, some misclassification is unavoidable. As a guess, we suppose that the false negative rate for parental smoking was 0.3 and the false positive rate was 0.15, independent of "exposure" status. Define p_{aE} to be the fraction of exposed controls with at least one smoking parent. Then, correcting for misclassification, our best estimates of p_{aE} and $p_{a\bar{E}}$ are 0.44 and

0.18, respectively (since $0.7\ p_{aE} + 0.15(1 - p_{aE}) = 0.39$ implies $p_{aE} = 0.44$).

For the exposure histories represented by $a = 1$, we used the uncorrected estimates 0.39 and 0.25, and otherwise used the corrected estimates. The uncorrected estimates were used in our sensitivity analysis because we do not know the true misclassification rates and, if false-positive and false-negative rates depend on "exposure" status, the true ratio of $p_{aE}/p_{a\bar{E}}$ may be less than or equal to 0.39/0.25. To develop estimates of f_{1a} and f_{2a} we proceed as follows. Jarvis et al. (1985) give mean salivary cotinine levels in children of 0.44, 1.32, 1.99, 3.39 ng/ml, depending on whether neither parent smoked (269), only father smoked (96), only mother smoked (76), or both parents smoked (128). (The numbers in parentheses give the number of children in each parental smoking category.) Now, Jarvis et al. conjecture that an average active smoker would have a salivary cotinine level of approximately 300 ng/ml. It follows that, as a rough approximation, the exposure to ETS of a child with nonsmoking parents is approximately $0.3d_0$ since Wald and Ritchie (1984) found the urinary cotinine levels of currently-"unexposed" individuals were approximately 1/200 that of an average active smoker and $0.44 \times 200/300 \cong 0.3$. (This result obviously depends on unverified assumptions about the comparability of nicotine metabolism in adults and children.) Furthermore, the ratio of ETS exposure in an average child with a smoking parent to an average child without a smoking parent is $[(1.32)(96) + 1.99(76) + 3.39(128)/(96 + 76 + 128)]/0.44 = 5.1$ (which is a dose of $1.53d_0 = 5.1(0.3)d_0$. Similar data from a study of Coultas et al. (1986) give a ratio of 3.07 rather than 5.1, under the assumption that the fraction of children with two smoking parents among children with at least one smoking parent is $128/(76 + 56 + 128)$, as in the Jarvis study. These results motivated the choice of f_{1a} and f_{2a} for a equal to 1 and 2.

One would expect that in the 1920s children living in homes with no parents smoking might well have less ETS exposure than such children currently have (since in the 1920s fewer caretakers, who were almost exclusively female, smoked). On the other hand, among children who lived in a home with a smoking parent, presumably a higher percentage had only a father who smoked. (Data on this question was not available from the Garfinkel et al. (1985) control population.) Thus, the ETS exposure in the 1920s of an average child with a smoking parent would also be less than that of a similar child in the 1980s. These observations led to our choice of f_{1a} and f_{2a} for $a = 4$. On the other hand, it is likely that, conditional on having had a smoking parent in childhood, "exposed" individuals are more likely than "unexposed" individuals to have had a mother who smoked. Furthermore, it may well be that "exposed" individuals without a smoking parent had, on average, higher exposures in childhood than "unexposed" individuals without a smoking parent. (Recall that a higher percentage of "exposed" individuals are known to report having at least one smoking parent.) These observations led to our choice of the exposure histories characterized by $a = 3$. The final choice, $a = 5$, reflects the ratio of 3.07 found by Coultas et al. and the possibility that in the 1920s, when few women smoked, this ratio was even less. The maximum value for the ratio of the childhood ETS exposure of "exposed" compared to "unexposed" subjects is 3.17 occurring when $a = 3$.

All 30 exposure histories presume that the ratio of ETS exposure in the 1970s and 1980s in currently-"exposed" subjects to that in currently-"unexposed" subjects is 3, as found by Wald and Ritchie. Thus, the sensitivity analysis may not be applicable to studies carried out in Greece and Japan, for reasons discussed above (although it is possible that in recent years the exposure of Japanese nonsmoking women outside the home has increased to United States' and British levels). Thus, one might wish to use both 1.3 and 1.14 as the summary observed rate ratio in a sensitivity analysis.

Remark 8: Estimating the True Relative Risk Under Assumptions for Method 2 Above Consider a group of individuals (i.e., the "exposed" individuals or the "unexposed" individuals in Garfinkel et al.'s (1985) study) such that each individual i has a constant exposure to ETS, d_{1i}, from age 0 to t_0, exposure d_{2i} from age t_0 to t_s, and exposure d_{3i} from age t_s to t. The d_{1i}, d_{2i}, d_{3i} may vary between individuals in the group. Then, the true relative risk at age t for the group compared to a completely unexposed group, when exposure affects the first and fourth stages of a five-stage multistage model, is:

$$RR(t) = 1 + \beta_1 d_0[H_1] + \beta_4 d_0[H_2] + \beta_1\beta_4 d_0^2[H_{12}], \qquad \text{D-8}$$

where β_1 and β_4 are unknown constants (reflecting the magnitude, on a ratio scale, of the exposure effect on the first and fourth stage, respectively), d_0 is as defined in Section D-2 and

$$
\begin{aligned}
H_1(t) =&(t^4 d_0)^{-1}[E(d_1)t^4 + [E(d_2) - E(d_1)](t - t_0)^4 \\
&+ [E(d_3) - E(d_2)](t - t_s)^4] \\
H_2(t) =&(t^4 d_0)^{-1}[E(d_3)t^4 + [E(d_2) - E(d_3)]t_s^4 \\
&+ [E(d_1) - E(d_2)]t_0^4] \\
H_{12}(t) =&(t^4 d_0^2)^{-1}\{[E(d_1)]^2 t_0^4(1 + m^2(d_1)) \\
&+ E(d_1)E(d_2)[1 + p(d_1, d_2)m(d_1)m(d_2)](t_s^4 - t_0^4 - (t_s - t_0)^4) \\
&+ [E(d_2)]^2(t_s - t_0)^4[1 + m^2(d_2)] \\
&+ E(d_1)E(d_3)[1 + p(d_1, d_3)m(d_1)m(d_3)][t^4 - t_s^4 - (t - t_0)^4 \\
&+ (t_s - t_0)^4] \\
&+ [E(d_3)]^2(t - t_s)^4[1 + m^2(d_3)] \\
&+ [1 + p(d_3, d_2)m(d_3)m(d_2)][(t - t_0)^4 - (t_s - t_0)^4 \\
&- (t - t_s)^4]E(d_2)E(d_3)\}
\end{aligned}
$$

where $E(d_1)$ is the average of $d_1, m(d_1) = \sqrt{\text{Var}(d_1)}/E(d_1)$, and $p(d_1, d_2)$ is the correlation between d_1 and d_2. For simplicity, we shall assume that all correlations are 0. This will have little effect on our analysis.

Now define

$$F_1(t) = H_1(t) + (\beta_4/\beta_1)H_2(t) \text{ and } F_{12}(t) = (\beta_4/\beta_1)H_{12}(t).$$

Then we have:

$$RR(t) = 1 + \beta_1 d_0 F_1(t) + (\beta_1 d_0)^2 F_{12}(t). \tag{D-9}$$

Now with $t_0 = 20, t_s = 55$, and $t = 70$, for any given choice for β_4/β_1 and for the exposure vector (a,b,c), we can compute $F_1(70), F_{12}(70)$ for both "exposed" and "unexposed" groups. Since 1.3 is assumed to be the ratio of the true relative risk in "exposed" subjects to that in "unexposed" subjects at age 70, we have

$$1.3 = \frac{1 + (\beta_1 d_0)F_{1E}(70) + (\beta_1 d_0)^2 F_{12E}(70)}{1 + (\beta_1 d_0)F_{1\bar{E}}(70) + (\beta_1 d_0)^2 F_{12\bar{E}}(70)}. \tag{D-10}$$

Equation D-10 is a quadratic equation in $\beta_1 d_0$. Thus, we can solve for $\beta_1 d_0$ even though we do not know β_1 or d_0 separately. We then substitute this value of $\beta_1 d_0$ along with the values of $F_{1E}(70)$ and $F_{12E}(70)$ into Equation D-9 to give an exposure-history-β_4/β_1-specific estimate of the true relative risk at age seventy in "exposed" individuals. If we substitute $F_{1\bar{E}}(70)$ and $F_{12\bar{E}}(70)$ instead, we get an estimate of the true relative risk at age 70 in "unexposed" individuals. Note that if we had an independent estimate of β_1, we could also estimate d_0. Given β_4/β_1 and (a, b, c) (and thus $\beta_1 d_0$ by Equation D-10), our estimate of d_0 is inversely proportional to our estimate of β_1.

Estimation of d_0

Remark 9: Interpretation of β_1 and d_0 β_1, when estimated from data on active smokers, is the fractional increase in the rate of the first cellular event per actively smoked cigarette. Since cigarettes differ in carcinogenic potency, neither β_1 nor d_0 are biological constants. Therefore, we must specify the type of cigarette to which we want our estimate of β_1 to refer. In this Appendix, we shall let β_1 be the functional increase in the rate of the first cellular event associated with one current nonfilter U.S. cigarette containing 20 mg tar as smoked by an average U.S. citizen. In Section D-2 we adjusted our estimates of β_1 from the Doll and Peto data (1978) with this definition of β_1 in mind. Even after adjustment, β_1 will still be defined in terms of the cigarettes smoked by the study subjects in the American Cancer Society (Hammond, 1966) and European case-control studies (Lubin, 1984), which, on average, contained more than 30 mg of tar (since most of the cigarette exposure in these studies occurred before the adoption of low-tar cigarettes). Thus, if we wanted to define β_1 in terms of actively smoked unfiltered cigarettes with a tar content of 20 mg, one might further divide all estimates of β_1 (and multiply all estimates of d_0) by a factor of 1.5 to 2, although we have not chosen to do so. One must still consider the possibility that the lower relative risk found in the European and ACS data compared to the British data is a consequence of the fact that there was less misclassification of smokers as nonsmokers among the British doctors than among the ACS or European case-control study populations. Since, presumably, doctors are accurate reporters, such an assumption may not be unrealistic. If so, the baseline rate among nonsmokers from the ACS study would be falsely inflated upwards and the values of β_1 of 2.93 and 0.803, as originally estimated for the British doctors, would be the more appropriate values to use. For these reasons, we report results for all five of the combinations of β_4/β_1 and β_1 given in Table D-3.

Remark 10: Adjusting for the ETS Exposure of Active Smokers In estimating β_1 and β_4 from active-smoker data neither we nor Brown and Chu (in press) took account of the fact that in those studies active smokers (and the comparison groups of nonsmokers) were themselves breathing other peoples' cigarette smoke. If $3d_0$ is of the order of 3 or more cigarettes per day (as in Table D-3), a proper analysis (and thus proper estimates of β_1, β_4, and d_0) would require refitting the active-smoking data taking account of ETS exposure. We have not done so here. We expect that the effect on our estimates of the true relative risk in "exposed" and "unexposed" subjects using Method 2 would not be great (because of the insensitivity of these estimates to uncertainty in β_1/β_4). On the other hand, the effect on our estimates of d_0 may be more pronounced. Further study is required.

Remark 11: Estimation of d_0 from Dosimetry The estimates of d_0 given in Table D-4 are obtained in step 5 of the following sequence of calculations.

1. For the ETS constituents B*a*P and NDMA we estimated the weight of each constituent inhaled directly by an active smoker from the mainstream smoke of a single cigarette by using the midpoint of the range given in the mainstream weight column in Table 2-10 (i.e., 25 and 30 ng for NDMA and B*a*P, respectively). (The weights entered in the mainstream weight column of Table 2-10 are averages based on cigarettes whose mainstream-smoke tar content, as measured by a smoking machine, varied between 16 and 30 milligrams.)

2. We estimated the weight of each of the above constituents inhaled daily by a nonsmoker with a nonsmoking spouse by multiplying by 1.07 the range of values given under the ETS weight column in Table 2-10. (1.07 is our estimate of the average number of hours of daily ETS exposure occurring in nonsmokers with nonsmoking spouses. Nonsmokers without smoking spouses report that they are exposed, on average, to ETS between 5 (Table 6, Friedman et al., 1983) and 10 hours a week (Wald and Ritchie, 1984). Our value of 7.5 hours/week (= 1.07 hours/day) is the average of the above estimates. We could have chosen to multiply

the value of 1.07 by a factor of up to 2, since most components of ETS decay with a half-life of approximately 1 hour when smoking ceases, assuming approximately one air change per hour and little plating out onto surfaces.)

3. For each constituent we divided the endpoints of the weight ranges calculated in Step 2 by the weight estimated in Step 1. The resulting range of values is, for each constituent, an estimate of the number of cigarettes that would have to be actively smoked in order that the weight of the constituent in the directly inhaled mainstream smoke would equal the weight of the constituent (attributable to ETS) inhaled daily by an average nonsmoker with a nonsmoking spouse. We shall call this number I_{0m}.

4. We next estimated for each constituent the number of cigarettes whose mainstream smoke would have to be directly inhaled by an active smoker to deliver to the lungs a dose of the constituent equal to the daily (biologically effective) pulmonary dose (attributable to ETS) of a nonsmoker with a nonsmoking spouse. We refer to this number as d_{0m}. For B*a*P we multiplied the endpoints of the range for I_{0m} by one-seventh. This reflects the fact that B*a*P is in the particulate phase and, as discussed in Chapter 7, a rough estimate of the deposition rates for particulates in ETS and in mainstream smoke is 10% and 70%, respectively. [This calculation ignores important differences between the ETS and mainstream particulate phases in terms of deposition site, clearance rates, and particle size. Thus, even if B*a*P were the active carcinogen in ETS and mainstream smoke, d_{0m}, as calculated above, could conceivably be quite different from the true value of d_{0m} defined in terms of the biologically effective dose for producing lung cancer.]

For NDMA we assumed $d_{0m} = I_{0m}$. The rationale for this decision is that NDMA is in the vapor phase in both ETS and mainstream smoke. We therefore assumed that the pulmonary absorption of NDMA per nanogram inhaled was the same for mainstream smoke and ETS. (This assumption may be inadequate, since NDMA is water soluble and thus will dissolve in mucous membrances before reaching the lungs. Therefore, the fraction of inhaled NDMA that reaches the lungs may well be up to several orders of magnitude greater in active smokers (whose intake is via deep inhalations taken through the mouth) than in nonsmokers (whose intake is largely via shallow inhalations taken through the nose). If so, our estimate of d_{0m} would need to be reduced by here. d_{0m} for RSP was calculated as follows. In Chapter 7 it was calculated that the amount of tar deposited in the lungs after 8 hours of ETS exposure would be about 0.005%-0.26% of that deposited in the lungs of an active smoker of 20 cigarettes containing 14 mg tar each. Thus, the upper limit of the range for d_{0m} (in terms of 20 mg tar cigarettes) equals $(14/20) \times 0.26 \times 10^{-2} \times 20 \times 1.07/8 = 8.2 \times 10^{-5} = 0.005$. The total range is 0.0001-0.005.

5. In what follows we estimate for each of the constituents NDMA, BaP, and RSP the number of cigarettes that would have to be actively smoked to deliver to the smoker a pulmonary dose of the constituent equal to the daily pulmonary dose (attributable to ETS) of a nonsmoker married to a nonsmoking spouse. This number we will call d_0^*. The $*$ as a symbol serves to distinguish this definition of d_0 from that in Section D-2. d_0^* for a given constituent is equivalent to d_0 as defined in Section D-2 if, as assumed in Table D-4, the constituent is the active lung carcinogen in ETS and mainstream smoke or, more generally, if d_0^* for the constituent is equal to d_0 for the unknown active carcinogen.

For the constituents RSP, BaP, and NDMA we first estimated the difference between the total pulmonary dose attributable to a single actively smoked nonfilter cigarette and the fraction of that pulmonary dose attributable to the directly inhaled mainstream smoke. This difference includes contributions from the plume of sidestream smoke, the plume of exhaled mainstream smoke, and the ETS subsequently derived from the plumes of sidestream and exhaled mainstream smoke. We shall call this difference the nonmainstream (pulmonary) dose of the constituent. How does the magnitude of the nonmainstream (pulmonary) dose to a smoker compare to the pulmonary dose of the constituent absorbed by a nonsmoker without a smoking spouse in the Wald and Ritchie study (1984) during that nonsmoker's 1.07 hours of daily exposure? We have no empirical data that directly bear on this question. Nonetheless, we shall assume that the ratio, f, of the dose to the smoker from the nonmainstream smoke of a single cigarette to the daily dose (attributable to ETS) to a nonsmoker with a nonsmoking spouse is between 0.1 and 2. We believe the ratio could be as high as 2 because the active smoker is much more likely to directly inhale the highly concentrated plumes of sidestream and exhaled mainstream smoke. (In fact, the ratio could possibly be a good deal higher than 2.) This ratio could be as low as 0.1 if active smokers rarely directly inhale the plumes of smoke and during the hour in which a nonsmoker with a nonsmoking spouse is exposed to ETS, the average smoker density is 4, with each smoker smoking 2.5 cigarettes per hour. (This is a rather high smoker density and 0.1 may therefore be somewhat too low an estimate.) It is a straightforward algebraic exercise to show that the relationship between d_0^* and d_{0m} is

$$d_0^* = \frac{1}{(1/d_{0m}) + f}.$$

The minimum of the range of d_0 (equivalently, d_0^*) values given in Table D-4 (for each constituent) was computed by plugging into the above formula the minimum of the range of d_{0m} estimated in step 4, and $f = 2$. The maximum of the d_0 range in Table D-4 was computed by plugging in the maximum of d_{0m} and $f = 0.1$. The ranges calculated for d_0^* essentially equal those for d_{0m}, with the exception that both endpoints of the d_{0m} range for NDMA were reduced by approximately 40% and the upper endpoint for B*a*P was reduced 25%.

Remark 12: Dosimetry Based on Urinary Nicotine or Cotinine In this remark we consider whether it is reasonable to take the ratio of urinary nicotine (or cotinine) in nonsmokers to that in active smokers as a proxy for the ratio of the biologically effective dose (attributable to ETS) of the active lung carcinogen in nonsmokers to the biologically effective dose in active smokers.

In aged ETS, nicotine is largely in the vapor phase. Nicotine is water soluble. Thus, presumably most of the nicotine in aged ETS dissolves in the mucous membranes of the upper airways and diffuses directly into the bloodstream. Thus, little of the inhaled nicotine from aged ETS reaches the lower respiratory tract. Therefore, urinary and blood nicotine in nonsmokers should roughly reflect the total amount of inhaled nicotine. In contrast, nicotine in mainstream and sidestream smoke and in fresh ETS is largely in the particulate phase. Therefore, most of the nicotine directly inhaled in mainstream smoke by a smoker reaches the lower respiratory tract (and from there the bloodstream) since the deposition fraction for particulates in mainstream smoke is 70% with most deposition occurring in the lower respiratory tract.

Therefore, if (1) the true carcinogen is in the vapor phase in both ETS and mainstream smoke, (2) the true carcinogen is in the particulate phase in both ETS and mainstream smoke, or (3) the true carcinogen is in the particulate phase in mainstream smoke, the vapor phase in ETS, and is, in addition, water soluble (so that the total dose of the carcinogen from ETS greatly exceeds the pulmonary dose), then serious questions must be raised about the appropriateness of using the ratio of urinary nicotine (or cotinine) in nonsmokers to that in active smokers to approximate the ratio of the biologically effective lung dose of the active carcinogens in nonsmokers to the lung dose in active smokers.

Remark 13: Estimating Lung Cancer Deaths Attributable to ETS Among Lifelong Nonsmokers in 1985 As in the Garfinkel et al. (1985) study, we use "exposed" to mean ever-"exposed", since one cannot calculate a population attributable number from case-control studies in which individuals who are ever-"exposed" but not currently-"exposed" are excluded. If we assume that Assumption 1a and Equation D-5 hold with $c(70) = 3$, then $RR(70|E)$ and $RR(70|\bar{E})$ are 1.54 and 1.18, respectively, based on a summary rate ratio of 1.3. We would then need to assume, for example, that $RR(t|E)$ and $RR(t|\bar{E})$ do not depend on t. Using this approach we obtain an attributable number of 2,010 in nonsmoking women. In contrast, the naive approach, which ignores the ETS exposure of "unexposed" individuals by assuming $RR(70|E) = 1.3$ and $RR(70|\bar{E}) = 1.0$, gives an attributable number of 1,150.

The second approach supposes that assumptions of Method 2 in Section D-2 hold. We then choose a value for exposure history (a, b, c) and β_4/β_1 which, given that $\gamma(70|E)/\gamma(70|\bar{E}) = 1.3$, allows us to calculate $\beta_1 d_0$ from Equation D-10. Knowledge of $\beta_1 d_0$, then, allows us to calculate, from equation D-9, $RR(t|E)$ and $RR(t|\bar{E})$ for all t (not just $t = 70$).

The third approach is to assume that the first assumptions under Method 2 concerning the multistage cancer model hold but not to assume that $RR(70|E)/RR(70|\bar{E}) = 1.3$. We then must select a value of β_1 and d_0 in order to estimate $\beta_1 d_0$ and, given (a, b, c) and $\beta_4/\beta_1, RR(t|E)$.

Remark 14: Estimating the Lifetime Risk of Lung Cancer Due to ETS $S(t|t_0) = \Pi_{u=t_0}^{t}[1 - \lambda(u)]$ where $\lambda(u)$ is the all-cause mortality rate in 1985 among nonsmoking women of age u (and we are following the standard convention of using current, i.e. 1985, mortality rate). We estimated $\lambda(u)$ for female nonsmokers by multiplying the all-cause age-specific mortality rates (for female nonsmokers) given in Hammond (1966) by the ratio of the overall U.S. age-specific female death rates in 1985 (all smoking categories) to those rates in 1962. Furthermore, $\gamma_{\mathrm{EXCESS}}(t) = \gamma_0(t)[RR_{\mathrm{EXCESS}}(t)]$, where $\gamma_0(t)$ is the incidence of lung cancer death at t in the absence of all exposure, and $RR_{\mathrm{EXCESS}}(t)$ is the excess relative risk for lung cancer due to exposure history M. $\gamma_0(t) = [1 - AF(t)]I_0(t)$ where $AF(t)$ and $I_0(t)$ are as defined above.

From Equation D-9 we can obtain an estimate of $RR_{\mathrm{EXCESS}}(t) = RR(t) - 1$ for given values of $\beta_1 d_0$ and β_4/β_1 and choice of exposure history M. It follows that, under the assumption that the observed rate ratio of 1.3 is causal, we can then obtain an estimate of $AF(M)$ for $t_0 = 45$ for each choice of exposure history (a, b, c) and value of β_4/β_1, since, using Equation D-10, we obtain an estimate of $\beta_1 d_0$ from which, in turn, we obtain an estimate of $AF(t)$ and $RR_{\mathrm{EXCESS}}(t)$.

Remark 15 In estimating $AF(M)$ in ex- and current smokers, $RR_{\mathrm{EXCESS}}(t)$ can be estimated from Equation D-9 for a given value of exposure history (a, b, c), β_4/β_1, and β_1 under the assumption that the rate ratio of 1.3 is causal. (Knowledge of β_1 is necessary so that we can estimate from Equation D-10 the value of d_0 rather than simply $\beta_1 d_0$.) $\gamma_0(t)$ is estimated as for nonsmokers. To estimate the all-cause mortality rate among exsmokers and continuing smokers we used the data in Hammond (1966) as described for nonsmokers, except for smokers of 20 cigarettes per day we used an average of the age-specific all-cause mortality rates in Hammond for smokers of 1-19 and >19 cigarettes per day; and for exsmokers we used both their smoking rates while smoking and the number of years since quitting (as a time-dependent covariate) to enter Hammond's table at the proper place. Missing values in Hammond's table were filled in by linear interpolation or extrapolation.

Remark 16 Under Assumption 1a, $RR_{\mathrm{EXCESS}}(t)$ would be the same for exsmokers and nonsmokers who had the same history of exposure to other people's cigarette smoke. But if we assume that cigarette smoke affects two stages of a multistage cancer model, then, for an exsmoker, the quadratic terms in Equation D-9 cannot be ignored. As such, a small increment in dose due to breathing other people's cigarette smoke will have a larger absolute effect on the age-specific-mortality rate of the exsmoker than of the nonsmoker.

Effects of Bias

We now consider the following three questions. In deriving our summary estimates of 1.3 we amalgamated studies that compared ever-"exposed" to never-"exposed" subjects with studies that compared currently-"exposed" to never-"exposed" subjects. Does this introduce an important bias? In Remark 17 below, we show that it does not. Second, under the assumption that our multistage model is correct, Assumption 1a is false, since Equation D-8 has a quadratic dose term. Nonetheless, for calculating the true relative risk in "exposed" and "unexposed" subjects, is Assumption 1a an adequate approximation? Third, should case-control studies of the relationship between childhood ETS exposure and lung cancer have greater power to detect an ETS effect than case-control studies of adult ETS exposure? In particular, does the failure of Garfinkel et al. (1985) to find an effect of childhood exposure cast doubt on the validity of our 13 epidemiologic studies of adult ETS exposure? We will show in Remark 19 that when one takes into account the inevitable misclassification of childhood ETS exposure occurring some 60 years previously, the observed relative risk expected from a case-control study of childhood ETS exposure could be as low as 1.01 and would be no greater than 1.3. Thus, it is not surprising Garfinkel et al. found no effect of childhood exposure.

Remark 17 It is clear that the same causal parameter is not being estimated in studies in which the "exposed" group is ever-"exposed" as in studies in which the exposed group is currently-"exposed" individuals. Yet, our summary value of 1.3 was based on amalgamating estimates of $RR(t|E)/RR(t|\bar{E})$ from these two different types of studies. To estimate the magnitude of the bias associated with this amalgamation, we proceeded as follows. Consider studies with exposure history of the form $(a,b,1)$. For each choice of (a,b) and β_4/β_1 we obtain, from Equation D-10, an estimate of $\beta_1 d_0$, say, $\beta_1 d_0(a,b,\beta_4/\beta_1)$, if we can assume $RR(t|E)/RR(t|\bar{E})$ is 1.3 for such studies. For each $\beta_1 d_0(a,b,\beta_4/\beta_1)$ we estimated, using Equation D-10, $RR(t|E)/RR(t|\bar{E})$ for a study with exposure history $(a,b,3)$. The maximum value of $RR(t|E)/RR(t|\bar{E})$ estimated in this way for studies with exposure history $(a,b,3)$ was 1.39 (associated with $\beta_4/\beta_1 = 1.8$, of course). Given the confidence interval of (1.12,1.49) reported in Chapter 12 for the amalgamated parameter $RR(t|E)/RR(t|\bar{E})$, it follows that any bias due to improperly amalgamating these two types of studies will be small compared to sampling error.

Remark 18 Conditional on the assumption that our multistage model holds for lung cancer, we can test the adequacy of Assumption 1a. Let $\beta_1 d_0'$ and $RR'(70|E)$ be the estimates of $\beta_1 d_0$ and $RR(70|E)$ obtained by removing the quadratic term (in $\beta_1 d_0$) from the numerator and denominator of Equation D-10. Now, since Equation D-9, modified so that the quadratic term in $\beta_1 d_0$ is eliminated, is a linear excess relative risk model, it follows that Assumption 1a is an adequate approximation if the estimates $\beta_1 d_0'$ and $RR'(70|E)$ do not differ greatly from the estimates, $\beta_1 d_0$ and $RR(70|E)$, based on the unmodified Equation D-10. We therefore estimated $\max[RR'(70|E) - RR(70|E)]$ as (a,b,c) and β_4/β_1 varied. The maximum was 0.05. Thus, the linear approximation of Assumption 1a is probably adequate.

Remark 19 We now estimate the maximum and minimum relative risk (at age 70) we would expect to observe in a case-control study of ETS exposure in childhood (controlling for ETS exposure in adult life) under the assumption that our multistage model for lung cancer is correct. To do so, we perform a sensitivity analysis over the possible exposure histories of the "exposed" and "unexposed" study subjects in such a case-control study. In particular, we assume that (1) for all study subjects the exposure rate from ages 20 to 70 years was $2d_0$; (2) the false-positive and false-negative rates for the exposure "at least one parent smoked" were 0.15 and 0.3, respectively; and (3) exposure rate from 0 to 20 in the truly "exposed" (i.e., among those who did have a smoking parent) to the truly "unexposed" was, in units of d_0, one of the following: 1.53 to 0.3, 0.75 to 0.15, 1.0 to 0.6, or 1.0 to 0.05. It only remains necessary to choose values for β_4/β_1 and $\beta_1 d_0$. For each of our three choices of β_4/β_1, we let $\beta_1 d_0$ range over the values found previously (using Equation D-10) as (a,b,c) varied.

The maximum relative risk was 1.26, which occurred with exposure rates of 1.53 and $0.3d_0$ in the exposed and unexposed, respectively, $\beta_4/\beta_1 = 0.0124$, and the value of $\beta_1 d_0$ (computed using Equation D-10) based on $(a,b,c) = (1,2,3)$. The minimum relative risk was 1.01. Even when we unrealistically assumed that both the false-positive and false-negative rates for exposure misclassification were 0, the maximum relative risk was only 1.51. Thus, it is not surprising that Garfinkel et al. (1985) failed to detect an effect of childhood exposure in his case-control study.

References

Brown, C.C., and K.C. Chu. Use of multistage models to infer stage affected by carcinogenic exposure: Example of lung cancer and cigarette smoking. J. Chron. Dis., in press.

Correa, P., L.W. Pickle, E. Fontham, Y. Lin, and W. Haenszel. Passive smoking and lung cancer. Lancet 2:595-597, 1983.

Coultas, D.B., J.M. Samet, C.A. Howard. G.T. Peake, and B.J. Skipper. Salivary cotinine levels and passive tobacco smoke exposure in the home. Am. Rev. Respir. Dis. 133:A157, 1986.

Day, N.E., and C.C. Brown. Multistage models and primary prevention of cancer. J. Natl. Cancer Inst. 64:977-989, 1980.

Doll, R.D., and R. Peto. Mortality in relation to smoking: 20 years' observations on male British doctors. Br. Med. J. 2:1525-1536, 1976.

Doll, R.D., and R. Peto. Cigarette smoking and bronchial carcinoma: Dose and time relationships among regular smokers and lifelong non-smokers. J. Epidemiol. Comm. Health 32:303-313, 1978.

Doll, R.D., and R. Peto. The Causes of Cancer: Quantitative Estimates of Avoidable Risks of Cancer in the United States Today. J. Natl. Cancer Inst. 66:1191-1308, 1981.

Friedman, G.D., D. Pettiti, and R.D. Bawol. Prevalence and correlates of passive smoking. Am. J. Public Health, 73:401-405, 1983.

Garfinkel, L. Time trends in lung cancer mortality among nonsmokers and a note on passive smoking. J. Natl. Cancer Inst. 66:1061-1066, 1981.

Garfinkel, L., O. Auerbach, and L. Joubert. Involuntary smoking and lung cancer: A case-control study. J. Natl. Cancer Inst. 75:463-469, 1985.

Hammond, E.C. Smoking in relation to the death rates of one million men and women. Nat. Cancer Inst. Monogr. 19:127-204, 1966.

Hirayama, T. Cancer mortality in nonsmoking women with smoking husbands on a large-scale cohort study in Japan. Prev. Med. 13:680-690, 1984.

Hirayama, T. Non-smoking wives of heavy smokers have a higher risk of lung cancer: a study from Japan. Br. Med. J. 282:183-185, 1981.

Jarvis, M.J., M.A.H. Russell, C. Feyerabend, J.R. Eiser, M. Morgan, P. Gammage, and E.M. Gray. Passive exposure to tobacco smoke: Saliva cotinine concentrations in as representative population sample of non-smoking schoolchildren. Br. Med. J. 291:927-929, 1985.

Jarvis, M.J., H. Tunstall-Pedoe, C. Feyerabend, C. Vesey, and Y. Saloojee. Biochemical markers of smoke absorption and self reported exposure to passive smoking. J. Epidemiol. Comm. Health 38:355-339, 1984.

Lubin, J.H., W.J. Blot, and F. Berrino, et al. Patterns of lung cancer risk among filter and nonfilter cigarette smokers. Int. J. Cancer 33:569-576, 1984.

Matsukura, S., T. Taminato, N. Kitano, Y. Seino, H. Hamada, M. Uchihashi, H. Nakajima, and Y. Hirata. Effects of environmental tobacco smoke on urinary cotinine excretion in nonsmokers. N. Engl. J. Med. 311:828-832, 1984.

Trichopoulos, D., A. Kalandidi, and L. Sparros. Lung cancer and passive smoking: Conclusion of Greek study. Lancet 2:677-678, 1983.

Wald, N.J., and C. Ritchie. Validation of studies on lung cancer in non-smokers married to smokers. Lancet 1:1067, 1984.